Medical Pluralism and Homoeopathy in India and Germany
(1810–2010)

Medizin,
Gesellschaft und Geschichte

Jahrbuch
des Instituts für Geschichte der Medizin
der Robert Bosch Stiftung

herausgegeben von
Robert Jütte

Beiheft 50

Medical Pluralism and Homoeopathy in India and Germany (1810–2010)

A Comparison of Practices

Edited by Martin Dinges

Franz Steiner Verlag Stuttgart
2014

Gedruckt mit freundlicher Unterstützung der Robert Bosch Stiftung GmbH

Coverabbildung: Hakim (Unani-Arzt), aus: „Früchte aus dem Morgenland"
von Johann Martin Honigberger, 1851, © Institut für Geschichte der Medizin
der Robert Bosch Stiftung Stuttgart

Bibliografische Information der Deutschen Nationalbibliothek:
Die Deutsche Nationalbibliothek verzeichnet diese Publikation in der Deutschen
Nationalbibliografie; detaillierte bibliografische Daten sind im Internet über
<http://dnb.d-nb.de> abrufbar.

© Franz Steiner Verlag, Stuttgart 2014
Druck: Laupp & Göbel GmbH, Nehren
Gedruckt auf säurefreiem, alterungsbeständigem Papier.
Printed in Germany
ISBN 978-3-515-10484-5

Contents

Martin Dinges
Introduction 7

Silvia Waisse
East Meets West: Johann M. Honigberger and Medical Pluralism
through the Eyes of a 19th Century Transylvanian Saxon in India 31

Shinjini Das
Innovating Indigeneity, Reforming Domesticity:
Nationalising Homeopathy in Colonial Bengal 53

Avi Sharma
Rethinking Asymmetries in the Marketplace:
Medical Pluralism in Germany, 1869–1910 71

Ameeta R. Manchanda
A Homeopathic Clinic in a Multispeciality Hospital.
Reflections from Practice 85

Raj Kumar Manchanda / Surender Kumar Verma / Leena V. Chhatre /
Harleen Kaur
Homeopathy in Urban Primary Healthcare Units
of the Delhi Government: An Assessment 91

Harish Naraindas
Nosopolitics.
Epistemic Mangling and the Creolization of Contemporary Ayurveda .. 105

Hugues Dusausoit
The Quest for Another Recognition.
Ethnography of an homeopath in Tamil Nadu 137

Marion Baschin
The Patients' Choice – How and Why Sick People
Used Homeopathy in 19th Century Münster 149

Rahul Tewari / Ramachandran Valavan
Patients' Trend in Choosing the Homeopathic Medical System in India .. 167

Philipp Eisele
Medical Pluralism and the Patients' Perspective in Germany –
Letters to "Natur und Medizin" (1992–2000) 183

Nupur Barua
Medical Pluralism in a Slum in Delhi:
Global Medicine in a Local Garb?... 203

Krishna Soman
Pluralism, Popularity and Propaganda:
Narratives of Lay Practices of Homeopathy in India 217

William Sax
Looking Behind and Ahead.. 245

Authors... 249

Introduction

Martin Dinges

Pluralism(s) of Medical Systems

There are various definitions of Medical Pluralism. A broad definition by the German medical ethnologist Pfleiderer focuses on the level of systems: She defines Medical Pluralism as the "juxtaposition of medical systems which is a historical result of cultural and social developments leading to institutionalized forms of medical care".[1] Medical systems may have more or less strict delimitations. They can be differentiated internally. And they may interact with other systems – which they evidently do continuously. The definition underlines the crucial role of social, political and cultural factors – such as for example diversities of class, ethnicity and gender within societies or nation states and external pressures such as colonialism. The importance of history is evident: In the case of health and medicine during the 19th and 20th centuries one must refer particularly to the rise of biomedicine. In the case of India, the role of homeopathy as a "naturalized" medical system is another issue[2], as is the very recent successful commoditization of Ayurvedic and – to a certain extent also – Unani medications, which enlarged the Indian market for these products a hundred times in the twenty years between 1980 and 2000[3].

Medical Pluralism is by now recognized as a reality in many countries. The "traditional systems of medicine" have even found their way into the documents of the WHO. The organization defines them as

> the sum total of the knowledge, skills and practices based on the theories, beliefs and experiences indigenous to different cultures, whether explicable or not, used in the maintenance of health, as well as in the prevention, diagnosis, improvement or treatment of physical and mental illnesses. The terms complementary/alternative/non-conventional medicine are used interchangeably with traditional medicine in some countries.[4]

In fact the WHO suggests the integration of these systems into the national health care schemes. What a remarkable development after decades of witnessing the ever increasing power of biomedicine! Since the end of WWII and the subsequent introduction of antibiotics, it seemed that there was nothing to stop the march towards a biomedical monopoly. Some medical historians would put the starting point of this triumphant development even further back to the beginnings of bacteriology in the 1880s or to the birth of the clinic at around 1800.

---

1 Pfleiderer (1995), p. 86; for other definitions s. Dilger/Hadolt: Überlegungen (2010).
2 Arnold/Sarkar (2002); cf. article of Das in this volume.
3 Bode (2008), p. 83. Sales rose from $ 7.5 million in 1980 to 800 million in 2001 and 1,000 million in 2005.
4 World Health Organization (2000), p. 1.

On this issue, history has to be brought into the debate again: The term medical pluralism in its most current meaning has several hidden implications, referring to two specific conditions, that need to be made evident for a critical use of the term: Firstly, it should only be applied to a period after the point of time when biomedicine was established as a distinctive medical system, and, secondly, it must have played or still play a dominant role. Depending on the country or point of view – or the preference of either the role of scientific progress or therapeutic effectiveness of biomedicine – one can locate this point of time somewhere between the 1880s and the 1950s in the case of Germany, and in India at a later time. For earlier eras before the establishment of such a hegemonic position of biomedicine I propose the term "old medical pluralism" (up until at least the 1880s, possibly even until the 1950s); for the "golden age of biomedicine" (from the 1950s at the earliest to the 1980s) I would call it "modern medical pluralism"; for the decades after the 1980s I propose the term "new medical pluralism".[5]

From a European point of view, developments began to take a different direction from the 1980s at the latest: the general public grew dissatisfied with certain aspects of biomedicine, such as the side effects of medications and the impression that physicians took too little time for the individual patient. Other points of concern included the power of the physicians as specialists and the growing dominance of diagnostics over treatment. What was probably even more important was that the limitations of biomedicine became more and more evident. After the end of most epidemics (at least in the rich Northern countries) the importance of chronical forms of disease increased. The ageing of the population – a common trend in rich and poor nations – will make these problems even more acute in the future.

As a reaction to these changes, some physicians in post-industrial countries began, from the 1980s onwards, to add "alternative medicine" to the biomedical treatments, which they continued to provide: they could be naturopathy, herbal medicine, Anthroposophic Medicine, "Traditional Chinese Medicine", Acupuncture, Homeopathy or, more recently, Ayurveda. An enquiry about the year 2000 shows the motivations of these German physicians as a mixture of personal dissatisfaction with biomedicine and the standardized patient care in hospitals. Sometimes they were driven by commercial considerations or a fascination with Asian spirituality or concepts.[6] From the 1990s onwards, between half and two thirds of all general physicians in France and in Germany have occasionally prescribed alternative medications or treatments, particularly homeopathy, and four fifth of the population are inclined to use it.[7] – And what is more: Non-academically trained practitioners supplied these

---

5   Jütte (2008), p. 382, referring to Cant/Sharma (1998), p. 189; and in more detail to Cheng (2003).
6   On the physicians' motivation see Frank/Stollberg (2006); Stollberg (2010), esp. pp. 241–246. See also Thanner (2010).
7   Stange (2010), pp. 37–38. "Basisdaten Homöopathie" of the DZVhÄ referring to a study of the CAM-Institute: http://www.dzvhae.de/dzvhae-presse/basisdaten/basisdaten-

and many other therapies which could include esoteric forms as well as magic. In other countries, such as the USA, over-the-counter (OTC) sales of non-conventional medical products flourished and showed the growing interest of patients for self-medication with alternative treatments.[8] We must keep in mind that the respective role of healthcare providers and of self-medication varies much between countries, continents and markets. In any case, self-medication hints at the idea of self-help – without consulting a medical specialist – which is another, cultural, element of the critique of biomedicine and the resurgence of alternative medicine during the 1980s.

Since that pivotal decade, alternative or complementary treatments have increased their share in the medical market in postindustrial societies.[9] The public debate forces the custodians of healthcare systems to take a stand and either reject or integrate these therapies – and to make up their minds as to whether to consider them as "complementary" or "alternative". One point is clear: the time of a monopolistic position of academic trained physicians offering "biomedicine" exclusively seems to be over – if such a situation ever existed.

Before looking further afield, I will continue this Eurocentric narrative for the moment. It is typical for this kind of narrative to overemphasize aspects that are tended to be seen as "modern" – in this case the dominant role of biomedicine when referring to Europe or North America. Such dichotomies between the "modern" and the "traditional" still play an important role in the background of public and even scientific debates on medical pluralism, particularly when referring to entire "medical systems".[10] This might be astonishing for scholars versed in postcolonial and postmodern critique. There is no doubt that these dichotomies tend to dwell on differences between medical systems while they neglect common features. It is also true that they conceive systems as being not only different but also stable and quite rigid.[11] One should, in contrast, underline the internal differentiation of systems. Finally, dichotomies are certainly linked more often to discourses about medical systems than to practice. But these dichotomies may be heuristically fruitful when used to deconstruct the Eurocentric narrative. A shared hypothesis in this volume is that there is much more "traditional medicine" in the North than we might have thought possible still twenty years ago! I use the term "traditional" here to signify healing practices that are not "biomedically proven".

During the last decades there is increasing evidence that invites us to doubt the monopolistic role of biomedicine in the "North" even during its

homoeopathie.html (last accessed on April 30, 2013).

For France: "L'homéopathie, un désaccord constant": http://elise10delannoy.free.fr/ desaccord.html (last accessed on April 30, 2013); cf. "Homéopathie classique/uniciste": http://www.inhfparis.com/homeopathie-uniciste/hom%C3%A9opathie-classique-uniciste-0 (last accessed on April 30, 2013).

8   Sales nearly doubled from $ 439 million in 2002 to $ 831 million in 2008: Riley (2011).
9   For Germany cf. Stange (2010), esp. p. 37.
10   For a critical discussion of dichotomies see Ernst (2002), pp. 3, 6.
11   Ebrahimnejad: Introduction (2009), p. 4.

"golden age" (from the 1950s to the 1980s): in Germany, for example, a huge market of all sorts of non-conventional health products flourished throughout the 20th century and continues to do so. Products were mailed by companies and pharmacies directly to the homes of people who were prepared to pay large sums for them.[12] They were advertised promising much, but without serious "scientific" credentials. Sometimes, the fake credentials showed at least an implicit subservient reference to the dominant scientific discourse. Too little research is unfortunately still available for other comparable countries. From recent scholarships on Belgium and Germany we know at least that the clientele of magic and religious healers was, and is, vast and included, and includes, users from the better-off strata of society.[13]

Further on, one must keep in mind that in the – specific – German case phytotherapy, Anthroposophic Medicine and Homeopathy have been recognized specialisations of physicians for a long time.[14] Over the last 30 years the demand for complementary and alternative medicine and for homeopathy has been continuously growing in all of Europe, whether one considers the number of physicians with this specialisation or the quantity of medications sold in pharmacies.[15] Whether all this is "traditional", "modern", "post-modern" or a sign of "second or reflexive modernity" might be a topic of academic debate, but it shows that the dominance of biomedicine was never complete. It may be a question of a larger or a smaller market share, but to better understand the significance and the importance of this proportion was one of the aims of the conference that gave rise to this volume.[16]

It is even possible that the growing demand of patients for "Traditional Chinese Medicine", acupuncture and, more recently, Ayurveda in many European countries or in the Americas is just another phase of this long-term "underground" medical pluralism, which is just beginning to come to public attention. The best evidence for this visibility is a national referendum of the Swiss people which decided in 2009 with a majority of two thirds of the population to include the support of alternative and complementary systems of medicine in their national constitution!

To finally move from the Eurocentric view to India, one certainly needs to start by calling attention to the enormous internal diversity of that country and its effects on the medical market.[17] What is even more important in this con-

---

12 Mildenberger (2011).
13 Schmitz: Médecines (2006); Schmitz: Soigner (2006).
14 For basic information on the German legal and institutional framework for medical pluralism see Walach (2012).
15 Dinges (2014); Dinges (2012).
16 Report at http://www.igm-bosch.de/content/language1/html/11643.asp (last accessed on April 30, 2013). The participants of this conference came from India and Germany, Brazil, the US and Belgium and had very different disciplinary backgrounds – they were physicians, scholars from anthropology, public health, medical and social history and the history of science.
17 English-language literature on the subject is vast and better known to the English-language reader, some of it is cited in Dinges: Versorgungsbeitrag (2011); Dinges: Patienten-

text is the kind of medical pluralism that seems to be quite different from what has been presented so far with regard to Germany and Europe: First of all, "modern medicine" has still a more particular prestige, as only a minority of the population has access to it and can afford it. This distinctive character of biomedicine might be a driving force in fostering the demand for it among the entire population. In this first perspective, the good image of biomedicine might even disadvantage "traditional systems of medicine". On the other hand, biomedicine encountered and may still encounter specific barriers – beyond the already mentioned economic threshold and the simple lack of allopathic healthcare providers in large parts of the country and in the less well-off neighbourhoods, one needs to consider the cultural barriers. One such barrier has to do with difficulties some patients have when they seek treatment in public institutions, because they worry about impurity if members of a lower caste are also attending.

Another distinctive element in many Asian countries such as India is a continuous and more evident tradition of medical pluralism.[18] This is in part a result of prevailing local traditions of rural or tribal medicine. Both are often transferred to the cities by migrants. On the other hand, the Indian medical pluralism is an effect of the history of long-distance immigration. Unani medicine is a good example: it originated as a result of the Islamic appropriation of Greek ("Ionian") medicine, transferred centuries later in a readapted form to South Asia where it was again modified. It continues to be linked to the Muslim community but tends to spread beyond these limits. Ayurveda has certain connections to Hinduism – some, in old Brahmin texts, are real, others are imagined and reinvented. Since the 19th century there have been nationalists who have tried to exploit this fact for political purposes.[19] Medical systems might certainly play a role in the identity building of religious communities, a fact that can contribute to stabilize medical pluralism.

The colonial period added "modern western medicine", which was – quite significantly – called "English (or Angrezi) medicine", to the existing traditional medical pluralism. "Scientific medicine" was appropriated in various ways by the people of the colonies. For a long time the impact of Western medicine was largely limited to the cities. As a reaction to the colonial influences and pressures, Ayurveda had to define its own genealogy, orthodoxy and canon and continues to do so as it keeps reinventing its history.[20] Comparable developments can be observed for Unani medicine.[21] The various medical systems are now under the umbrella of the administrative department of

präferenzen (2011), p. 122, literature referring more directly to medical pluralism is cited below.

18   Studied since the 1970s first by Leslie (1976); on his pioneering role see Pfleiderer (1995), pp. 87, 90, and more recently Johannessen (2006), p. 3.

19   Sivaramakrishnan (2006), p. 242; on these inventions of tradition also for TCM Ernst (2002), pp. 6, 8; on the case of Sri Lanka see Jones (2009).

20   Cf. Wujastyk/Smith (2008).

21   Bode (2008); Liebeskind (2002).

AYUSH (an acronym for Ayurveda, Yoga and Naturopathy, Unani, Siddha, Homeopathy), which is part of the Indian ministry of health and family welfare. This selection of medical systems, their clear cut delimitation and the exclusion of other "traditional systems" is to a large extent a long term effect of the professionalization and biomedicalization that first gained momentum around 1900.[22] Given the particular regional, tribal, communal and social fragmentation of the Indian society and its corresponding medical market with very uneven chances of access, medical pluralism continues to have a more important impact in this country than in postindustrial societies such as Germany.

Some authors have even strongly criticized the idea of medical pluralism and suggested to introduce the concept of a "forced medical pluralism": They refer to the fact that Western biomedicine is unaffordable for large social strata in poorer countries.[23] As a consequence, less well-off citizens in these countries are simply obliged to use cheaper forms of medicine. This applies to the medical system used – such as folk-medicine or religious healing (which is, by the way, not necessarily and generally cheap) – as for the type of provider, who is often non-academically trained or simply entirely self-educated. To employ the friendly sounding term "medical pluralism" for this situation of deficient healthcare provision would contribute to dissimulate the social inequalities in access to medical services. From this point of view, the WHO with its recent interest in "traditional medical systems" would simply participate in a neoliberal attempt to add euphemism to social injustice. One implicit assumption of this criticism of the WHO is that "alternative" forms of medicine are less efficient than biomedicine. This assumption is – in such a general way – definitely not true. This idea of the general superiority of biomedicine might be just another Eurocentric bias in this debate.

Nevertheless, the socio-economic core of this criticism needs to be taken seriously. It must be remembered that "pluralism" in the Western intellectual tradition is a term which was coined against privilege, especially the privileges of noblemen. The concept is linked to the bourgeois critique of absolutism and suggests the fundamentally liberal idea of equal chances of access to wealth and happiness. The term "medical pluralism" keeps this normative egalitarian connotation, which always resonates when used against the monopolistic claims of biomedicine. Using the concept of "medical pluralism" implicates heuristically the challenge to conceive at least the normative idea of an equal access to medical care – which in fact does not exist.

This difference between the potentialities and the given reality exists even in national healthcare schemes based on statutory health insurance for literally everybody, as they exist in Germany or, in a different way, in the British National Health System. It is less evident in India. This concerns not only the access to health services but also the quality of these services: if one considers, for instance, the structure of the local medical market in an urban agglomera-

---

22   Wujastyk/Smith (2008), p. 7; Liebeskind (2002); Pahari (2005); Sivaramakrishnan (2006).
23   A good overview of the recent debate is given by Sheehan (2009).

tion such as Delhi, the qualification of the same kind of providers – private physicians, physicians in PHC, Registered Medical Practitioners – is significantly better in well-off neighbourhoods than in the poorer ones, as recent research has convincingly demonstrated.[24]

We have so far focused on the level of systems which allowed us to make the point about the limitative and productive impact that internal and external political power can exert on medical pluralism in given societies. Some effects of the social inequalities with the possible use of the pluralistic medical offer have come to the surface. The differentiated role of the administrative and institutional framework of medical pluralism was also addressed. The acknowledgement of the somewhat euphemistic connotation of the term "medical pluralism" may be used to critically indicate that it is better not to expect salvation from the market or overestimate its capacity to automatically bring about a more equal access to healthcare.

At any rate, these implications should not encourage us to reject the concept lock, stock and barrel.

But it reminds us not to fall into the trap of a casual culturalism, when focusing on the interactive and cultural aspects which are also part of the concept of medical pluralism. From the 1970s onwards, these aspects have often been the main focus of research in medical anthropology and ethnology.[25] The patients' ideas of the body and of medicine and their attempts to make sense of it all were at the main focus.[26]

Homeopathy as part of Medical Pluralisms

A particular focus of this collection of essays is the specific position of homeopathy within the German and the Indian medical pluralisms. From its very beginnings at around 1800, this medical system has struggled to find recognition among "allopathic" physicians. This is not the place to enter into the epistemological, nosological, historical and other reasons for this. Suffice it to call to attention one socio-professional aspect that makes the ambivalent position of homeopathy particularly clear: homeopathy has in most countries been mainly, if not exclusively, provided by physicians. The fact that lay practitioners played a certain role added to the difficulties of recognition inside the community of physicians and allocated to homeopathy a marginal role within the medical system.

The debate on homeopathy is in actual fact quite heated again around the globe.[27] A key argument is the allegation that homeopathy is not evidence-based – despite a growing number of outcome-studies with quite differentiated

---

24 Das/Hammer (2007).
25 Dilger/Hadolt: Überlegungen (2010), p. 15.
26 Nichter (1980) is still very instructive.
27 This is more the case in the English speaking world than elsewhere, cf. Dinges (2014).

results about the efficiency of homeopathy in practice.[28] This current campaign must be seen in the context of the steadily rising demand for homeopathy by patients in Europe, the Americas and a number of Asian countries during the last generation. The counter-attack from supporters of biomedicine, sponsored by pharmaceutical companies, is certainly an expression of their fear to lose markets. Homeopaths reckon that the amount of money pharmaceutical companies would lose if homeopathy could propose an efficient treatment for diabetes would constitute a real financial disaster for them.

Apart from the particular success in the open medical market of the USA, mainly during the 19th century, the position of homeopathy was relatively favourable since its inception in Germany.[29] Homeopathy gained recognition from the board of physicians as a medical specialization in several stages, in 1928, 1937 and 1956. Homeopathic consultation is in fact paid for by the national health insurance scheme – as are medications as long as they are prepared as low potencies. The continuously growing demand over the last 30 years led to a historic peak in the number of homeopathic physicians: The more than 6,200 homeopaths of the first decade of the new millennium represent roughly 1.5 % of all active physicians also in hospitals, research, and administration (342,000) and 5 % of all physicians in private practice (124,000 in 2011).[30] This is more than the highest levels attained in Germany in 150 years. Between 1860 and the 1970s the proportion of homeopathic physicians was always between 0.6 % and 1.2 % of all physicians. Considering the ordinary activity of homeopathic physicians the best indicator of their role in German healthcare provision is the comparison with GPs. Here, the proportion of homeopaths was up to 16.2 % in 2010, while it was only 5 % in 1993.[31] In Germany one must add to this historically high number of physicians the lay practitioners offering homeopathic treatment. These lay practitioners called "Heilpraktiker" are licensed healthcare providers who have passed a medical exam, with physicians on the examination board. Their market share is very difficult to evaluate as they practise homeopathy beside other healing methods and patients' expenditure is – in general – not refunded by the national health

---

28 Most recent overview in Bornhöft/Matthiessen (2011).
29 On Germany: Dinges: Patienten (1996); on other countries: Dinges: Weltgeschichte (1996); Jütte/Risse (1998).
30 Data from http://www.gbe-bund.de (last accessed on April 30, 2013): "Bei den Ärztekammern registrierte Ärztinnen und Ärzte mit Gebiets- und Facharztbezeichnung (absolut, je 100.000 Einwohner und Einwohner je Arzt). Gliederungsmerkmale: Jahre, Region, Alter, Geschlecht, Gebiets-/Facharztbezeichnung, Tätigkeitsbereich".
31 1993: 317,737 (all physicians – active and not active); 44,075 GPs; 2,212 Homeopaths; corresponds to 0.7 % of all and 5 % of all GPs;
2007: 413,000 (all physicians – active and not active); 42,000 GPs; 6,268 Homeopaths; corresponds to 1.52 % of all and 15.2 % of all GPs;
2010: 439,090; 42,050 GPs; 6,809 Homeopaths, corresponds to 1.55 % of all and 16.2 % of all GPs.
Gesundheitsberichterstattung des Bundes, http://www.gbe-bund.de/, various websites (last accessed on April 30, 2013).

scheme.[32] Patients pay most of this expenditure out of their own pocket, something traditionally very uncommon to Germans as they have been used to a comprehensive insurance for more than a century. The fact that the sub-profession of *Heilpraktiker* nevertheless flourishes is therefore a strong indicator of patients' demand – and for some of the patients of a declared distrust in physicians. On the whole, the entire homeopathic choice on offer in Germany – 16.2% of the GPs and the *Heilpraktiker* together – is still a smaller proportion of the market share than in India.

In India, homoeopathy has been well received as the "other modern medicine" since the 1830s. In this volume Waisse revisits an early historical moment, presenting the Transsylvanian physician M. Honigberger as an observer of applied medical pluralism in Lahore (now Pakistan) during the 1840s. Despite a certain degree of socio-cultural prejudice against the local healing traditions which one must expect for that time, Honigberger praises the institutionalized freedom of choice of the patients who could attend traditional, Hindu and Unani healers in the same hospital. He was also ready to learn about the specific treatments and the materia medica of these other systems, which he appreciated on practical grounds to such an extent that he published a trilingual dictionary, contributing further to medical pluralism in the making.

Homeopathy gained momentum first in Bengal, from where it spread mainly in the Northeast.[33] The contributions of Das and Soman elaborate on this particular important development of homeopathy in Bengal which started during the later 19th century. Das considers the political and intellectual discourses and Soman focuses on lay healing in Bengal. Das calls the Bengal reception a "domestication" of the western category of 'homeopathy', which was based on its claims to indigeneity in the late nineteenth to early twentieth century. She remarks on the overlap of discussions on homeopathy and those on the nationalist reform of Indian families. Homeopathy came to be posited as an efficient disciplining mechanism to reform colonial domesticities – a remedy to cure the institution of 'family' from the corruptions inflicted by colonial rule on the pristine ways of Bengali life. Homeopathic science was even projected as a way of life, capable of producing the ideal family for the nation – a very particular "nostrification" of a medical system imported from abroad.

The contribution of Sharma shows a specific pattern of medical pluralism for the German Empire before World War I. During this period even the elites insisted on the important role of alternative systems and providers for various reasons – liberty of choice, science (!) and national identity – which shows that the hegemony of biomedicine was far from being established. This differs markedly from the contemporary situation, where biomedicine seems to have gained a hegemonic role at least when considering the results of three contributions to this volume on India: it is present in the diagnostic episteme of practitioners of Ayurveda, as Naraindas shows, as well as in the ideas about

---

32   According to Stange (2010), p. 40, in 2007, € 1 billion of practitioners' fees (of € 517 billion health expenditure) were reimbursed – and € 800 million for medication.
33   Poldas (2010).

research of the south Indian homeopath studied by Dusausoit or the daily practice of a homeopath prescribing allopathic drugs, studied by Barua.

Especially during the 1920s homeopathy spread all around the country. After independence it attained the most advanced state of recognition in India worldwide, being ultimately institutionalized as an integral part of the national health system in 1973. The Central Council of Homoeopathy and the Central Council of Research in Homoeopathy accredit the nearly 190 colleges and organize research in 30 publically funded institutes nationwide. In 2007, 15.4% of all physicians in India were homoeopaths. Growth seems to be very slow and their market share seems to have attained a certain threshold during the last generation, as, already in 1982, homeopaths represented 13.7% of all physicians.[34] Ayurveda with some 32.1% of all physicians had a faster path of institutionalization during the last 30 years. The fabulous market share of alternative medical systems amounts to more than 50% of all physicians including some minor systems such as Unani with 3.3%. The contribution of "complementary" systems to healthcare provision in general is probably even larger when one takes into account the non academically trained healthcare providers for whom statistical evidence is missing.

Table 1: Number of Physicians in India (in 2007, in thousand)[35]

System	number	percentage
Allopathic	696	49.2
Ayurvedic	454	32.1
Homeopathic	218	15.4
Unani	46	3.3
Total	1,414	100

Beyond the market offer, legal frameworks are important for the patients' possibilities to choose. The Indian institutional setting is particularly interesting as a way to promote more equal chances for various medical systems and to give the patient equal access to this differentiated medical offer. Since 1973 the department of "Indian Medical Systems and Homeopathy" (IMS&H), under the umbrella of the Ministry of Health, keeps its own register of physicians, decides on training requirements, organizes research and accredits colleges. It is remarkable that homeopathy was integrated with the "Indian Medical Systems", which shows its intermediate position between traditional medicine and biomedicine, belonging somehow neither to the one nor to the other. At the same time this position is a sign of "nostrification" of homeopathy into the

---

34 Cf. Dinges (2008); the share of homeopaths for 2007 shown is slightly higher than in my earlier publications which were based on figures for allopaths from 2004 – at the time the latest available to me.

35 Human resources in health sector. In: National Health Profile (NHP) of India – 2007, p. 136, http://cbhidghs.nic.in/writereaddata/linkimages/Health%20Human%20Resources 4484269844.pdf (last accessed on April 30, 2013).

Indian medical context. In 2003 the name of this health administration department has changed to the more explicit acronym AYUSH (=Ayurveda, Yoga and Naturopathy, Unani Sidda, Homoeopathy). To my knowledge, such an institutionalisation of alternative medical systems is unique. In other countries the legal requirements for physicians of all systems are exactly the same and they are decided by a unified national body once and for all. This is also the case in Germany: practitioners first have to pass medical exams before they can specialize, for instance in internal medicine or balneology, homeopathy or surgery. In India, on the other hand, the systems have more freedom of decision, for example on whether to prescribe four or five years of medical training for physicians. They also have independent training institutions (medical colleges) for homeopathy, biomedicine, Ayurveda and so on.

Taking public funding into consideration it is evident that the department of AYUSH is not on a par with biomedicine: it receives nine times less research funds than the latter. This is in sharp contrast to the fact that only 49.2% of all physicians in India officially practise biomedicine. For a similar situation – the status of Ayurveda in comparison with biomedicine in Sri Lanka – Jones proposed the useful term "bounded pluralism" to express a formal but not real equality.[36] It is certainly evident that a realistic appreciation of health politics in the field of medical pluralism is only possible if the cash flow is taken into consideration. The relatively limited research of the various medical systems inside AYUSH is another cause as well as effect of inequalities – for the simple reason that some departments of AYUSH do not even spend all the funds allocated to them.

With this organisational structure in place, the various systems have, at least in principle, the chance to gain equality. The institutional potential for equality is even more evident when considering the importance of public institutions of primary healthcare in countries such as India and Brazil: in both countries, the public administration has many possibilities to act and to impose medical pluralism as long as it can recruit qualified personnel in sufficient numbers. Germany has no such system. Here, exclusively private GPs are sharing the market within certain boundaries set by the national health insurance scheme. GPs can choose to qualify as homoeopathic physicians (see above) and provide homeopathic care. Most homeopathic medications are not reimbursed by the health insurances in the general system, which covers around 90% of the population. Some of the private insurance companies covering the remaining 10% do reimburse these medications.

Looking at the question of equality inside the Indian system with regard to the preferences of physicians and lay healers a different picture presents itself: observing the daily practice and the aspirations of some "homeopathic" or "ayurvedic" physicians, Naraindas and Dusausoit argue in this volume that the attractiveness of biomedicine seems irresistible even to non-allopathic physicians. This leads to a kind of practice which combines elements of bio-

36 Jones (2009), p. 118.

medicine – or at least its diagnostic and nosological components – with elements of complementary medicine in an astonishing variety of ways. The result is a kind of hybrid medicine which is neither biomedical nor strictly homeopathic or Ayurvedic.

Another practical problem of medical pluralism in India seems to be patients' dissatisfaction with the practical functioning of the public health institutions. Naturally, this concerns representatives of all medical systems inside the
public health infrastructure. Let me illustrate this with the outcome of German
research into a Tamil Nadu rural district, Madukottai, recently published by
Alex: in Madukottai, the low caste patients are prepared to use all systems of
treatment without giving priority to either biomedicine, AYUSH-systems or
other – from a quantitative point of view – even more important folk-systems
such as magic or religious healing.[37] The health-seeking behaviour was illness-
specific: in case of fever, people preferred private and government clinics, for
problems with the bronchial tubes they preferred non-biomedical treatments.[38] In practice, 60% used biomedicine, 26% non-biomedical methods,
13% self-medication (with no further specification).[39] All in all – an ideal starting point for medical pluralism. And what is more: physicians of all medical
systems working inside the public health institutions are generally considered
to be well trained, of good quality and in general even friendly or neutral.
Four fifth of the 150 persons who were extensively interviewed shared these
opinions. Nevertheless, 70% of the same population prefer private practitioners: The two main reasons are
–   the physical distance to Primary Health Care Units or hospitals,
–   the long waiting lists and overcrowding of the institution.
These two critical points are again shared by four fifth of the respondents.[40]
One must see these results in context with the different findings of Barua on
Delhi slum dwellers, which provide a different set of dissatisfactions.[41] The
point here is that one should differentiate between the potential of the impressive Indian institutional setting and its practical achievements as long as it is
considered by many locals as so little satisfactory. Below the level of institutions, medical pluralism seems to function perfectly in Madukottai on the patients' side. They use all sorts of (traditional) healers, local private practitioners, OTC-medicines, the private homeopathic physician or any other means
of helping themselves.

---

37   Alex (2010), pp. 167–168, 295.
38   Alex (2010), p. 302.
39   Alex (2010), p. 275–276.
40   Alex (2010), p. 278–279.
41   Such as bureaucratic paper work before treatment, non-gentle treatment of poorer pa-
     tients and bribes, to name just a few.

Patients' Preferences and Physicians' Practices

This is the moment to look more closely at practices as the main focus of this volume. The first focus is on the health-seeking behaviour of patients in countries like India as it has been highlighted in medical anthropology. According to recent scholarship one can attempt to reconstruct the "pragmatic patients'" list of motivations:[42]

– most important of all is the local offer of health services and their accessibility;
– second in line is the medical success of a healer or a group of healers;
– in third place are the sort of actual symptoms and their seriousness, which seem to have priority over preferences for medical systems or even for specific healers;[43]
– fourthly, the potential further serious social effects of the illness on the personal network of the ill person is considered;
– fifthly, the explanatory model of medical systems seems to play a minor role for the patients – it might be slightly more important for upper class patients in India and in Germany because of a greater possibility of deliberate choice;[44]
– social norms and social relations on the basis of ethnic backgrounds may be important under certain circumstances;
– habitual user patterns which may be linked to specific family traditions may also have an impact.[45]

This – not exhaustive – list from research exclusively about Asia provides a few interesting points of comparison between the German and the Indian situation.

The actual demand of patients for complementary and alternative medicines (CAM) in Germany is known due to market research, representative polls and in-depth studies. The main outcomes of recent surveys are the following:[46] it is unfortunately not possible on the basis of this evidence to propose a strict ranking beyond the first two reasons for choice of patients.

In Germany, the patients' demand for CAM is

– first of all driven by dissatisfaction with former biomedical treatment, a frustration which plays a crucial role in the rising demand for CAM,
– the assumption that CAM-methods have little side effects, an idea which plays also an important role in India and many other countries[47],

---

42   This is based on the most recent review of literature by Alex (2010), p. 78, and complemented with further readings; cf. Bourdier (1996), pp. 447–448.
43   Alex (2010), p. 288, which gives in detail the bibliography for each argument.
44   Cf. Dinges (2002), p. 18.
45   Alex (2010), p. 78.
46   Leonhard (1984); Günther/Römermann (2002); Köntopp (2004); Kahrs (2002); Stange (2010).
47   See the studies on India cited in Dinges: Patientenpräferenzen (2011) and on India and many other countries, Dinges (2012).

-   the idea of a gentle mode of action – significantly more often mentioned by women than men, and more valued by persons with higher formal education[48],
-   the patient-oriented relationship between therapist and patient,
-   the accordance of CAM with personal life-styles also plays a role. Empowerment of the patient to take responsibility for his health is positively associated with CAM by many patients.[49] This includes a reference to self-medication and to the idea of relative independence from the help of a (professional) healer.
-   In general the trend towards CAM is stronger in cases of less serious illnesses in Germany; this is in line with results of a representative poll about Indian patients, whereas the findings of Raj K. Manchanda for the use of Primary Health Care Centres in New Delhi show a preference of the patients to use biomedicine in acute, homeopathy in chronic and sub-chronic illness.[50]

To a certain extent India seems to be a different medical world, when trends towards life-style-medicine are considered.[51] One might even suggest – and Barua does it in this volume – that there are stark contrasts between the two medical pluralisms which we are comparing – but there are also evident similarities. The choices of the Indian Upper and urban upper middle classes seem to show more resemblances with the German pattern of preferences for CAM than with the general Indian pattern, which is based to a large extent on medical anthropological observations on lower class or caste groups. This might bias the outcome.

The contribution of Baschin addresses a historical case of patients' demand in the German city of Münster during the second and third quarter of the 19th century, considering the practice of father and son Bönninghausen, the first being a lay healer, the second a physician. From around 21,000 patient files Baschin reconstructs the medical treatments used before patients consulted the homeopath, and the various healers consulted who were often allopaths. Consultation frequency and other aspects are analysed. Homeopathy was often a last resort and patients were not necessarily convinced of it. Homeopathy was not used for economic reasons and it is impossible from the source to decide, whether the patients were "shopping around" or whether they were cured after a single visit.

Eisele's contribution analyzes the interest of a particularly active group of German patients in complementary and alternative medicine during the last decade of the 20th century. He focuses on persons who wrote letters to the independent patient association "Natur und Medizin". Using 1,655 inquiries he can identify these patients' motivations for writing a letter, their social back-

---

48   Kahrs (2002), p. 147.
49   Kahrs (2002), pp. 145–146.
50   Kahrs (2002), pp. 150–151; R. K. Manchanda in this volume; Singh/Yadav/Pandey (2005), p. 138.
51   Wolff (2010).

ground, the illness episodes that are the reason for writing, the third party that benefitted from the letter and the way patients obtained information about CAM. More than two fifths of the patients wanted to replace biomedical treatment with CAM, nearly as many used it as a last resort, and a smaller group used it as a complement to allopathy.

The paper of Tewari and Valavan on the Indian patients focuses on people who choose homeopathy nowadays. The authors are interested in the social, economic and educational background of these people, their gender profile, the different patterns in cities and in the country, trends in follow-up and the question as to whether they were referred to homeopathic physicians and by whom. The paper also analyzes how patients found their way to the homeopathic healer.

The motives of German physicians for choosing to offer CAM or homeopathy mainly or as a supplement have been addressed above.[52] CAM-therapies have become an integral part of the therapies offered by a large majority of GPs.[53] This corroborates the assumption that these methods are far more wide-spread within the general medical system than one might think if one only considers the number of physicians with a specialisation in homeopathy, phytotherapy, anthroposophic medicine and so on. It also shows that many GPs without a special training prescribe CAM-medications, evidently lacking the necessary qualification.[54] Especially in the case of regular and repetitive users of "alternative medicine" the physicians must accept a relationship between patient and healer that is based on equality rather than on the traditional role of the physician as specialist and the patient as a follower of his advice.[55]

With regard to India one has to consider the motives of students for choosing a training other than the biomedical one. The reasons for this choice are under discussion. Some students are more or less convinced followers of a particular "alternative" system such as Unani, Ayurveda, Siddha or homeopathy due to family tradition or good healing experiences. For others, attending a college of one of the AYUSH systems is a second choice. They wanted to study allopathy but did not attain the necessary grades in their school-leaving certificate. It is impossible to quantify the proportion of these two groups. In later practice the treatment used is not necessarily a logical consequence of the training received in the medical school attended as for example many graduates of Ayurvedic colleges go on to do what they originally wanted to do: practice allopathy! The examples of physicians crossing the boundaries of medical systems show an unintended effect of the strictly differentiated system of academic teaching in India. Here again, we have evidence of a lack of qualification.

52 Thanner (2010), p. 190.
53 Marstedt (2012).
54 Stange (2010), p. 40.
55 Marstedt (2012), esp. p. 145.

Beyond the "free market", provision of healthcare in public institutions is important for the structure of medical pluralism and for the access to what it has to offer. In some Indian states the "cafeteria approach" allows the patient to choose his or her preferred medical system inside the same public primary healthcare units, where homeopaths are present at the same level as allopaths and Ayurvedic physicians. This choice inside a public service is only possible in sufficiently densely populated areas, where more than one physician can be employed in each primary healthcare centre. Locally, the choice may be between allopathy and Unani or allopathy and Ayurveda or homeopathy. It is rare that three or more systems are available.[56] The paper of R. K. Manchanda, which is based on the statistical analysis of millions of consultations in Delhi, shows how intelligent patients make use of this medical offer. He analyzes their preferences for either allopathy or homeopathy, depending on the type of illness. He compares this with the morbidity profiles, and this enables him to discover the rational pattern of the patients' choices. He also demonstrates the cost effectiveness of homeopathic treatment.

Homeopathic healthcare provision inside hospitals is another important issue in the institutional practice of medical pluralism. A. Manchanda studies in this volume the case of the Holy Family Hospital, a multi-speciality centre in south Delhi, run by the Delhi Catholic Arch-Diocese. In 1987, the ayurvedic and homeopathic departments were established in this hospital as a pilot project to provide holistic health services. Homeopathic consultation was initially provided by a lay practitioner, succeeded by two qualified homeopathic doctors, one of whom was the author. From her practical experience she describes the economical expectations of the responsible authority, the cooperation with the physicians of other medical systems and the possibilities of a homeopathic physician to influence the medical offer of the hospital as a whole. The experience at this hospital – which was successful for the homeopaths – was instrumental in spreading this form of institutionalized medical pluralism to other hospitals. As the integration of homeopaths into hospital care is practised in less than a dozen hospitals in Germany, the Indian experience might inspire German institutions to reconsider their refusal to accept them.

After the presentation of these examples of the integration of homeopathy into institutional healthcare one has to consider a very different kind of "medical pluralism": biomedical treatment under a homeopathic label. Barua uses the case of an urban homeopath who has established his practice in a Delhi slum.[57] He is not one of the "less-than-fully-qualified" practitioners currently offering their services in poor neighbourhoods but a qualified homeopathic physician. As a private provider he is on the spot in a slum that lacks a primary healthcare centre for its 25,000 habitants. The doctor's presence makes it possible for the slum dwellers to avoid the loss of time and money that go with using the distant public services. The interesting point with this doctor in

56   Cf. figures for Delhi.
57   On health conditions in the slums cf. Chaplin (2011), p. 135.

our context is that he is diagnosing and practising biomedicine, not document-
ing the cases and prescribing allopathic medications (antibiotics, multivitamins etc.). No pattern for prescription can be discerned. He explains that he
feels obliged to give these pills and leave homeopathy aside because his patients need immediate help and have no understanding for homeopathic initial aggravation that might even incite them to turn to a competitor.

Dusausoit presents another case of a homeopath who does not seem to be
very convinced by his own system. Having attended during three months the
daily consultations of a South Indian homeopath, the author underlines the
differences between the consultations in theory and in practice. The homeopath takes very little time for patients but a lot for friends, case taking is super-
ficial, the personality of the patient takes priority over the symptoms. The
main point in this context of medical pluralism is not the deficient practice of
this – not necessarily very typical – homeopath, as Dusausoit concedes, but his
orientation towards biomedicine as the pattern of "real" medicine – as science
and as therapy. He would have liked to become an allopathic doctor and gain
the prestige of that profession. Again, considering daily practice, the institutional equality of the medical systems is no guarantee against the lesser recognition of homeopathy in an age when biomedicine pretends to be the bench-
mark of science.

Naraindas presents a comparable case of applied medical pluralism, "the
modern doctor of traditional medicine" as he calls it. He focuses on the episteme of this medical practice. The physicians in question, trained in Ayurveda, Unani or Siddha, do in fact something very different from what they
have learnt during their training. They use biomedical diagnostics and translate them subsequently somehow into the therapeutic categories of their traditional systems. The result is an asymmetric creolization based on a dominant
biomedical understanding of the body and of illness and combined with Ayurvedic therapeutics.

Unfortunately, too little is still known about the continuing role of lay
practitioners in healthcare provision, particularly in slums and in the rural
parts of India.[58] Studies normally concern exclusively the district level, such as
the one of Sen and colleagues about Koppal in Karnataka with 60 villages and
a population of 82,000.[59] Their survey of healthcare providers generated the
following results:

---

58 Some information is compiled in Sheehan (2009), p. 140; on the utilization of health ser-
    vices by tribal people cf. Dhandapani (2010), p. 195; on their choice of medical systems
    p. 177.
59 Cf. Sheehan (2009).

Table 2: Health care providers in Koppal

35	spiritual healers
133	traditional healers
178	traditional birth attendants
47	registered medical practitioners
1	qualified Ayurvedic doctor
152	provision stores
2	medical shops
548	providers

The authors conclude: "Although there are a few private specialists in the largest towns, the rural reality of Koppal is 'dominated by informal providers'."[60] The situation seems to be similar in small market towns in Maharastra and in slums. All in all, too little is known, even about the number of non-academically trained providers as they are – per definition – not registered. Only ethnographic research may disclose more about their preferred therapies and allow a closer look at their actual practice. This type of research is much needed particularly considering the fact that seemingly casual criticism from the point of view of urban biomedical physicians reflects their professional interests and is, secondly, spread by worldbank reports which still tend to neglect the particular contribution of these healers to healthcare provision in disadvantaged areas.[61]

This volume contributes to a better knowledge of these non-registered healers with a paper from Soman about the West-Bengal rural districts. She presents a very rich picture of this practice over the last 150 years, taking as one of the examples the case of Rabindranath Tagore and leading the reader all the way to the actual practice of lay healing in the country. Her narrative of three generations of homeopathic healing activities which started inside her family, the Chatterjees, is particularly interesting. Mothers and fathers were playing varying roles, which adds the important and often not sufficiently studied aspect of gender. Using family papers and personal souvenirs she is able to situate the medical choice of her ancestors in the contexts of (non) availability of other medical offers, personal choice and political ideas such as self-reliance and Bengal nationalism. Soman allows new qualitative insights into this part of applied medical pluralism. The importance of this contribution is evident when considering that 73% of all physicians practise in the cities for the 15% of urban population of India, whereas only 27% of the physicians have to care for the 85% of rural population.[62] Therefore the role of these lay practitioners remains a crucial issue for healthcare in India.

---

60 Citation taken from Sheehan (2009), p. 140.
61 On research about the reasons for continuous underutilization of biomedicine in the country see Pfleiderer (1995), p. 81; cf. Dhandapani (2010), pp. 195, 177.
62 Manchanda/Kaur (2012).

Conclusion

To compare these two very different countries, their institutional framework and the patients' choices inside these economical, social and political conditions allows interesting insights into the functioning of medical pluralism in practice. It was a voluntary choice of the conference, from which this volume has arisen, to go beyond the description of systems and infrastructure of medical pluralism and to focus on practices. This allowed for new insights into the historical development as well as into the current situation. Already the first glance at medical pluralism in South-Asia by Honigberger during the 1830s shows a mixture of rejection and acceptance of medical pluralism in practice. Medical pluralism as the determined choice of German elites before World War I initiated a medical specialisation that went on until medical pluralism experienced a renaissance after the 1980s. There is no teleological march towards a monopoly or hegemony of biomedicine – even if the Indian evidence in some of the contributions shows this attitude in a small number of physicians. Medical pluralism, in its old, modern and new form, seems to be a much longer-lasting phenomenon than one might have expected a generation ago. The Indian "nostrification" of homeopathy in Bengal before Independence shows a particular set of arguments which invite to compare it with other such processes of indigenization.

In terms of an institutionalized pluralistic medical provision, India provides interesting experiences inside the Primary healthcare system and inside private hospitals. Referral practices show that cooperation between different systems that is in the patients' best interest may function well under the conditions prevailing there. The German setting – although friendly towards medical pluralism when compared to other welfare states – could be reconsidered in the light of these examples of successful practice. That, at least, is the opinion of the patients.

Considering patients' demands, the contributions shed new light on patients' motives for choosing a treatment in line with a system of complementary medicine. Such motives are not easy to detect. Even considering the long-term situation since the 19th century, patterns seem less different in the two countries than it might appear at first sight, but there are also a few particularities, since economic constraints are different and had less impact in Germany even a century ago. Patients are very pragmatic in their choices, have good reasons for choosing and sticking to a certain medical approach, but they are rarely sufficiently convinced of a system to not give another system a try. "Convinced" patients are probably as rare as medical "shoppers" are.

The practice of healthcare providers shows in some of the studied cases remarkable switches from one system to another – either between diagnosis and therapy or in taking biomedicine as an idealized image of medicine for research in homeopathy or just as a way to make a living. This might be an indication for an identity crisis in some representatives of "alternative" systems of medicine that should be studied further. If there is such a crisis its extent would be another question.

The practices of homeopathic lay healers have rarely been studied in such depth as in this volume. They show the intention of these healthcare providers to be autonomous but one also has to remember the constraints that they experience. Comparable studies on Germany could cast more light on this much too little known part of the medical market.[63]

Other issues will have to be addressed later: we left out most of the transnational interactions inside systems, a fashionable research topic these days. The role media play in the development of medical pluralism is another point: how and with what kind of impact did and do they foster ideas of autonomy, self-help, self-healing, lay practice or medical consumerism? And how has this changed with the internet? Another question about the background of the burgeoning medical pluralism around the world should not be ignored: What is the role of pharmaceutical companies and their publicity inside the developing medical pluralism? Another task would be to analyze how homoeopaths and the representatives of other "alternative" healing methods succeed to assure their position inside the medical system with its asymmetric distribution of power. The practice of public and political lobbying would be one aspect. The impact of lay healers on medical pluralism at certain moments of history would be another interesting issue. Is it really only a sign of decay if they are dominantly active in favour of a certain system?

Bibliography

Internet Links

http://www.dzvhae.de/dzvhae-presse/basisdaten/basisdaten-homoeopathie.html (last accessed on April 30, 2013)

http://elise10delannoy.free.fr/desaccord.html (last accessed on April 30, 2013)

http://www.inhfparis.com/homeopathie-uniciste/hom%C3%A9opathie-classique-uniciste-0 (last accessed on April 30, 2013)

http://www.igm-bosch.de/content/language1/html/11643.asp (last accessed on April 30, 2013)

http://www.gbe-bund.de (last accessed on April 30, 2013)

http://cbhidghs.nic.in/writereaddata/linkimages/Health%20Human%20Resources4484269 844.pdf (last accessed on April 30, 2013)

Literature

Alex, Gabi: Medizinische Diversität im postkolonialen Indien. Berlin 2010.

Arnold, David; Sarkar, Sumit: In search for rational remedies. Homoeopathy in nineteenth century Bengal. In: Ernst, Waltraud (ed.): Plural medicine, tradition and modernity, 1800–2000. London 2002, pp. 40–57.

---

63   Cf. Naraindas (2011); Faltin (2000).

Becker, Raymond; Sertel, Serkan et al. (eds.): "Neue" Wege in der Medizin: Alternativmedizin – Fluch oder Segen? Heidelberg 2010.

Bode, Marteen: Taking Traditional Knowledge to the Market. The Modern Image of the Ayurvedic and Unani Industry, 1980–2000. Hyderabad 2008.

Bornhöft, Gudrun; Matthiessen, Peter: Homeopathy in Healthcare, Effectiveness, Appropriateness, Safety, Costs. Berlin; Heidelberg 2011.

Bourdier, Frédéric: Rencontres thérapeutiques dans l'Inde méridionals ou l'art d'élaborer une medicine masala dans les strategies de soins. In: Benoist, Jean (ed.): Soigner au pluriel. Essais sur le pluralisme medical. Paris 1996, pp. 425–460.

Cant, Sarah; Sharma, Ursula: A new medical pluralism? Alternative medicine, doctors, patients and the state. London 1998.

Chaplin, Susan E.: The politics of sanitation in India: cities, services and the state. New Delhi 2011.

Cheng, Huei-chu: Medizinischer Pluralismus und Professionalisierung – Entwicklung der chinesischen Medizin in Taiwan. Diss. soz.wiss. Bielefeld 2003.

Das, Jishnu; Hammer, Jeffrey: Location, location, location: Residence, Wealth and the Quality of Medical Care in Delhi, India. In: Health Affairs 26 (2007), no. 3, pp. w338-w351.

Dhandapani, C.: Household expenditure pattern of tribals on health in India. New Delhi 2010.

Dilger, Hansjörg; Hadolt, Bernhard (eds.): Medizin im Kontext: Krankheit und Gesundheit in einer vernetzten Welt. Frankfurt/Main et al. 2010.

Dilger, Hansjörg; Hadolt, Bernhard: Medizin im Kontext: Überlegungen zu einer Sozial- und Kulturanthropologie der Medizin(en) in einer vernetzten Welt. In: Dilger, Hansjörg; Hadolt, Bernhard (eds.): Medizin im Kontext: Krankheit und Gesundheit in einer vernetzten Welt. Frankfurt/Main et al. 2010, pp. 11–29.

Dinges, Martin (ed.): Homöopathie. Patienten, Heilkundige und Institutionen. Von den Anfängen bis heute. Heidelberg 1996.

Dinges, Martin (ed.): Weltgeschichte der Homöopathie. Länder – Schulen – Heilkundige. München 1996.

Dinges, Martin: Patients in the history of homoeopathy: Introduction. In: Dinges, Martin (ed.): Patients in the History of Homoeopathy. Sheffield 2002, pp. 1–32.

Dinges, Martin: Homöopathie in Indien. Ein Absteiger innerhalb des indischen Gesundheitssystems? In: Zeitschrift für Klassische Homöopathie 52 (2008), no. 2, pp. 60–68.

Dinges, Martin: Patientenpräferenzen und die öffentliche Gesundheitsversorgung in Indien Der Versorgungsbeitrag der Homöopathie (Zweiter Teil). In: Zeitschrift für Klassische Homöopathie 55 (2011), no. 3, pp. 122–133.

Dinges, Martin: Der Versorgungsbeitrag der Homöopathie in Indien (Erster Teil). In: Zeitschrift für Klassische Homöopathie 55 (2011), no. 1, pp. 4–18.

Dinges, Martin: The next decade for homoeopathy: Any lessons from the last decades? In: Homoeopathy for Public Health: Proceedings of 66th LMHI Congress. Delhi 2014 [forthcoming].

Dinges, Martin: Entwicklungen der Homöopathie seit 30 Jahren. In: Zeitschrift für Klassische Homöopathie 56 (2012), no. 3, pp. 137–148.

Ebrahimnejad, Hormoz (ed.): The Development of Modern Medicine in Non-Western Countries. Historical Perspectives. London 2009.

Ebrahimnejad, Hormoz: Introduction: for a history of modern medicine in non-Western countries. In: Ebrahimnejad, Hormoz (ed.): The Development of Modern Medicine in Non-Western Countries. Historical Perspectives. London 2009, pp. 1–22.

Ernst, Waltraud (ed.): Plural medicine, tradition and modernity, 1800–2000. London 2002.

Faltin, Thomas: Heil und Heilung: Geschichte der Laienheilkundigen und Struktur antimodernistischer Weltanschauungen in Kaiserreich und Weimarer Republik am Beispiel von Eugen Wenz (1856–1945). Stuttgart 2000.

Frank, Robert; Stollberg, Gunnar: German medical doctors' motives for practising homoeopathy, acupuncture or ayurveda. In: Johannessen, Helle; Lázár, Imre (eds.): Multiple medical realities: patients and healers in biomedical, alternative, and traditional medicine. New York 2006, pp. 72–89.

Günther, Martina; Römermann, Hans: The Homoeopathic Patient in General Practice: Findings of a Comparative Poll of Patients in Conventional Medical Practices and Homoeopathic Private and Health Insurance Scheme Practices. In: Dinges, Martin (ed.): Patients in the History of Homoeopathy. Sheffield 2002, pp. 281–299.

Johannessen, Helle: Introduction. In: Johannessen, Helle; Lázár, Imre (eds.): Multiple medical realities: patients and healers in biomedical, alternative, and traditional medicine. New York 2006, pp. 1–17.

Jones, Margret: A bounded medical pluralism: Ayurveda and Western medicine in colonial and independent Sri Lanka. In: Ebrahimnejad, Hormoz (ed.): The Development of Modern Medicine in Non-Western Countries. Historical Perspectives. London 2009, pp. 108–122.

Jütte, Robert: Pluralismus in der Medizin aus historischer Perspektive. In: Michl, Susanne; Potthast, Thomas; Wiesing, Urban (eds.): Pluralität in der Medizin. Werte – Methoden – Theorien. Freiburg/Brsg.; München 2008, pp. 381–393.

Jütte, Robert (ed.): Medical Pluralism: Past – Present – Future. Stuttgart 2013.

Jütte, Robert; Risse, Guenter B. et al. (eds.): Culture, knowledge, and healing: historical perspectives of homeopathic medicine in Europe and North America. Sheffield 1998.

Kahrs, Marcus: Ansprüche an medizinische Versorgung im Spannungsfeld zwischen Angebotsstruktur und individuellen Bedürfnissen: quantitative Befunde zur Artikulation von Ansprüchen an medizinische Versorgung und deren Befriedigung. Diss. rer. pol. Bremen 2002.

Köntopp, Sabine: Wer nutzt Komplementärmedizin? Theorie, Empirie, Prognose. Essen 2004.

Leonhard, Joachim: Motive zum Heilpraktikerbesuch: eine empirische Untersuchung über die sozialen Aspekte und die Krankengeschichte als Hintergrund eines Entscheidungsprozesses. Teningen 1984.

Leslie, Charles (ed.): Asian Medical Systems: A Comparative Study. Berkeley 1976.

Liebeskind, Claudia: Arguing Science: Unani tibb, hakims and biomedicine in India, 1900–1950. In: Ernst, Waltraud (ed.): Plural medicine, tradition and modernity, 1800–2000. London 2002, pp. 58–75.

Manchanda, Raj Kumar; Kaur, Harleen: Medical Pluralism in Health Care – Experiences from New Delhi. In: Jütte, Robert (ed.): Medical Pluralism: Past – Present – Future. Stuttgart 2013 [forthcoming].

Marstedt, Gerd: Die steigende Popularität alternativer Medizin – Suche nach medizinischen Gurus und Wunderheilern? In: Böcken, Jan; Braun, Bernard et al. (eds.): Gesundheitsmonitor 2012. Die ambulante Versorgung aus Sicht der Bevölkerung und Ärzteschaft. Gütersloh 2012, pp. 130–149.

Mildenberger, Florian: Medikale Subkulturen in der Bundesrepublik Deutschland und ihre Gegner (1950–1990): die Zentrale zur Bekämpfung der Unlauterkeit im Heilgewerbe. Stuttgart 2011.

Naraindas, Harish: Of relics, body parts and laser beams: the German Heilpraktiker and his Ayurvedic spa. In: Anthropology and Medicine 18 (2011), pp. 67–86.

Nichter, Mark: The laypersons perception of medicine as perspective into the utilization of multiple therapy systems in the Indian context. In: Social Science and Medicine 14 B (1980), pp. 225–233.

Pahari, Subrata: The Travails of Traditional Medicine. In: Palit, Chittabrata; Dutta, Achintya Kumar (eds.): History of Medicine in India. The Medical Encounter. Delhi 2005, pp. 219–232.

Pfleiderer, Beatrix: Medizinische Systeme Südasiens. In: Pfleiderer, Beatrix; Greifeld, Katarina; Bichmann, Wolfgang: Ritual und Heilung. Eine Einführung in die Ethnomedizin. 2nd ed. Berlin 1995, pp. 67–110.

Poldas, Samuel Vijaya Bhaskar: Geschichte der Homöopathie in Indien: von ihrer Einführung bis zur ersten offiziellen Anerkennung 1937. Stuttgart 2010.

Riley, David: Homeopathy in the United States (1824–2011), talk at the DHU-meeting "Homeopathic Medicinal Products at the Beginning of the 21st Century: Opportunities and Challenges", 50 Years DHU, Karlsruhe 9.-10. Juni 2011, referring to: http://www.research andmarkets.com/reports/648969/complementary_and_alternative_medicines_in_the (last accessed on August 2, 2012).

Schmitz, Olivier (ed.): Les médecines en parallèle: multiplicité des recours au soin en Occident. Paris 2006.

Schmitz, Olivier: Soigner par l'invisible. Enqûete sur les guérisseurs aujourd'hui. Paris 2006.

Sheehan, Helen E.: Medical Pluralism in India: patient choice or no other options. In: Indian Journal of Medical Ethics 6 (2009), no. 3, pp. 138–140.

Singh, Padam; Yadav, R.J.; Pandey, Arvind: Utilization of Indigenous Systems of Medicine & Homoeopathy in India. In: Indian Journal of Medical Research 122 (August 2005), pp. 137–142, URL: http://www.ncbi.nlm.nih.gov/pubmed/16177471 (last accessed on April 30, 2013).

Sivaramakrishnan, Kavita: Old Potions, New Bottles. Recasting Indigenous Medicine in Colonial Punjab (1850–1945). Hyderabad 2006.

Stange, Rainer: Naturheilkunde und komplementäre Medizin in der heutigen Gesellschaft: Eine Bestandsaufnahme zu Relevanz und Akzeptanz. In: Becker, Raymond; Sertel, Serkan et al. (eds.): "Neue" Wege in der Medizin: Alternativmedizin – Fluch oder Segen? Heidelberg 2010, pp. 35–50.

Stollberg, Gunnar: Welche Motivation haben deutsche Ärztinnen und Ärzte, Homöopathie, Akupunktur oder Ayurveda auszuüben? Welche Vorstellungen von einem "guten Arzt" haben sie und ihre Patientinnen und Patienten? In: Witt, Claudia (ed.): Der gute Arzt aus interdisziplinärer Sicht. Ergebnisse eines Expertentreffens. Essen 2010, pp. 239–257.

Thanner, Mirjam: Geld oder Glaube? Warum Schulmediziner alternative Heilverfahren anbieten. In: Becker, Raymond; Sertel, Serkan et al. (eds.): "Neue" Wege in der Medizin: Alternativmedizin – Fluch oder Segen? Heidelberg 2010, pp. 187–202.

Walach, Harald: Medical Pluralism in Germany. In: Jütte, Robert (ed.): Medical Pluralism: Past – Present – Future. Stuttgart 2013 [forthcoming].

Wolff, Eberhard: Alternativmedizin und Gesundheitsgesellschaft – kulturelle Hintergründe einer anhaltenden Popularität. In: Becker, Raymond; Sertel, Serkan et al. (eds.): "Neue" Wege in der Medizin: Alternativmedizin – Fluch oder Segen? Heidelberg 2010, pp. 177–185.

World Health Organization: General Guidelines for Methodologies on Research and Evaluation of Traditional Medicine. Geneva 2000, URL: http://whqlibdoc.who.int/hq/2000/WHO_EDM_TRM_2000.1.pdf (last accessed on April 30, 2013).

Wujastyk, Dagmar; Smith, Frederick M.: Introduction. In: Wujastyk, Dagmar; Smith, Frederick M. (eds.): Modern and Global Ayurveda. Pluralism and Paradigms. New York 2008, pp. 1–28.

East Meets West: Johann M. Honigberger and Medical Pluralism through the Eyes of a 19th Century Transylvanian Saxon in India

Silvia Waisse

Introduction

Johann Martin Honigberger's (1795–1869) claim to fame has two main sources: on the one hand, he was the protagonist of a famous and enigmatic short story by Mircea Eliade – "Secretul doctorului Honigberger", and on the other, he is traditionally acknowledged as having introduced homeopathy to India.[1]

"The Secret of Doctor Honigberger" has been surrounded by mystery, from its original publication in 1940 to this day, giving rise to a remarkable corpus of hermeneutical literature.[2] Not less remarkable is the fact that until very recently, Romanians considered Honigberger a fictional persona, namely a doctor who had travelled to India, where he had engaged in esoteric practices. Twenty years later, Eliade mentioned Honigberger again, this time as the source on Haridas, an Indian fakir reported to have survived being buried for 40 days.[3]

Haridas' story, indeed, is told by Honigberger in his major work, "Thirty-Five Years in the East"[4], mostly known for the account of 35 (of the 50) years its author spent travelling across the East and the West. In addition to presenting lively descriptions of people and places, political upheavals, and social and cultural aspects, the book is largely devoted to medical matters, for Honigberger, a pharmacist by training, toured half the world as a medical practitioner. Indeed, the book is divided into three major parts: an Introduction, mostly devoted to a discussion of the contemporary state of Western medicine; Part I, which includes the description of his travels between 1815 and 1851; and Part II, comprising an actual repertory and a materia medica of the medicines he used, including the Western traditional and more recent ones, the Eastern medicines about which he learned from local doctors and other kinds of healers as well as other medicines that he designed and tested. As an appendix, this book concludes with a medical lexicon in eight different East-

---

1   I am not concerned with and thus do not discuss in this article who first introduced homeopathy to India. However, this article may contribute to dispel some common misconceptions as the ones stated by Poldas (2010), Ghosh (2010), p. 130, and Singh (2003), p. 163, for instance.
2   For an appraisal of this debate, see Ciurtin's study appended to his translation of Honigberger (2004).
3   See Grinshpon (2002), p. 22.
4   Originally published in German in Vienna, in 1851, an English translation was published in London the following year. In this study I used the German 2nd edition (1853), the first English edition (1852) and a critical Romanian translation (2004); quotations correspond to the English edition except when explicitly indicated otherwise.

ern and Western languages – Latin, English, French, German, Turkish, Arabic, Persian, Indian & Kashmiri.

Thus, "Thirty-Five Years in the East" offers the modern scholar a glimpse of a particular crossroads in the history of medicine characterized by an epistemological void, during the 18th and first half of the 19th century, between the fall of traditional Galenism and the emergence of contemporary Western medicine, which allowed for multiple medical approaches to develop, including homeopathy. This perspective is further enriched by the (not always sympathetic) inclusion of Eastern medicine and pharmacy resulting in a synthesis rarely seen in works on materia medica, and in early models of medical pluralism, perhaps not surprisingly – by multiculturalism.

The first part of this article discusses the cross-cultural environment that characterizes Honigberger's homeland in Transylvania, which exerted deep influence on his personality and intellectual makeup and enabled him to adjust to multiple cultural environments (Figure 1). The second part is devoted to a discussion of the state of Western medicine in Honigberger's times, and more particularly to his views on it, which resulted in the formulation of a medical approach of his own, which he named the 'medial system'. The next section discusses his encounter with the multicultural environment of the Punjab, focusing on some attempts at medical pluralism. Finally, the last section discusses some examples from Honigberger's studies of medicines.

Figure 1: Honigberger at different moments of his life

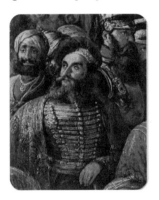 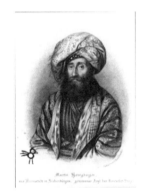 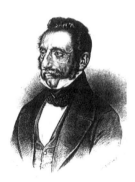

A Transylvanian 'Saxon' travels the world

Born on 10 March 1795 in Brașov/Kronstadt/Brassó[5], not a great deal is known about Honigberger's early years of life. He studied at the local German

---

5   Because of the cross-cultural features I discuss in this section, it is customary to name the Transylvanian towns with their three names, namely, Romanian, German and Hungarian.

Honterus grammar school[6] and later on was an apprentice first in a local pharmacy and then at Bistriţa/Bistritz/Beszterce. For reasons unknown, in 1815, he decided to travel to India. This was in fact to be the first of five trips to Asia, three journeys across Europe and one to Africa (Table 1) which took more than 50 years, until 1869, when he passed away on 18 December, in the town of his birth.

Table 1: The six journeys of Honigberger[7]

1.1815–34	Romania; Bulgaria; Turkey; Syria (7 years); Lebanon; Israel; Egypt; Iran; Oman; India/Pakistan: Karachi, Hyderabad, Multan, Lahore, 4 years in Punjab and Kashmir;[8] Afghanistan; Russia; Ukraine; Braşov.
2.1835–36	Vienna; Italy; France (met Hahnemann in Paris); London; Germany; Poland; Ukraine; Braşov.
3.1836–51	Bucharest; Turkey, Istanbul (2 years); Alexandria; India/Pakistan: Bombay, Delhi, Lahore, 10 years in Lahore and Kashmir, Kolkata; Cape Town; London; Paris; Vienna; Braşov.
4.1852–61	Istanbul; Cairo; India/Pakistan: Mumbai, Delhi, Lahore, 3 years in Kashmir, Lahore, Kolkata (3 years); Cairo; London; Paris; Algiers; 2 years across Africa; Sardinia; Italy; Vienna; Braşov; Vienna; Russia; Denmark; London; Paris.
5.1861–65	Marseille; India/Pakistan: Mumbai, Kolkata, England, Italy, Vienna, Switzerland, Naples, Pyrenees, England.
6.1865–69	India: Nainital; Himalaya; Marseille; Braşov.

6   Oişteanu (2009), p. 275. Johannes Honter (1498–1549) was a Braşov 16th century city councilman, printer and humanist, strongly associated with the movement emphasizing the German identity of the Transylvanian Saxons. By this time the movement had also become defined in religious terms, so that German came to be spoken also at schools and churches. As throughout the Lutheran world strong efforts were devoted to reorganizing the school system so as to encompass the whole community (*ecclesia Dei nationis Saxonica*), both urban and rural, the young grammar school graduates were sent to Protestant universities in the German lands. See Gündisch (1998); for a general overview on the Protestant reform of education, see Hunter (2008).

7   Geographical names and political divisions have changed dramatically since Honigberger's times; for this reason, and to make spatial orientation easier for readers, I have chosen to mention locations and countries according to present-day usage. Whenever necessary, I have added explanatory notes.

8   At the time of the partition in 1947, Punjab was split into East and West, becoming respectively part of India and Pakistan. The political situation of Kashmir has not yet been decided. By the time of Honigberger's visit, both areas were under the rule of Maharaja Ranjit Singh (1780–1839), a period of intense conflict. Honigberger was a witness of the struggles for power and describes them in full detail in "Thirty-Five Years". One cannot fail to be impressed by the similarity of political, religious and nationality issues between

Transylvania – which together with Wallachia and Moldova has constituted modern Romania since the end of the 19th century – has been characterized by multiculturalism since the earliest of times.[9] The particular development of ethnic, social, religious and cultural plurality that interests us begins at the end of the 9th century, when the Magyars successively invaded Europe, were vanquished by Otto I, the Holy Roman Emperor (955), and converted to Christianity. Occupying a strategic position between the German and Byzantine Empires, Hungary, to make its position more secure, extended its territory to the East, to the 'Land beyond the Forest', *Ultra silvam*, Transylvania. This vast territory, which reached as far as the Carpathians, needed protection and development, therefore the Hungarian kings encouraged immigration. This is how Székelys on the one hand[10], and miners, farmers, tradesmen and lower nobility of German and Flemish extraction came to settle in Transylvania (Ardeal/Siebenbürgen/Erdély) from the mid-12th century onwards[11]. This was the origin of the Transylvanian multicultural elite, composed of three different ethnic groups that later on developed also linguistic and religious – and consequently, also political – differences and whose independent status was assured by legislation and special privileges.[12] A thorough discussion of all these groups would require too much space. Up to the present time, Honigberger was known to be a 'Transylvanian Saxon', therefore to have closer insight into the peculiar autonomy enjoyed by the ethnic groups that composed the Transylvanian multicultural elite, I discuss only the status of the so-called 'Saxons'.

Originally, settlers with various religious and ethnic backgrounds from all over the Holy Roman Empire, once they were in Transylvania became a group with its own identity, based on the German language and culture. In 1224, the Transylvanian Saxons were given a "Golden Bull" by the Hungarian king Andrew II that ensured them the right of land ownership and inherit-

---

Honigberger's original and his adopted homeland and this similarity may lie behind a curious assertion he made, '[…] medicine […] a republic (*Freistaat*), founded for the well-being and prosperity of humankind', see Honigberger (1853), p. 7.

9   Transylvania was an outpost of the Roman Empire originally inhabited by the Thracians (which the Romans called Dacians). By the 3rd century CE, only a population speaking Vulgar Latin remained that was exposed through seven centuries to multiple invasions from Gothic, Asian and Slavic tribes, and then Pechenegs and Bulgars in the 9th and 10th centuries. This was the origin of the region's ethnic and cultural diversity that, however, left no traces besides linguistic relics and some archaeological findings. The data on the history of Transylvania and Transylvanian multiculturalism in this article was taken from Haraszti (1971); Cadzow/Ludanyi/Elteto (1983); Dragoescu (1997); Gündisch (1998); Zach (2004); Keul (2009); Davis (2011).

10   Also known as Szeklers, a Hungarian people that is, however, ethnically distinguished from the Magyars.

11   The origins of the "Transylvanian Saxons" are not exactly known; they migrated continuously and in small groups beginning at some time between 1141 and 1158. By 1191, documents mention the *ecclesia Theutonicorum Ultrasilvanorum*, and in 1206 the general appellative 'Saxon' is used to name any individual enjoying the privileges conceded by the "Golden Bull", as it is discussed next.

12   See Bahlcke & Gündisch preface to Zach (2004), p. 1.

ance, personal freedom, freedom to move, their own administration, an autonomous judiciary, religious autonomy with free election of priests, controlled taxes, the privilege to build castles and cities and the right to keep half of the output of the mines, among other privileges.[13]

Constantly facing the threat posed by the Hungarian aristocracy in the late 14th century, the Transylvanian Saxons formalized their status through the creation of the *Sächsische Nationsuniversität*, a political, administrative and judicial entity ensuring their own legal status within the medieval Hungarian state.

Autonomy was only strengthened when Hungary was conquered by the Turks, in 1526, and Transylvania was made an independent principality within the Ottoman Empire. Identity, in turn, was reinforced by the formal adoption of Lutheranism, which further distinguished the Transylvanian Saxons from the mostly Catholic Hungarians and Székelys. And this is the place to introduce two further ethnic groups that are also part of the Transylvanian multiethnic patchwork.

Whereas the larger towns were inhabited mostly by Hungarians and Saxons, who developed urban middle classes and a bureaucratic administration, including an intellectual and professional elite, the largest ethnic population, namely the native Romanians, composed a socially marginalized, Greek Orthodox peasantry, fully excluded from the legally defined political estates, to the point that they were not even allowed to enter the cities. Their political role, therefore, was minimal until the end of the 17th century, when following a demographic explosion, the Romanian population slowly began to mobilize eventually acquiring political expression from the second half of the 19th century onwards.

Then, there was the Jewish community, which needs to be addressed in this context, since Austrian biographer Constantin von Wurzbach attributes explicit Jewish ancestry to Honigberger.[14] In any case, the example of the Jews lends us further insight into Transylvanian multiculturalism.

The origins of the Jews in Transylvania can be traced back to the times of the Roman Empire, but since – as in the case of the original population – several centuries are lost due to the constant invasions, they are only mentioned again in Latin and Slavic documents from the 12th and 13th centuries.[15] Like the Romanian population the Jews did not belong to the elites, but unlike the former, they were fully integrated in the economic, social and political life due to their function as traders and suppliers of credit to the rulers and to urban and rural communities. Jewish doctors, meanwhile, were particularly sought after. Therefore Jews were, as early as the Middle Ages, entitled to own prop-

---

13 See Wagner (1998), pp. 16–19.
14 Wurzbach (1863), p. 255. It must be noted that Ciurtin, in Honigberger (2004), p. 22, observes that archives only allow the reconstruction of the genealogical history of the Honigberger family from mid-18th century onwards, which is consistent with a possible Jewish origin.
15 For data on the history of Transylvanian Jews, the main sources in this article are Gyémánt (2000; 2002; 2004) and Vago/Krausz/Gold (2005).

erty, they paid taxes, participated in the courts of justice (as accused, defendants or witnesses), had freedom to move, and even had influence on the choice of rulers, besides providing an essential chain of communication between Central and South-eastern Europe and also with the Near East. This status did not exempt them from hostility, as was manifest in widespread prejudice (also among the educated classes) and in restrictive laws. Just as the Transylvanian Saxons, the Jews, too, were granted privileges by the Hungarian kings and local rulers, such as, Prince Gábor (Gabriel) Bethlen (1580–1629), who guaranteed the Jews freedom to settle and to move, to practise trade and observe their religion, and to deal autonomously with community matters.

This was the situation when the Habsburg Empire reclaimed Hungary, including Transylvania, from the end of the 17th century. Initially, Austria appealed to the German-rootedness of the Transylvanian Saxons, and promised to maintain all their privileges, including religious autonomy. However, during Maria Theresia's and more especially, Joseph II's rule, intense efforts were made to transform Transylvania into a regular province of the Empire. The territory was now mostly populated by Hungarians and Romanians, whereas the Transylvanian Saxons had become a minority with no special privileges and, in time, they were reduced to a sort of 'Saxon aristocracy' characterized by economic power and an even stronger identification with the German culture. Some of them, as the Transylvania governor Samuel of Brukenthal (1742–1803) – known in homeopathic history for hosting Hahnemann in Sibiu/Hermannstadt/Nagyszeben between 1777 and 1779 – became powerful members of the Habsburg administration by pretending to have converted to Catholicism.

On the Jewish side, the traditional status also deteriorated under Habsburg rule, reaching a climax in 1776, when Maria Theresia proclaimed a highly restrictive *Judenordnung*, drastically limiting the number of Jews, their mobility and their trading rights, while establishing special districts for residence and limiting the social and economic relationships between Christians and Jews to the bare minimum. These measures were further strengthened between 1779 and 1780, when the Jews were banned from all activities but trade, and lost all rights to freedom of movement. However, this legislation was never enacted due to the Empress' death, whereas a new era of tolerance was inaugurated by Joseph II whose edict of tolerance for Hungary also included the Jewish population.[16]

In regard to medicine, the Habsburg's powerful 'medical police', according to T. D. Sechel, gave the initial push for the institutionalisation of the health care professions in Transylvania, beginning at the end of the 18th century. This

---

16   Indeed, under Joseph II's rule, Jews not only recovered all previous privileges, but were also granted the right to enter guilds and access to public education including the universities. However, in the period that concerns us here, the situation of the Jews was so oppressive, that it is safe to assume that it might have triggered conversions. In the particular context of Braşov, it is worth to observe that as late as 1715, a Jew was quartered when accused of ritual murder, see Gyémánt (2004), p. 29; Vago/Krausz/Gold (2005), p. 151.

was not only to improve public health as a whole, but also to enrol the intelligentsia in counteracting the local political elites.[17] Up to that time, doctors had a somewhat uncertain social position, becoming eventually marginalized and occupying the lowest socioeconomic levels. The Habsburg administration transformed the Jesuit College at Cluj/Klausenburg/Kolozsvár into a Royal Academy with the faculties of Philosophy, Theology and Law, to which Medicine was added in 1775.[18] In spite of these developments, the number of doctors remained very small. Moreover, as highlighted by B.Zs. Török, there were patent inequalities as a function of ethno-confessionalism.[19]

This is the cross-cultural context into which Honigberger was born and where he lived until the age of 20. Apart from his ability to adjust to different environments and to synthesize seemingly conflicting medical approaches, this complex context helps us to understand not only why he had no formal training as either a physician or a pharmacist, but also why, up to the present time, he has been seen as a Hungarian by some authors (Márton János), by Romanians (naturally) as a national character, and by others even as a Frenchman (Jean-Martin) or an Englishman (Martin).[20]

Western medicine in the early 19th century

As A. Cunningham and R. French remarked, the medical landscape in the 18th century was so chaotic that even modern historians have tended to eschew it.[21] To summarize, traditional Galenism fell apart in a gradual process, partly accompanying the parallel overthrow of Aristotle´s natural philosophy, but also due to heavy criticism of its foundations (it suffices to mention the names of Andreas Vesalius and William Harvey), the introduction of the chemical and mechanical medical philosophies and, last but not least, the introduction of new drugs coming from the Americas, whose actions and effects directly contradicted the prevailing therapeutic views.[22] Within the context of

17 Sechel (2008), pp. 97 et seq.
18 It must be noted that the medical school only had chairs of surgery, anatomy and obstetrics. Veterinary teaching started in 1787. Joseph II downgraded the faculty to the status of a surgical lyceum; in the 1790s it became a Royal Academy Lyceum, and in 1816, it was raised to a Medical-Surgical Institute. With all these changes it did, however, keep its major goal of training surgeons and midwives. Sechel (2008), p. 106.
19 Török (2008), p. 118.
20 See e.g. Verma (1983); Honigberger (2004), p. 23; Popescu/Mogoşanu/Praţa (2010), p. 109. The biographical information in this paper was taken from Ciurtin's study, in turn based on Roşu (1962). I agree with this author that Sigaléa's (2003) study offers no new information. For an appraisal of the current state of scholarship on Honigberger, see Bordaş (2005).
21 See their "Introduction" to Cunningham/French (1990), p. 1; with the exception of the German and French traditions of historians of medicine, as they make a point of emphasizing.
22 I dealt with the factors associated with the fall of Galenism and the void it created in Waisse (2005), sections 1.3, 1.4. 2.1, and 2.2.

the contemporary emergent early modern science, all throughout the 18th century doctors attempted to give an answer to the problems posed by medical theory, practice, teaching and learning.

Perhaps the most successful of the earliest attempts was the one performed by Hermann Boerhaave (1668–1738), as it is reflected by the judgment of none less than Albrecht Von Haller (1707–1777), 'The Great': "*Europae* [...] *communis preceptor*".[23] Such projects eventually came to be seen and condemned as 'system-framing', possibly due to their sound epistemological foundations and their joining of medical theory and practice[24], but their inefficacy in actual clinical practice. This led to the complete lack of consistent and, once again, effective therapeutic approaches, that was deplored by the vast majority of doctors at the end of the century and that eventually led Pierre J. G. Cabanis (1757–1808) to ask openly whether there was any certainty whatsoever in medicine.[25]

On the other hand, the same lack paved the way for several competing approaches to medical practice. In the German-speaking world – the one concerning us in this study – following Boerhaave and with Kantian roots, Johann C. Reil (1759–1813) – the first dean of the medical school of the new Berlin University – concluded that medicine would only become truly rational after acquiring scientific status.[26] At the same time, his co-dean, Christoph W. Hufeland (1762–1836) emphasized the practical, essentially art-like nature of medicine, requiring a strictly individual approach in each case of disease.[27] The utilitarian and pragmatic side of the *Aufklärung* existed side-by-side with the ideal of individual growth and accomplishment (*Bildung*), which in its extreme version led to so-called *Naturphilosophie* and Romantic medicine.[28] Among Brownianism, Mesmerism, hydrotherapy and – naturally – homeopathy, there were also more conservative approaches that upheld the inherited tradition, of which an exemplary case is the one of August F. Hecker (1763–1811).

Honigberger's medicine

Honigberger addresses these matters explicitly and even more comprehensively since he includes in the discussion also the medical traditional lore of the many areas he visited – which he systematically made a point of learning from local healers – and the more formal medical systems then prevailing in

---

23 Haller (1774), p. 756.
24 Among other projects with the same goal, it is worth mentioning those of Georg E. Stahl (1659–1734), Friedrich Hoffmann (1660–1742) and a little later, of Montpellier so-called "vitalist doctors", see Waisse/Amaral/Alfonso-Goldfarb (2011).
25 See e.g. Sauvages (1751); Cabanis (1798); Hufeland (1805); Pinel (1810).
26 Broman (1996), p. 136.
27 Broman (1996), pp. 113–119.
28 For an up-to-date review of the literature on the notions of *Naturphilosophie* and Romantic medicine, see Waisse (2010), ch. 2, and the sources quoted there.

India. Although he criticizes the "spirit of system-framing"[29], this proves to be
– like in everybody else's case – nothing but plain lip service, since he also
announces his own 'medial system' as supposedly intermediary between allopathy and homeopathy. It must be emphasized that for Honigberger, the
difference mainly concerns the amount of medicine prescribed at one time.
This is: allopathy is an ages-old sanctioned medical system grounded on the
use of powerful drugs in large amounts, whereas homeopathy exclusively em-
ploys small doses.

After admitting that both systems had their advantages and disadvantages,
and that he had used them successfully and unsuccessfully, he rates his own
'medial system' – which combines the beneficial parts of allopathy and homeopathy – "the best, and I recommend it as the most efficient".[30]

As a fact, Honigberger never gives a full account of such a 'system,' rather
its components have to be extracted from his writings and can be summarized
as follows:[31]

1) A strong pragmatic base, illustrated by guidelines such as "One must al-
    ways avoid large doses and administer only those that, if not beneficial, at
    least cannot do any harm".[32] In order for patients to comply with treat-
    ment, among other advantages, "the medicine is administered in a pleas-
    ant form"[33], that is, dissolved in sugar. Furthermore,

    In order to avoid mistakes in the application of medicines, I used boxes of different sizes
    and colours. In each one, I placed a paper with the main symptoms of the disease, the
    name of the medicine, its amount, how to take it and the date when it was filled.[34]

2) The emphasis on the use of small doses arises from the empirical observa-
    tion that

    Minute doses alone can produce real medicinal action. Properly employed, they operate benefi-
    cially; because their action is confined to that part of the body which is the seat of disease,
    while the remainder of the system is not attacked or weakened; if improperly employed,
    they cannot, from their minuteness, be very injurious.[35]

Consistent with this, he proposes a classification of medicines and doses (Table
2).[36]

---

29 Honigberger (1852), Introduction, p. iii.
30 Honigberger (1852), Introduction, p. x; vol. 1, p. 143.
31 Honigberger (1852), vol. 2, p. 1.
32 Honigberger (1852), Introduction, p. xi.
33 Honigberger (1852), Introduction, p. ix; preparation is described in vol. 2, p. v: one drop
    of tincture in one sugar-loaf; however, the use of lozenges (pastilles, cakes) is simpler and
    easier.
34 Honigberger (1852), Introduction, p. xx.
35 Honigberger (1852), Introduction, p. xxvi; emphasis is Honigberger's.
36 Honigberger (1852), vol. 2, pp. iii, iv.

Table 2: Classification of drugs and corresponding doses

Class	Substances	Dose
I: usually employed in allopathy in very large doses (scruples, drachmas or even ounces).	Mildest plants, earths, coals, salts, metals, mildest vegetal acids. E. g.: bitter almonds, poppy, mercury.	1/25 to 1/5 of a grain.
II: usually employed in grains.	Acrid plants, some crystallised vegetal acids, mild chemical preparations. E. g.: potash prussiate, opium, calomel.	1/50 to 1/25 of a grain.
III: usually employed in doses smaller than 1 grain	Venoms (animal, vegetal and mineral), strong acids. E. g.: hydrocyanic acid, morphia[37], corrosive sublimate.	1/100 to 1/50 of a grain.

3) As for proper theory, there is not too much in this book, but it clearly echoes the medical tradition from Boerhaave onwards. According to Honigberger, nature acts destructively on the one hand and productively on the other, and therefore, it continually strives to keep a state of balance. Such continual exchange of matter also gives rise to "subtle elements", which sometimes exert damaging influence on living beings and originate disease. The doctor must therefore assist the "preserving and healing powers", even when he does not know how they act. In this regard, the only possible guide is (clinical) experience.[38]

Regarding actual practice, the book shows him applying the widest eclectic approach, resorting to medicines from any source (chemical, vegetal, including Galenic) as well as blood-letting and other time-sanctioned surgical procedures, as, for instance, those employed to expel kidney stones.[39] This can be only natural if we remember that Honigberger never studied medicine, but had some practice in apothecary shops, and that he started his journey at the age of 20, i. e. with very little actual therapeutic experience. A further subject

---

37 Morphine.
38 Honigberger (1852), Introduction, p. xxv.
39 See, e. g., the discussion on his method of extracting stones compared to the one used by Arabic "Stone-operators" in Honigberger (1852), vol. 1, p. 7. A typical example of Honigberger's eclectic approach is his "antiflogistic plan" for an epidemic infection of the eyes, including the use of bloodletting, blistering, leeches, calomel, small doses of emetic tartar, purgatives and Dover's powders (ipecacuanha and opium) systemically, together with eye-drops made of corrosive sublimate, lead acetate, laudanum, camphor and rose-water, Honigberger (1852), vol. 1, p. 14.

that patently caught Honigberger's full attention was vaccination against small-pox, which he made a point of applying as much as he could throughout his years of travelling.

Honigberger first heard about homeopathy in Orenburg, Russia, on his journey back from his first trip to India. In Orenburg he met German generals serving in the Russian army, who were accompanied by German doctors. The latter told him about a "new method of healing recently discovered that was diametrically opposed to the one in use until that moment".[40] Naturally, due to his inborn curiosity, the first thing he did when visiting Paris, in 1836, was to go and visit Hahnemann, in order "to learn from the very source itself".[41] Honigberger is surprisingly laconic in his description of his meeting with Hahnemann – when one compares, for instance, the description of his talk with "Ibrahim, the shoemaker", who taught him how to diagnose and treat *habbet-ul-kei* (possibly trachoma).[42] He merely states that he was very well received by "the magnanimous old man and his lovely young wife", that Hahnemann disclosed to him several interesting facts about homeopathy and "of particular importance", referred him to his colleague and assistant in Köthen, Dr Lehmann, who also prepared homeopathic medications.[43]

Honigberger first tested homeopathy on himself, when he caught cholera in Vienna in 1836, and employed the *Ipeca* he had bought from Lehmann, one dose every half an hour, reporting himself to be fully healed after 6 hours.[44] This success made him eager to expand homeopathy as much as possible, and for this purpose, he chose Constantinople.

Upon arriving, there was an on-going epidemic of plague, and he treated successfully with homeopathy poor patients who had been abandoned at a plague hospital in Pera. Notably, he chose to prescribe *Ignatia amara,* having observed that Armenians wore a thread with St. Ignatius' beans (*Strychnos ignatia* Lindl.). This earned him a great reputation – so that he was called to treat some of the most prominent families of the capital of the Empire – but also the animadversion of the local doctors.

At any event, he remained two years practising medicine in the Ottoman Empire, apparently with much success, until in 1838 he heard that Maharajah Ranjit Singh was asking for him to go back to Lahore.[45] It was therefore on this second trip that he took homeopathic medicines to India.

Unfortunately, upon arriving in Lahore, the Maharajah was severely ill and the local doctors did not initially trust in the "wonderful new method of healing", homeopathy, and refused Honigberger's services. In time, however, since there was no improvement, he was finally allowed to prescribe for the Maharajah, who nevertheless passed away a few days later – Honigberger at-

40   Honigberger (1852), vol. 1, p. 73.
41   Honigberger (1852), vol. 1, p. 81.
42   Honigberger (1852), vol. 1, pp. 14–15.
43   Honigberger (1852), vol. 1, p. 81.
44   Honigberger (1852), vol. 1, p. 82.
45   Honigberger (1852), vol. 1, pp. 83–88.

tributed this sad outcome to an 'overdose' of *Dulcamara* in the 3rd dilution (the Maharajah had taken two drops instead of the one prescribed!) and an electuary of precious stones prescribed by a consensus of Muslim and Hindu doctors and astrologers.[46]

Incidentally, it was at this time that Honigberger was told the story of fakir Haridas, which was the one that caught Eliade's imagination.[47] Another episode involved a fakir able to escape snakebites unharmed thanks to the use of arsenic; Honigberger's report had loud repercussions among the medical circles of London.[48] As for Honigberger, this episode awakened a deep interest in snakes in him, more particularly in their potential medicinal uses.[49]

Ranjit Singh's death was the direct trigger for Honigberger to give up homeopathy and start devising his own 'medial system', precisely as the midpoint between the huge doses of allopathy and the infinitesimal doses of homeopathy.[50] He further performed some tests with "galvano-electric" rings, made of copper, as a preventive for cholera[51], and with chloroform as a surgical anesthetic[52].

Apart from medicine, other feats worthy of notice are the collection of antiques that he gathered literally "by opening graves"[53] and that financed his travels, as well as the Eastern plants that he sent to Joseph F. Jacquin (1766–1839), the son of the famous Nikolaus, who succeeded his father as professor of botany and chemistry in Vienna[54].

A multicultural medical marketplace

Honigberger is highly critical of both Muslim and Hindu medicine; the former because it "derived from the ancient Greeks and Egyptians" and the latter because it had little advanced from the state "described in their old manuscripts; their treatment guidelines are extravagant and superstitious and also appeal to astrology. Since it is further mixed with religion" one can have no hope of it ever making any progress.[55] Conversely, Honigberger, throughout the text, praises his own (European) medical skills. It is therefore not surpris-

---

46 Honigberger (1852), vol. 1, pp. 92–95.
47 Honigberger (1852), vol. 1, pp. 127 et seq.
48 Honigberger (1852), vol. 1, pp. 134 et seq. See the exchange in the British Medical Journal among Kesteven: Effects of bites (1858), Kesteven: Prophylactic for the bites (1858), Braid (1858), and Balfour (1858).
49 Honigberger (1852), vol. 1, pp. 138–139; see below.
50 Honigberger (1852), vol. 1, p. 144. There is no mention either of homeopathy in two later writings by Honigberger on the treatment of cholera (1859, 1865).
51 Honigberger (1852), vol. 1, pp. 146–147.
52 Honigberger (1852), vol. 1, p. 148.
53 Honigberger (1852), vol. 1, p. 59; the catalogue was published in 1835 by the Asiatic Society of Paris.
54 Edited by Endlicher/Fenzl (1836).
55 Honigberger (1852), Introduction, p. iii.

ing when he tells us that, upon his arrival in Lahore, he was immediately called upon to serve as practising physician in the circles of Maharajah Ranjit Singh.[56]

The first facility made available to Honigberger as a medical practice, on his first trip to Lahore, was the *gulab-haneh*, the place where rosewater and *be-demusk* (water of flowers of willow[57]) were distilled. There, apart from teaching pharmacy and chemistry to the Maharajah's advisors, the fakirs Aziz Uddin and Nur Uddin, he prepared opiates, including morphine, and several metallic oxides. Honigberger remarks that several substances were unknown there, including milk, sugar and coffee, and he elaborates extensively on cantharides and other methods of blistering, a procedure that he strongly favoured.[58]

In time, a hospital was established, which was shared by Honigberger, Muslim doctors (*Hakims*) and Hindu surgeons (*Jerahs*) (Figure 2). Honigberger's department was placed at one side of the building, while the other side was occupied by the *Hakim* appointed by the *Durbar* (state council) to assist him, who was free to treat according to his system. In this way, patients were also free to choose between both medical systems. In between, there were three *Jerahs*, also appointed by the *Durbar,* who performed external cures (remember that this was the proper field of surgeons in Europe at Honigberger's time). Honigberger observes that while this arrangement made the hospital look like "a marketplace morning to night", it was not uncommon for patients to seek the help of all three kinds of healers.[59] In his opinion, this was due to the fact that medicines were given gratis: not only the *Hakims*, but also the *Jerahs* were in his view quite unskilled and only possessed a few rudimentary tools – some ointments, razors and lancets, pincers for tooth-extraction and glasses for cupping. On the other hand, Honigberger notices the ability of these doctors to learn very quickly how to perform tapping and vaccinations.[60]

---

56   Honigberger (1852), vol. 1, pp. 44 et seq., where he describes his first contact with the Maharaja and the early cures of the son of General Jean-François Allard (1785–1839), the Maharaja's younger brother Suchet and a group of British soldiers affected by hydrophobia.
57   Carmichael-Smyth (1847), Appendix, p. 24.
58   Honigberger, (1852), vol. 1, pp. 49–50.
59   Honigberger (1852), Introduction, p. xviii.
60   Honigberger (1852), Introduction, p. xxviii.

Figure 2: Hakim and Jerah[61]
Hakim taking the pulse; urine bottle behind;   Jerah shaving a customer
simple electuaries and pills in wooden boxes.

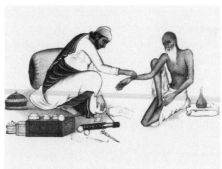 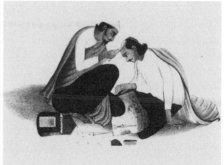

Among the local doctors in India Honigberger mentions having also met
Muslim "stone-operators", who used exactly the same procedure as the ones
used in Syria and whose origin Honigberger attributes to Celsus.[62] Regarding
Muslim eye-doctors, he tells that they sat on the street where they performed
surgical operations with coarse tools, concluding that "despite their undeniable theoretical knowledge, they make more people blind than they heal".[63]

Honigberger observes that consultations were always carried out in the
presence of patients, so that they could choose what treatment they preferred.
In the assembly of *Hakims* the official language was Persian, whereas the technical medical terms were Arabic, which was not understood by patients. Conversely, when Hindu doctors or astrologers were present – "which it is always
the case when consultations are held at the home of respectable families [...]
the Indian language was spoken, because they usually do not know Persian".[64]
Another difference Honigberger highlights is that he could only fill prescriptions for Muslims, since Sikhs and Hindu refused medicines prepared in liquid
form by European hands. They therefore obtained them in dry form and prepared them for themselves.[65]

Honigberger's curiosity was awakened by a form of exorcism, which he
describes as "a kind of animal magnetism", called *Jara* or *Manter* used for in-
flammatory, rheumatic or nervous pains. The operator (a man or a woman)
stood in front of the patient, holding a green branch or a small stick in hand
and thus took the evil spirit from the affected parts by occasionally striking the
body of the patient with the stick in a downward direction, while murmuring
"strange words" and blowing on the affected area.[66]

---

61 Honigberger (1852), vol. 1, Plates VIII and XVI.
62 Honigberger (1852), vol. 1, p. 149.
63 Honigberger (1852), vol. 1, p. 148.
64 Honigberger (1852), vol. 1, p. 149.
65 Honigberger (1852), Introduction, p. 150.
66 Honigberger (1852), Introduction, p. 156.

On the other hand, he is highly critical of the local interest in the pulse and in uroscopy, which made him "sometimes unable to forebear laughter".[67] However, Honigberger believes these to be purely Eastern practices and is seemingly unaware of their relevance in Western medicine since the Middle Ages and within Galenic medicine.[68]

He is lengthy in his description of preparations and ways of using marijuana (*Cannabis indica* Lam.), pointing out that it was purely recreational, and never therapeutic (Figure 3). For this reason, he carried out several experiments that are described in the materia medica.

Figure 3: Marijuana users[69]

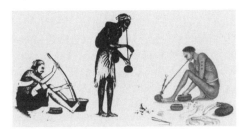

Honigberger's Materia Medica

Indeed, Honigberger paid particular attention to *C. indica,* and his descriptions and experiments might help us understand more accurately his approach to the study of medicines. A plant used in Turkey, Arabia, Persia, India and Egypt, Honigberger promptly observes that it is quite similar to the *C. sativa* known in Europe, albeit their properties differed. Notably, he describes both the use made by natives, and his own testing of the substance. He states that it is an agreeable intoxicating beverage, used particularly by the poorest classes (since they have no access to more powerful drugs). On the other hand, it does not cause dependence and is the "least prejudicial among toxics".[70] For these reasons, the government of Lahore had arranged for its preparation and free distribution to the lower classes.

Next, Honigberger describes the effects of experiments performed on himself, friends and on household employees, which he compares to the description in the "Bengal Dispensatory". This section is followed by a much larger one, where Honigberger describes with painstaking detail how to prepare the beverage and its proper dose, observing that for medical purposes he

---

67 Honigberger (1852), vol. 1, p. 149.
68 See e.g. McVaugh (1997); Bynum/Porter (2005).
69 Honigberger (1852), vol. 1, plate X.
70 Honigberger (1853), vol. 1, p. 154.

prescribes them as lozenges or candies. He concludes by discussing smoked *C. indica* (*churrus*), which he also tested on himself.

The medical indications of this plant are described in the 'repertory' section of "Thirty-Five Years" Part II, which is prefaced by a section where Honigberger describes the experimental status and 'degree of evidence', so to speak, as well as supplementary sources for the medicines he describes. He explains that all medicines described were tested and proved beneficial at least once for a given disease or symptom. However, when a drug so tested later failed only once, it is marked with the letter 'N'; when a drug failed more than once, it was not included in the book. The letter 'P' means that a medicine produced a given symptom or disease in a healthy subject; by itself, it means that it has not yet been tested therapeutically; 'P G' means it healed the same condition it induced, and according to the law of similarity, this is the most reliable class of medicines; 'P G N' indicates that later on it failed once; the letter 'R' means that the drug has not yet been tested in a particular indication, but it is recommended for trial. Finally, when the abbreviation 'TOHF' is added, the source is the *Tohfet*, a Persian materia medica.[71]

The proper indications are described in 'repertory' mode, as shown above, and therefore spread out, and the codes indicating the experimental status are added. For instance, four indications are rated R, three P, one G, and one G N. Honigberger's testing of *C. indica* yields about 65 clinical indications, corresponding to mental, general and local conditions, however, without the detailed descriptions of modalities that is typical of the homeopathic literature on materia medica.[72] Conversely, he pays more attention to traditional Eastern indications such as "powdered, prepared with goat's milk and applied to the soles of the feet is said to provoke agreeable sleep".[73]

A similar synthesis of Western and Eastern medicinal knowledge also permeates the section properly devoted to the materia medica (and thus entitled), which comprises hundreds of medicines, from which I have selected a few as illustrative examples.

Abrus precatorius

Not all medicines in Honigberger's materia medica are equally complete, but the instance of *Abrus precatorius* illustrates the type of project Honigberger had in mind:

---

71 According to Ainslie (1826), vol. 2, p. 511 – a source Honigberger quotes often and to which he suggests several additions – *Tohfet Khāny* was a "book containing the whole science of medicine" attributed to Mahmud ben Mohammed, a physician from Shiraz, and written in 1496. This book is still extant, but available exclusively in Persian; personal communication by A. M. Alfonso-Goldfarb and S. A. A. C. Jubran. *Tohfet al Momĭnin*, another "whole science of medicine", compiled from several sources by Persian author Mohammed Momin Vuld Mohammed Dilimy.

72 See the example set by Hahnemann (1811–1821).

73 Honigberger (1852), vol. 2, p. 147.

–   Geographical data: a plant native to India that due to geographical fea-
    tures might be transplanted to Europe.
–   Botanical data: the seeds are enclosed in a pericarp, have the size of small
    peas, are exceedingly hard, glossy and of two colours, red and white.
–   Eastern sources: the Hakims rank the white ones, which are the strongest,
    with arsenic; the Punjab midwives used them in combination with other
    drugs to effect abortion. The red ones are employed for necklaces and are
    eaten like other leguminous plants in Egypt. The roots are sweet and
    called Indian liquorice, because they are used as such.
–   Western sources: Linnaeus describes them as poisonous, and Gmelin –
    quoting Sloane – says that when swallowed, they induce violent vomiting,
    pains, convulsions and even death.
–   Honigberger emphasizes the remarkable difference between the root and
    seed, one used as liquorice and the other toxic as arsenic, and thus classi-
    fies their indications:
    ·   Root: class I.
    ·   Seed: class III; indicated in cholera, diarrhoea, and pains in the arms,
        chest and shoulders.

Alexipharmacum

This example is interesting, because Honigberger mentions that this root from
the hills was presented to him by the astrologer at the Court of Lahore (the
kind of local healers Honigberger so constantly claimed to despise) as an anti-
dote that he came to test in several experiments.

Asphaltum persicum

Also known as *Mumiai Persica*, is a specific for fractured bones and therefore
deserves its name of *Osteocolla.*
–   Physical properties: a solid, hard, black and glistening mass, with no par-
    ticular odour. These properties distinguish the genuine product, which is
    extremely rare, even in its native Persia. An adulterated form with similar
    appearance is found in all Eastern bazaars under the name of *Persian
    Mumiai.*
This description evokes traditional concerns about balsams[74] that are also very
frequently adulterated and to which both wonderful healing properties and
regal and mythical traits are attributed, as in the following report Honigberger
gives about *Asphaltum persicum*:
–   The whole yearly production is collected by the King of Persia, who keeps
    it in silver chests to distribute it as presents to family and friends.

---

74   See Alfonso-Goldfarb/Ferraz/Beltran (2010) and Alfonso-Goldfarb/Ferraz/Waisse (2010).

-   Honigberger also seeks information from reliable Western sources, such as
    R. Seligmann, who published three ancient Persian manuscripts referring
    to this substance.[75]
-   From this, and oral Persian sources, Honigberger tells us that *Mum* means
    wax and *Jai* or *Ajin* is the name of a village close to which there is a water
    spring containing this *Mumiai* or *Mumiajin*, which was discovered in a
    mysterious way. King Feridun was in a hunting party, when one of his at-
    tendants shot a gazelle with an arrow. The gazelle escaped and after drink-
    ing from this spring it was healed.
-   Honigberger reports two cases[76], where he used this substance in its raw
    state, but adds that he also tested it according to the rules of his own 'me-
    dial system', finding it useful for fractures and wounds.

Guia Khutai

For all Honigberger's misgivings regarding local doctors, he did not shun the
information they supplied on medicinal substances, as illustrated by the following case. Honigberger tells us he was presented a hard, pitch-like plaster
by a Hakim from Bukhara, who claimed it was able to relief any kind of pain,
and Honigberger describes at length its mode of preparation and application.

Harmala ruta

This plant represents a further instance of the knowledge Honigberger ac-
quired from local doctors, and its use is also characterised by cultural considerations. Honigberger tells that this plant, also known as *Hoormul*, grows plen-
tifully at Lahore, where it is devoted to the caste of Pariahs, who use it to fumi-
gate the room where a wounded person is in order to protect him or her from
noxious exhalations, but Sikhs and Hindus do not dare to touch it. It is also
popularly used for weakness of sight and retention of urine, whereas following
his own experience, Honigberger indicates it in spinal pain extending down-
wards.

75   Romeo Seligmann, author of "Codex Vindobonensis sive Medici Abu Mansur Muwak-
     kak Bin ali Heratensis Liber Fundamentorum Pharmacologiae" (Vienna 1859) and "Liber
     Fundamentorum Pharmacologiae Auctore Mansur Mowafik bem Ali al-Herui" (Vienna
     1830), see Levey (1973), p. 148.
76   One case of kidney stone, where it failed, Honigberger (1852), vol. 1, p. 66; the other, a
     bone fracture that healed in three days, Honigberger (1852), vol. 1, pp. 133–134.

Hypericum

This is a medicinal plant known independently in both the East and the West, albeit with very different indication. In Arabian sources, for instance, it is recommended to expel intestinal worms, and to heal haemorrhoids and prolapse of the womb and the rectum, whereas in Europe it is regarded as a mild stimulant, diuretic and emmenagogue, and in external use, as an anti-rheumatic agent.

Laminaria saccharina

This example, besides reuniting Eastern and Western knowledge, also takes into account chemical analysis, as Honigberger attributes its healing properties to its high iodine content, and indeed, it is indicated in conditions where iodine is effective, such as thyroid affections (goitre).

A last instance that is worth mentioning comprises some curious medicines originally developed by Honigberger, such as *Anguineum* (snake poison)[77], *Cataracteum* (human crystalline lens), *Leporineum* (blood from a hare), *Locusteum* (locust), *Nycteridium* (blood of a bat or fried bat extract), *Piscineum* (fish), *Scorpioneum* (scorpion), and *Tigrineum* (tiger whiskers),

Final remarks

L. Bordaș is very categorical in his judgment of Honigberger's attitude towards Eastern medicine. According to this author, Honigberger looked down from the heights of European science to Muslim and Indian doctors, and instead of discovering and learning Ayurveda, "he returned to the West to become initiated in homeopathy", of which he had heard from German compatriots.[78]

This, however, seems to be an anachronistic view that does not take socio-historical factors into account, namely that Honigberger could only do what his cultural makeup allowed him to do. On the other hand, his books allow us a glimpse on how a 19th century European approached an alien medical culture, almost as if we were looking 'through his eyes:' eyes naturally vitiated by socio-cultural prejudices that, on the other hand, also tell us much about a particular crossroads in time.

This glimpse introduces us, for instance, to a hospital where three different medical systems were available (and gratis) for patients to freely choose the one that suited them best. Or to different arrangements for making different types of medicines available to all, with deep respect for cultural and religious aspects. Furthermore, Honigberger did not eschew any potential source of

---

77   The first homeopathic proving of a snake, *Naja* (also tested by Honigberger) is attributed
      to Rutherfurd Russell, in 1853, see Hughes (1867).
78   Bordaș (2005), p. 509.

medical, therapeutic, pharmacological and pharmaceutical knowledge. On the contrary, he tried to integrate all these disparate sources in his practice and writings, and made a huge effort to translate the technical terms into as many languages as necessary.

A child of cross-cultural universes, Honigberger, in "Thirty-Five Years in the East", gives us a picture of multiculturalism and medical pluralism that can only be useful in times like ours, where globalisation threatens to do away with the innumerable differences that can only enrich human experience as a whole.

Acknowledgements

I thank Prof. Ana M. Alfonso-Goldfarb PhD, Prof. Safa A. A. C. Jubran PhD, Prof. Eugen Ciurtin PhD, Dr Gheorghe Jurj, MD, PhD; and Victoria Priven, for their help with this study; Prof. Robert Jütte PhD and Prof. Martin Dinges PhD, for this unforgettable conference. My participation was partially funded by Brazilian CAPES.

Bibliography

Ainslie, Whitelaw: Materia Indica; or some account of those articles which are employed by the Hindoos, and other Eastern nations, in their medicine, arts and agriculture. 2 Vols. London 1826.

Alfonso-Goldfarb, Ana Maria; Ferraz, Marcia Helena Mendes; Beltran, Maria H. R.: Substitutos do 'Novo' Mundo para as antigas plantas raras: um estudo de caso dos bálsamos. In: Química Nova 33 (2010), no. 7, pp. 1620–1626.

Alfonso-Goldfarb, Ana Maria; Ferraz, Marcia Helena Mendes; Waisse, Silvia: Studies on the balsams in the 18th century: a modern experimental approach. In: Annals of the History and Philosophy of Biology 15 (2010), pp. 123–140.

Balfour, George W.: Arsenic as a remedy for the bite of tsetse. In: British Medical Journal (March 13, 1858), p. 215.

Bordaş, Liviu: Memoriile orientale lui Johann Martin Honigberger. Posteritate istorică şi actualitate ficţională. In: Acta Musei Porolissensis 27 (2005), pp. 507–532.

Braid, James: Arsenic as a remedy for the bite of the tsetse, etc. In: British Medical Journal (March 13, 1858), p. 214.

Broman, Thomas: The transformation of German academic medicine, 1750–1820. Cambridge 1996.

Bynum, William; Porter, Roy (eds.): Medicine and the five senses. Cambridge 2005.

Cabanis, Pierre J. G.: Du degrée de certitude de la medicine. Paris 1798.

Cadzow, John; Ludanyi, Andrew; Elteto, Louis J. (eds.): Transylvania. The roots of ethnic conflict. Kent, OH 1983.

Carmichael-Smyth, G.: A history of the reigning family of Lahore. Calcutta 1847.

Cunningham, Andrew; French, Roger: Introduction. In: Cunningham, Andrew; French, Roger (eds.): The medical enlightenment of the eighteenth century. Cambridge 1990, pp. 1–3.

Davis, Sacha: East-West discourses in Transylvania: Transitional *Erdély*, German-Western *Siebenbürgen*, or Latin-Western *Ardeal*? In: Maxwell, Alexander (ed.): The East-West discourse. Symbolic geography and its consequences. Bern 2011, pp. 127–154.

Dragoescu, Anton (ed.): Istoria României. Transilvania. Cluj-Napoca 1997.

Endlicher, Stefan L.; Fenzl, Eduard: Sertum Cabullicum: Enumeratio plantarum quas in itinere inter Dera-Ghazee-Khan et Cabul, mensibus Maio et Junio MDCCCXXXIII, collegit Dr. Martinus Honigberger. Vindobonae 1836.

Ghosh, Ajoy K.: A short story of the development of homeopathy in India. In: Homeopathy 99 (2010), pp. 130–136.

Grinshpon, Yohanan: Silence unheard. Deathly otherness in Patañjala-yoga. Albany 2002.

Gündisch, Konrad: Siebenbürgen und die Siebenbürger Sachsen. München 1998.

Gyémánt, Ladislau: Evreii din Transilvania în epoca emancipării 1790–1867. Bucureşti 2000.

Gyémánt, Ladislau: The Romanian Jewry. Historical destiny, tolerance, integration, marginalisation. In: Journal for the Study of Religions and Ideologies 3 (Winter 2002), pp. 85–98.

Gyémánt, Ladislau: Evreii din Transilvania. Destin historic. Cluj-Napoca 2004.

Hahnemann, Samuel: Reine Arzneimittellehre. 6 Vols. Dresden 1811–1821.

Haller, Albrecht von: Bibliotheca Anatomica. Vol. I. Tiguri 1774.

Haraszti, Endre: The ethnic history of Transylvania. Astor, FL 1977.

Honigberger, Johann M.: Thirty Five Years in the East. Adventures, Discoveries, Experiments and Social Sketches, relating to the Punjab and Cashmere, in connection with Medicine, Botany, Pharmacy, etc., together with an original Materia Medica, and a Medical vocabulary in four European and five Eastern Languages. London 1852.

Honigberger, Johann M.: Früchte aus dem Morgenlande, oder Reise-Erlebnisse, nebst naturhistorisch-medizinischer Erfahrungen, einigen hundert erprobten Arzneimitteln und einer neuen Heilart, dem Medial-Systeme. 2nd ed. Wien 1853.

Honigberger, Johann M.: Heilung der Indischen Brechruhr durch Einimpfung des Quassins. Wien 1859.

Honigberger, Johann M.: Die Cholera, deren Ursache und unfehlbare Heilung und die Epidemien im Allgemeinen. 3rd ed. Wien 1865.

Honigberger, Johann M.: Treizeci şi cinci de ani în Orient. Pref. Arion Roşu. Ed., stud., note, addenda, posf. Eugen Ciurtin. Trad. E. Ciurtin, C. Lupu şi A. Lupaşcu. Iaşi 2004.

Hufeland, Christoph W.: Makrobiotik oder die Kunst das menschliche Leben zu verlängern. 4th ed. Berlin 1805.

Hughes, Richard: Manual of Pharmacodynamics. London 1867.

Hunter, Ian: The secularisation of the confessional state. The political thought of Christian Thomasius. Cambridge 2008.

Kesteven, W.B.: Is arsenic eating prophylactic against the effects of bites of venomous reptiles? In: British Medical Journal (Feb. 27, 1858), p. 174.

Kesteven, W.B.: Arsenic eating as a prophylactic for the bites of venomous reptiles. In: British Medical Journal (March 27, 1858), p. 251.

Keul, István: Early modern religious communities in East-Central Europe. Ethnic diversity, denomination plurality and corporative politics in the Principality of Transylvania, 1526–1691. Leiden 2009.

Levey, Martin: Early Arabic pharmacology. An introduction based on ancient and medieval sources. Leiden 1973.

McVaugh, Michael R.: Bedside manners in the Middle Ages. In: Bulletin of the History of Medicine 71 (1997), no. 2, pp. 201–223.

Oişteanu, Andrei: Narcotics and hallucinogens. Scholars from Romanian territories travelling to the East (Spathary Milescu, Demeter Cantemir, Johann Martin Honigberger, Mircea Eliade). In: Stvdia Asiatica 10 (2009), no. 1/2, pp. 263–285.

Pinel, Philippe: Nosographie philosophique, ou la method de l'analyse apliquée à la medicine. 4th ed. Paris 1810.

Poldas, Samuel V.B.: Geschichte der Homöopathie in Indien: von ihrer Einführung bis zur ersten offiziellen Anerkennung 1937. Stuttgart 2010.

Popescu, Honorius; Mogoșanu, George D.; Prața, Raluca: Some pharmacists from the history of homeopathy in Romania. In: Farmacia 58 (2010), pp. 108–118.

Roșu, Arion. Sur les traces du Transylvain Martin Honigberger, médecin et voyageur en Inde. In: Janus 50 (1962), pp. 198–225.

Sauvages, François B.L. de: Dissertation dans laquelle on recherché s'il ya des médicamens Qui affectent certaines parties du corps humain plutôt que d'autres et quelle seroit a cause de cet effet. Bordeaux 1751.

Sechel, Teodora D.: The emergence of the medical profession in Transylvania (1770–1848). In: Karady, Victor; Török, Borbála Zs. (eds.): Cultural dimensions of elite formation in Transylvania, 1770–1950. Cluj-Napoca 2008, pp. 95–110.

Sigaléa, Robert: Johann Martin Honigberger. Médecin et aventurier à l'Asie. Paris 2003.

Singh, Mahendra: Pioneers of homeopathy. New Delhi 2003.

Török, Borbála Zs.: The ethnic design of scholarship. Learned societies and State intervention in 19th century Transylvania. In: Karady, Victor; Török, Borbála Zs. (eds.): Cultural dimensions of elite formation in Transylvania, 1770–1950. Cluj-Napoca 2008, pp. 115–137.

Vago, Raphael; Krausz, Judy; Gold, Karen: The history of the Jews in Romania. Vol. 1: From its beginnings to the nineteenth century. Tel Aviv 2005.

Verma, Devinder K.: Johann Martin Honigberger. A Hungarian at the Court of Maharajah Ranjit Singh. In: Punjab Past and Present 17 (1983), no. 1, pp. 211–215.

Wagner, Ernst: Quellen zur Geschichte der Siebenbürger Sachsen, 1191–1975. 2nd ed. Köln 1998.

Waisse, Silvia: Hahnemann: Um médico de seu tempo. Articulação da doutrina homeopática como possibilidade da medicina do século XVIII. São Paulo 2005.

Waisse, Silvia: The science of matter and the autonomy of life. Vitalism, antivitalism and neo-vitalism in the German long 19th Century. Saarbrücken 2010.

Waisse, Silvia; Amaral, Maria T.C.G. do; Alfonso-Goldfarb, Ana Maria: The roots of French vitalism. Bordeu and Barthez between Paris and Montpellier. In: História, Ciências, Saúde – Manguinhos 18 (2011), pp. 625–640.

Wurzbach, Constantin von: Biographisches Lexikon des Kaiserthums Oesterreich, enthaltend die Lebensskizzen der denkwürdigen Personen, welche seit 1750 in den österreichischen Krönlandern geboren wurden oder darin gelebt und gewirkt haben. Wien 1863, digital version available at http://www.literature.at/viewer.alo?objid=11812&page=1&viewmode=fullscreen (last accessed on May 8, 2013)

Zach, Krista: Konfessionelle Pluralität, Stände und Nation. Münster 2004.

Innovating Indigeneity, Reforming Domesticity: Nationalising Homeopathy in Colonial Bengal

Shinjini Das

'Indians believe in the power of infinite, imperceptible and imponderable spirit or "para-matma", therefore India is the real land of homeopathy.'[1]

'[…] if the householders have to visit a doctor or a kaviraj on every domestic complaint, it would be extremely taxing on the familial budget.'[2]

'It is more than probable that the Indian flora contains specimens which would best be adapted to cure diseases peculiar to this country. Will there not be found, in that very same country, specimens of men, ready to subject themselves to proving of the drugs of their own soil?'[3]

Introduction

The colonial career of homoeopathy is distinct from the state-imposed dominant medical practice commonly referred to as allopathy in Bengal. Homoeopathy did not enjoy straightforward legislative patronage or an overt infrastructural support of the colonial state especially in the nineteenth century. The state endorsed apparatus of 'western' medicine including the Calcutta Medical College as well as the appointments of the Indian Medical Service were meticulous in excluding practitioners associated with homoeopathy from their ambit.[4] In this respect, homeopathy was perceived as yet another 'unorthodox'/ 'heterodox' therapeutic sect of European origin, like the mesmerists, bio-chemists, herbalists or electro-magneticians.[5] However, as is well known, unlike these 'other' western practices, homeopathy thrived as a medical ideology in Bengal since the mid-nineteenth century and was an extremely popular form of therapeutics by the early twentieth century. The historiography dealing with the 'initial entry'[6], 'gradual spread'[7] or with the figure of 'the chief protagonist'[8] of the system have consistently referred to its popularity in Bengal.

---

1 Dirghangi (1920), p. 406.
2 Anonymous: Atma Nirbharata (1899), pp. 204–205.
3 Anonymous: Atma Nirbharata (1899), pp. 204–205.
4 For an account of the exclusion of the homeopaths from the Medical Faculty of the University of Calcutta in 1870s see Arun Kumar Biswas (2003).
5 The history of such western heterodoxies in India has remained relatively uncharted over the years except for a few sporadic initiatives. For an interesting account of mesmerism and its enmesh with notions of colonial psychiatry see Ernst (2004).
6 Kishore (1973).
7 Kumar (1998).
8 Palit (1998).

To account for this popularity, it is important to look at the processes of 'indigenisation' and 'domestication' of the western category homeopathy in Bengal over the late nineteenth and early twentieth centuries. This essay seeks to primarily understand the historical constitution of notions of the 'indigenous' in colonial Bengal. It as well examines the relation between the 'indigenous' and the 'national' with relation to homeopathy.

In exploring this widespread popularity of homeopathy, David Arnold and Sumit Sarkar have drawn attention to homeopathy's cultural appeal to the Bengalis.[9] Highlighting homeopathy's modern, rational claims they argued that its professed German origin added to the cultural nationalist aspirations of the Bengalis.[10] However, they refrained from elaborating on the specific modalities of such aspirations. This paper, at one level, explores the ways in which actors associated with homeopathy systematically upheld it as the legitimate 'indigenous' remedy most appropriate for Indian households. It draws upon a range of writings by Bengali homeopaths from the mid-nineteenth century onwards. These were published regularly in a range of popular journals, manuals and monographs meant for the 'grihasthas' or householders dealing with issues of quotidian health. Apart from a range of domestic health manuals these included journals exclusively devoted to the homeopathic cause, including the *Calcutta Journal of Medicine, Indian Homeopathic Review, Hahnemann, The Hahnemannian Gleanings* etc.

At the same time, one observes a remarkable overlap between discussions on homeopathy and those on the nationalist reform of Indian families. It demonstrates how the efforts towards promoting homeopathy as the ideal cure for Bengali domesticities were intricately linked to emerging discourses on homeopathy's indigeneity. In so doing, it complicates the recent historiographic conceptualization of homeopathy's appeal among the 'bhadralok'[11] as primarily 'a search for rational remedies' free from colonial impositions.[12] The paper explores how physicians writing on homeopathy succeeded in projecting it as the most effective indigenous remedy for Indians over Ayurveda. Rather than taking the 'traditional' or the 'indigenous' as given, the paper engages with the literature that looks into the nineteenth century makings or 'inventions of traditions'.[13] Secondly, it illustrates how, based on such claims of indigeneity, homeopathy was posed as extremely compatible with the Bengali familial set

---

9   Arnold/Sarkar (2002).
10   Arnold/Sarkar (2002), p. 41.
11   The term 'bhadralok' literally means "respectable people." It is a broad generic term widely used in Bengal to refer to the English educated, though not necessarily affluent, middling to upper stratum of society. Works of S. N. Mukherjee or John McGuire suggest that the term bhadralok referred to both a class of aristocratic landed Bengali Hindus as well as to those of more humble origins who belonged to the salaried sector or the various independent professions. See for instance Mukherjee (1993). Referring primarily to the salaried section, Partha Chatterjee calls the 'bhadralok', the mediators of nationalist ideologies and politics. See Chatterjee (1993), pp. 35–75.
12   Arnold/Sarkar (2002), pp. 41–43.
13   See for instance Hobsbawn/Ranger (1992).

ups. The practice and consumption of homeopathy was presented as a powerful remedy to the late nineteenth to early twentieth century nationalist apprehensions over the possible dissolution of existing familial structures in Bengal. At one level, homeopathy was written about as the most cost-effective, efficacious and 'indigenous' solution to domestic health problems. Simultaneously, its consumption apparently ensured the most efficient functioning of Bengali domesticities.

The institution of family was the central focus of a larger nationalist literature concerned with the preservation of the identity of Indians in the face of growing westernization of values and lifestyle. Indeed, families were repeatedly acclaimed as the blueprints, the foundational units of the emergent nation.[14] Central to this literature was a concern for the declining health of the Indian people. A growing concern over the structure and vitality of the Indian families characterized as the 'joint family' or the 'ekannoborti poribaar' also resonated through this literature. Potential disintegration of the traditional Indian joint families in the face of colonial rule was a crucial theme in this literature. This paper argues that authors advocating homeopathy could strategically intervene and weave these two discourses together to uphold the practice of homeopathy as an ideal 'indigenous' response to nationalist apprehensions regarding the decline of Bengali health and disintegration of Bengali joint families. Homeopathy, as characterized by its late nineteenth century Bengali proponents, was projected not merely as a health care regime but a particular way of life commensurate with fundamental nationalist ideals of economy and self-help. This article studies the processes through which homeopathy came to be posited as an efficient disciplining mechanism to reform colonial domesticities – a remedy to cure the institution of 'family' of the corruptions inflicted by a colonial modernity. Beyond the mere materiality of drugs, homeopathic science was projected and perceived as a way of living, capable of producing the ideal family for the nation. As distinct from the self-centred, Europe-inspired, individualized consumption, the use of homeopathy signified an acceptable, desired, and indigenous form of consumption, compatible with the commitment towards a moral economy of family.

In the process, homeopathy established an alternative domain of institutionalization in Bengal through its entanglement with the nationalist literature on family. The discourse on consuming homeopathy was complemented with that on production. Homeopathy, as the world of Bengali manuals and journals reveal, was a science that could be mastered at home, by all, through the simple act of reading. Mastery in homeopathy involved expertise in not only reading homeopathic tracts and consuming drugs but also the ability to (re)produce homeopathic knowledge. The notion of professionalization as understood in twentieth century India stood fractured and diluted in this homeopathic discourse. In almost defying the need to learn homeopathy through

---

14 For a comprehensive discussion of the link between debates on Bengali domesticity with the civil-political society of the emerging nation see Chakrabarty (1993).

formal professional institutions, 'family' promised an alternative domain of
affective institutionalization to homeopathy.

The first section studies the processes through which homeopathy constituted itself as 'indigenous' through extensive negotiations with Ayurveda in
the overlapping markets for medicine and print. In this respect the paper illustrates how 'medical pluralism' was as much about mutual interactions between differing forms of medicine as it was about delineating a unique space
for each medical tradition. It explores how homeopathy secured multiple
identities for itself through such negotiations: it claimed to be modern and
traditional, western and Indian at the same time. The second section illustrates
how, based on such claims of indigeneity, the practice and consumption of
homeopathy was shown to be best suited for the Bengali familial set ups. The
third section is about the distinctive promise of homeopathy to create democratic citizen doctors of the future, capable of participating in the production
of knowledge and adding to the homeopathic pharmacopoeia.

Innovating Indigeneity

In a range of Bengali texts since the mid nineteenth century, authors asserted
homeopathy's Indian roots. These included primarily homeopathic domestic
health manuals and articles in journals published by the leading homeopathic
enterprises of Calcutta.They unanimously highlighted homeopathy as the
most natural and legitimate form of healing for the Indians in view of its ancient Indian roots. These assertions included elaborate negotiations with si-
multaneous nineteenth century publications that claimed ayurveda or kaviraji
medicine as part of an authentic Indian classical past. This paper is informed
by the literature that has studied the historical construction of labels as 'indigenous' and 'classical' from myriad registers including language[15], music[16] or
gender identity[17]. It scrutinizes and nuances the historiography that simply
noted that despite its western origin, homeopathy was 'naturalized' and 'indi-
genized' in India. Writing in the early 1980's Surinder M. Bharadwaj had argued that the terms of homeopathy's indigenization in India derived from its
remarkable affinity with the therapeutic principles of ayurveda.[18] This paper
refrains from taking such 'affinities' and 'overlaps' between the two medical
doctrines for granted. Rather, it looks at the practices and agencies through
which such claims of 'affinity' came to be constituted. It argues that the assertions of being 'indigenous' and 'natural' to the Indian context were consciously
and systematically propounded in the vernacular print market by physician/
authors making careers out of writing on homeopathy. Hence, this section
draws attention to the discursive production of the label of 'indigeneity' for

15 Ramaswamy (1997).
16 Bakhle (2005). Also see Subramanian (2006).
17 Mani (1998).
18 Bharadwaj (1981), pp. 31–35. Also see Warren (1991).

homeopathy through interactions between plural medical systems in the overlapping markets of print and medicine. It illustrates how such negotiations
helped homeopathy delineate a unique identity for itself – of being simultaneously modern and traditional, of being western with deep Indian roots.[19]

In nineteenth century homeopathic writings, ayurveda was unanimously
recognized as the authentic, traditional medical knowledge of India. They emphatically condemned the consumption of western drugs advocated by physicians inspired by western allopathic tradition. Respectful as they were of ayurveda's potential and suitability in India, the homeopaths, through their writings, continuously remarked on the declining status of ayurvedic knowledge
in contemporary India. The article 'Bharatbarshe Homeopathy' or 'Homeopathy in India' in the journal *Hahnemann* for instance began by describing the
lost glory of ancient Indian civilization where ayurveda had flourished.[20] The
texts lamented the fading importance of ayurveda under the impact of mind-
less westernization initiated by colonialism. In an article on the homeopathic
treatment of fever in the journal *Chikitsha Sammilani*, the author unequivocally
stated, that 'under the aegis of allopathy our own customary medical science is
suffering. Earlier kaviraji [or ayurveda] was especially suitable for the cure of
all kinds of fever. It is not so any more.'[21] It was argued that although ayurvedic knowledge was particularly suitable for Indians, there was an increasing
absence of experienced reliable physicians. The article 'Rog o Paschatya Sabhyata' or 'Disease and Western Civilisation' pointed out,

> presently, ayurveda is in such a state that no one can be sure if it will still exist in another
> century from now. On the one hand there has been a drastic decrease in the number of
> physicians. Among those who still practise, there are hardly any outstanding physicians
> left.[22]

Homeopath Haranath Ray argued in the journal *Chikitsha Sammilani* that the
modern practitioners of ayurveda were thriving solely on the fine reputation
of the earlier generations.[23]

The homeopaths emphasized that the failing reputation of ayurveda had
necessitated the intervention of western medicine. In a series of articles in the
journal *Chikitsha Sammilani* the homeopaths for instance elaborated on the
inadequacies of ayurveda in contemporary society.[24] Physician Haranath Ray
asserted that in an age of overwhelming influence of science, it was inadvisa-
ble to rely only on traditional principles. He argued that

> under foreign domination there has been tremendous change in our social context and
> with the advent of several new diseases there is dire need for modern medical knowl-

---

19 For a similar articulation of homeopathy's in-between status between being 'indigenous'
    and 'scientific' in the Indian milieu see Hausman (2002).
20 Dirghangi (1920), p. 401.
21 Haranath Ray (1886), pp. 217–218.
22 Chakrabarti (1920), p. 217.
23 Haranath Ray (1886), pp. 217–218.
24 See for instance Shashibhushan Mukhopadhyay (1891), pp. 269–272.

edge. We cannot take it for granted that the way the Susrut, Charak, Bhagbat and Dhan-
wantary devised ayurveda, will be as effective in all times and in all social contexts.[25]

In short, these texts highlighted the outdated, weakened condition of ayurvedic knowledge in a colonized society.

In that context, homeopathy was being upheld as the natural choice for
Indians. Highlighting its modern, western roots, the homeopaths elaborated
on the reasons why homeopathy still had legitimate claims to indigeneity. At
one level, authors emphasized the deep similarity between the inherent philosophy of homeopathy and that of Hindu philosophy. The article 'Homeopathy in India' in the journal *Hahnemann*, for instance, emphasized that the rich
heritage of Hindu philosophy had always appreciated the power of the infinite
that was beyond human perception, which the Hindus had termed 'Brahma'.[26]
The authors urged their readers to look beyond the contemporary celebration
of materialism inspired by British rule. They argued that Hahnemann was the
most prominent western philosopher who had indicated the tremendous potential of the infinite, the spiritual, when he declared that diseases were caused
by immaterial vital forces. The article 'Kromo Nirnay ba Matra Bijnan' or
'The Science of Determining Potency' in the journal *Hahnemann* also asserted
that 'the basis of true homeopathy is spirituality. It is very apparent from the
texts of Hahnemann and those of his principal disciple Kent, that there is a
distinct overlap between their thoughts and Hindu philosophy.'[27] Given the
proximity of their thoughts, it was considered a pity that Hahnemann was not
born in India. Indeed, a number of homeopaths like the author of the article
'Bharatbarshe Homeopathy' found it preposterous that the people whose ancestors worshipped Brahma should find it difficult to appreciate the power of
the immaterial and the concept of infinite dose.[28] These authors repeatedly
emphasized that since 'Indians believe in the power of the infinite, imperceptible and imponderable spirit or "paramatma", therefore India is the real land
of homeopathy.'[29]

Parallel with these claims of similarity with Hindu philosophy, a group of
homeopathic authors further argued that 'the main principle of homeopathy
was inherent within the large ayurvedic corpus.'[30] In fact, there were contend-
ing claims by the practitioners of ayurveda too regarding the 'true' origin of
homeopathy. In their defence against the attack from other medical systems,
ayurvedic practitioners consistently upheld the antiquity of their doctrine.
With respect to the homeopaths, this was especially true. These ayurvedic authors frequently asserted the ancient Indian past as the 'authentic' origin of
homeopathy. In a representative long article written in 1885 in the journal
Chikitsha Sammilani, kaviraj Madhusudan Roy explicitly stated, 'the law which

25   Haranath Ray (1886), p. 222.
26   Dirghangi (1920), pp. 401–402.
27   Haricharan Ray (1918), pp. 322–323.
28   Dirghangi (1920), p. 401. Also see Raya: Garhasthya (1917), p. 250.
29   Dirghangi (1920), p. 406.
30   Dirghangi (1920), p. 407.

has made Hahnemann world famous had originally been invented by the now-fallen Aryans.'[31]

Such ayurvedic claims were hardly contested by writers propagating homeopathy. In a range of texts dealing with homeopathy's past and its claims of belonging to India, they referred to these assertions by ayurvedic practitioners and expressed solidarity with such a position. Through complicated historical narratives, a number of early twentieth century homeopathic texts argued that the fundamental tenet of homeopathy was indeed inherent in ayurveda. A typical Bengali text as 'Susrut o Hahnemann', published in 1906, developed a detailed account of the historical origin and trajectory of ayurveda and homeopathy.[32] Referring to Indian civilization and ayurveda as the oldest body of medicine, the author described how such doctrines travelled west primarily with the spread of Buddhism. On reaching Greece, some of the ayurvedic tenets were translated into Latin by the Romans that influenced Hippocrates. It was argued that these 'historical truths' explain why homeopathy has indeed deep roots in India. The author of 'Susrut o Hahnemann' firmly asserted that although the possibility of cure by similars was included in ayurveda, it had not been elaborated in a 'systematic and disciplined manner' before Hahnemann.[33] These homeopaths in colonial Bengal acknowledged that the greatness of Hahnemann lay in developing the fundamental principle already given in ayurveda into a coherent body of knowledge.

Through their participation in discussions on contentious historical pasts, the promoters of homeopathy claimed to have irrefutably established homeopathy's indigenous roots. In his 1924 article 'Light of Hope' author Kalikumar Bhattacharya concluded that, 'homeopathy is our own Vedic property which has recently come back to us dressed in western attire. If we make it our own, with time it will be most efficient in maintaining the power, health and resources of independent "swaraj" India.'[34] The homeopaths were so consistent in their assertion of homeopathy's indigeneity, that such an understanding was almost universal among them by the end of the nineteenth century. So much so, that English manuals like 'European Guide and Medical Companion in India' published in Britain advised homeopathic remedies as ideal even for the European families travelling to India.[35] Written in 1895 with the 'chief object of giving instructions to European comers and sojourners in India for maintaining good health and avoiding tropical disease, which so often cut short their lives', the manual firmly declared that 'the treatment of the diseases is based on the homeopathic principle which is most suitable for Indian conditions.'[36]

31   Roy (1885).
32   Ghosh (1906), pp. 2, 6–11.
33   Ghosh (1906), pp. 6–11.
34   Kalikumar Bhattacharya (1924), p. 80.
35   Gangadin (1895).
36   Gangadin (1895), pp. i-vi.

To substantiate these claims, the homeopathic practitioners also made sincere, consistent efforts to demonstrate the proximity and compatibility of homeopathy and ayurveda. In a remarkable display of medical pluralism, these authors made repeated attempts to synthesize fundamental features of the two doctrines. In the manual entitled 'Sadrisa Byabastha Jwar Chikithsa' or 'Homeopathic Treatment of Fever', published in 1871, the author highlighted the importance of consulting ayurvedic texts for the most relevant classification of Indian fevers unavailable in most European texts.[37] He stated that he had prepared his manual by synthesizing the knowledge of such classification from the ayurvedic texts of Susrut, Madhab etc. with the treatments suggested in the texts of homeopaths as Tsar, Gaurency, and Kent in order to prescribe the most effective remedy.[38]

Attempts at synthesis had myriad manifestations. Appropriate and disciplined diet was considered a critical aspect of homeopathic cure. In the third chapter of his manual 'Pathya Nirbachan' or 'Selection of Diet' written in 1925, the homeopath H. N. Mukhati elaborated on the ayurvedic notion of 'tridosha' or the three bodily humours 'bayu', 'pitta' and 'kaph'.[39] He argued that 'it is advisable to adopt the ayurvedic idea of diet along with homeopathic drugs as the former is ideally suited for our country.'[40] It is important to note that such trends of assimilation and 'harmonization' of the principles of both doctrines continued on the part of the homeopaths. The culmination of this trend may be seen in the book 'The Science of Tridosha' written by homeopath Benoytosh Bhattacharya in the 1950s, in which he held that 'in order that this dynamic system may be made full use of, it is absolutely necessary that the Tridosha methods should be applied to homeopathy for the benefit of mankind.'[41]

A Necessary Tool for the 'Ideal Hindu domesticity'

Based on their claims of indigeneity, homeopathic authors participated in intense nationalist discussions on the crisis of the institution of the family in Bengal. The crisis of domesticity and familial structure was a recurrent theme reflected in various texts including socio-medical journals as well as contemporary sociological anthologies. The themes and explanations of an impending domestic crisis elaborated in this literature were the very ones picked up by the homeopaths in their own manuals and journals. Citing homeopathy's indigenous roots, unique features and compatibility with Indian situations, the texts recurrently highlighted it as the ideal remedy for such crisis over ayurveda. Its peculiarity lay in its being able to simultaneously and most efficiently

---

37   Mallika (1871), Preface, page number not cited.
38   Mallika (1871), Preface, page number not cited.
39   Mukhati (1925), p. 17.
40   Mukhati (1925), p. 17.
41   Benoytosh Bhattacharya (1951), Preface, page number not cited.

manage the health of Bengali individuals while protecting the vitality of Bengali joint families.

The nationalist literature on families celebrated the traditional Indian joint family system while simultaneously discussing its potential disintegration in the face of a modernity imposed by British rule. These texts were unanimous in their explanation and concern about the dangers threatening the institution of the family in India. The encounter with the west, blind imitation and incorporation of western social values were considered immensely detrimental to the Hindu familial life. Exposure to western ideas was thought to be causing dislocation in the fundamentals of everyday life including childrearing, food habits, medication, education and the like. A representative article titled 'Baje Kharach' or 'Unjustified Expenditure' in the journal *Grihsthamangal* lamented,

> the Indians seemed to have made up their mind regarding the fact that everything western – the ways, customs, social norms, systems are all good, while everything indigenous is bad. All things they [the westerners] do are scientific while everything Indians ever did is superstitious […] by denying indigenous weather, food, clothes, recreation, music etc and trying to emulate the English in all these spheres, we are being weak, cowardly, unhealthy and poor by the day.[42]

An alarming increase in human need coupled with intense consumption and extravagance was characterized as an obvious consequence of this gratuitous westernisation. The contemporary time was suggested to be in the 'bhog marg' i.e. in a stage that could be defined solely in terms of consumption.[43] 'Bilash', or luxury, and 'Bhog', or consumption, were identified as the two most potent evils of the western modern lifestyle. Preservation of indigenous identity and judicious management of familial wealth and economy therefore emerged as crucial themes in almost all texts. It was argued that a serious threat faced by the Indian joint families was economic in nature. A number of texts dealt with the theme of the difference of income between brothers causing widespread familial tension. Indeed, Bengali literature of the time is replete with instances of authors elaborating on such themes of disintegration.[44] The authors, in that context, repeatedly emphasized the importance of thoughtful expenditure and saving. Bhudeb Mukhopadhyay's authoritative tract on the institution of family in late nineteenth century Bengal for instance had an entire chapter devoted to 'Artha Sanchay' or 'Codes of Saving'.[45]

The homeopaths engaged extensively with this pervasive discourse on familial degeneration. Consuming homeopathy, it was argued, took care of the domestic suffering of the people through efficacious indigenous remedies. Simultaneously, it also addressed the fundamental problems faced by the insti-

---

42 Choudhury (1931), p. 35.
43 Kanjilal (1921), pp. 1–21.
44 Joint familial troubles were at the heart of a range of novels written by the eminent Bengali novelist Sarat Chandra Chattopadhyay (1876–1938). Set in colonial Bengal, the novels dealing centrally with such joint familial crisis based on financial management were 'Nishkriti' (1917), 'Bindur Chhele', 'Ram er Sumati', 'Mejdidi' etc.
45 Bhudeb Mukhopadhyay (1889), pp. 186–191.

tution of the family by being extremely economical. Directed specifically to the 'grihasthas' or the householders, the homeopathic texts recurrently emphasized a series of advantages that made homeopathy indispensable within every household over any other form of medicine. Consumption of homeopathic drugs was characterized as absolutely 'safe and painless with literally no or only very mild side effects.'[46] They were considered so harmless that they 'could be safely consumed by all – from new born babies to old people.'[47] The mild and gentle nature of the drugs made them suitable for consumption by women too. It was argued that in 'diseases related to pregnancy as well as for infants, even physicians professing other medical systems often advised homeopathic drugs.'[48] In addition, some of the texts pointed out that 'since the Bengalis are becoming debilitated by the day, they can hardly stand the stronger remedies of other heroic therapies. Therefore, the tasty, minute, useful homeopathic medicines are the most suitable for them.'[49]

Apart from being safe, tasty, painless and gentle, homeopathic drugs were, as the texts noted, extremely economical. Not only were they cheaply priced, they were also advertised as long lasting to the extent that it was believed that 'if kept with care, fresh homeopathic drugs last for years.'[50] It was further emphasized that only a very small amount of the drug needed to be consumed at a time.[51] Thus it was explicitly pointed out that 'whereas a simple fever mixture for a week prescribed by other physicians costs a patient around Rs. 4–5, homeopathic drug worth Re. 1 can easily cure 5–6 such patients.'[52]

However, the texts argued that the greatest advantage associated with the practice of homeopathy was the virtue of being self-sufficient in terms of one's health. A range of homeopathic family medicine manuals promised to make amateur physicians out of ordinary householders in Bengal – who would be competent in taking care of their own selves and their families. Such texts promised to bestow enough curative power on the grihasthas to make expensive allopathic physicians redundant in everyday life. Written for the 'grihasthas and the literate women' these texts promised to be 'easy guides to various diseases, their special symptoms and the relevant drugs.'[53] Texts as 'Garhasthya Swasthya o Homeopathy Chikitsha Bigyan' or 'Domestic Health and Homeopathic Medicine' mentioned that these manuals were specifically written for lay householders by deliberately excluding 'complicated scientific explanations'.[54] The homeopathic domestic chest or box was presented as the most glaring symbol of the self-sufficiency associated with the consumption of homeopathy. Most texts advertized a range of boxes of various shapes and

46 Laha (1914), page number not cited.
47 Anonymous (1896–97), page number not cited.
48 Anonymous (1914), page number not cited.
49 Bandopadhyay (1926), Dedication page, page number not cited.
50 Anonymous (1926), pp. 13–14.
51 Anonymous (1896–97), page number not cited.
52 Anonymous (1900), p. 238.
53 Raya (1917), 'Preface', page number not cited.
54 Raya (1917), 'Preface', page number not cited.

contents. These boxes along with the domestic medicine manuals were considered essential in enabling the householders to heal themselves. Sarat Chandra Dutta's 'Primary Guide to Homeopathy' for instance promised that, 'with the said medical chest and a prescriptive manual, those who know absolutely nothing about medicine can also treat general cases.'[55] Most domestic manuals like 'Homeopathic Griha Chikitsha' written by Satyacharan Laha in 1914 guaranteed its readers that through meticulous reading they could become practising physicians of homeopathy.[56]

These texts are indicative of a profound overlap between the nationalist anxieties around domesticity and the homeopathic promises of relief. The virtues of 'Shwabolombita' (self-reliance) and 'Mitabyayita' (sense of judicious spending) were shown to be intricately related.[57] Hence, manuals as 'Byaktigato Arthaneeti' argued that the economic problem of nations had to be essentially negotiated in the 'nityo jibon' or everyday life of its people within their domestic spaces.[58] Such texts often recommended homeopathic knowledge as useful in taking care of the family's health without the intervention of physicians.[59] Writing in 1901 an article entitled 'Atma Nirbharata' or 'Self Sufficiency' in the journal *Swasthya,* for instance, pointed out that if the householders had to visit a doctor or a kaviraj for every domestic complaint, it would be extremely taxing on the familial budget.[60] Familial economy and notions of self-help in that sense were considered integrally related.

Given these advantages, the authors claimed that it was only natural that the homeopathic family medical guides were extremely popular with Bengali families plagued with economic crises induced by colonial rule. The introduction to the seventh edition of the manual 'Homeopathic Mowt e Saral Griha Chikitsha' or 'Simple Home Treatment according to Homeopathy' noted: 'that we are compelled to publish repeated editions of this book so often, clearly indicates that it is widely accepted by all.'[61] The author of the manual 'Homeopathic Family Physician' was therefore confident that the 'book will circulate just like an almanac, among poor Indians as well as among the rich residing in palaces.'[62] Indeed, the texts unanimously argued that the greatest advantage associated with the practice of homeopathy was the virtue of being self-sufficient in terms of one's health. It was the most appropriate response to the nationalist anxiety relating to loss of self-respect and the attitude of dependency that characterized the Indians.

---

55 Dutta (1899), Advertisement of Indian Homeopathic Hall, page number not cited.
56 Laha (1914), page number not cited.
57 Kanjilal (1921), pp. 1–21.
58 Kanjilal (1921), pp. 1–21.
59 Kanjilal (1921), pp. 1–21.
60 Anonymous: Atma Nirbharata (1899), pp. 204–205.
61 Anonymous (1926), Introduction, page number not cited.
62 Bandopadhyay (1926), Dedication page, page number not cited.

Celebrating Indigeneity: From Consumption towards an Ethic of Production

The previous section has dwelt upon the overlapping discourse of crisis-ridden ailing domesticity in colonial Bengal and the quotidian practice of homeopathy as its potential remedy. Asserting its deep indigenous roots, the practice of homeopathy was shown to present the ideal form of consumption for Indian households. Regular practice and consumption of homeopathy was shown to be commensurate with the values and ethics represented by the emerging nation. This section notes a subsequent shift in the homeopathic literature in the twentieth century from mere consumption to dealing also with the ethics surrounding production. Since the early twentieth century, it has intermittently been pointed out that despite its emphasis on self-reliance, India has remained largely dependent on the supply of homeopathic drugs from Europe or America. Accordingly, homeopathic literature on domestic health increasingly encouraged its consumers to shift their focus also to the processes of production. The appeal was directed primarily at the same householders or the Bengali grihasthas who had been encouraged to consume homeopathy since the mid-nineteenth century. The texts emphasized the crucial roles that every household in Bengal could play in the experiments relating to the preparation of drugs. One finds an unmistakable resonance with the Gandhian ideology of production and consumption around 'khadi' except that it was adopted even in the production of scienticised commodities.[63]

The publications elaborated on the incentives for experimenting with indigenous or local plants of India. The process of discovering new drugs or 'proving' was considered a critical aspect of homeopathic knowledge. As the author of the tract 'Bharat Bhaishajya Tattwa: Materia Medica of Indian Drugs' pointed out, apart from the homeopathic law, the other crucial contribution of Hahnemann was the methodology of testing drugs on healthy human body.[64] Indeed, it was argued that testing and proving drugs on healthy individuals as opposed to 'clinical verification' was a distinctive feature that set homeopathy apart from other medical systems, notably allopathy.[65] Homeopathic drug proving involved ingestion of different forms of plants in a specified manner by healthy individuals. The 'provers' had to maintain a record of all the minute reactions that were generated in their body following ingestion. The knowledge of their reactions to various quantities of the plant consumed was considered critical for their use in the preparation of homeopathic drugs. The authors regretted the fact that while many Bengali physicians adopted the ho-

---

63 For a discussion on the relation between the Gandhian ideology of spinning Khadi and nationalism see Bean (1989).

64 Pramada Prasanna Biswas: Materia Medica (1924), 'Note to Indian Physicians', page number not cited.

65 See Pramada Prasanna Biswas: Letter (1924), p. 332. Also see Pramada Prasanna Biswas: Materia Medica (1924), pp. 466–467.

meopathic law in their practice, they were sadly lacking in their efforts with the other important aspect i. e. proving.

The authors gave a clarion call to fellow homeopaths and their readers to address this problem by engaging in extensive proving with Indian. A letter to the editor of the journal *Hahnemann* in 1925 for instance stated this urgency saying that proper proving of indigenous plants would be beneficial not only for the Indians but the entire world.[66] Directly referring to the growing nationalist ideology of swadeshi[67] and self-reliance, the authors held that the production of indigenous drugs should be the logical culmination of the cult of swadeshi nationalism.[68] The authors reminded the readers of the difficulty faced in procuring homeopathic drugs during the First World War. Published in 1924, the 'Materia Medica of Indian Drugs' explicitly stated that

> it was impossible to get drugs from Germany during the war. Simple drugs like Aconite, Bryonia and Belladonna that are prepared from German plants were difficult to procure. The American dealers supplied those drugs at their will at the end of the war.[69]

Twentieth century physicians further argued that the imported drugs fell short of curing peculiarly Indian diseases. Hence, drugs made of indigenous plants were considered more useful compared to the imported ones. Sarat Chandra Ghose, a biographer of Mahendralal Sircar, noted

> it is daily marked by us that the plants growing in a particular locality bear a remarkable affinity to the temperament and constitution of the individuals inhabiting that locality. It is, therefore, apparent that Indian drugs will be found most suitable to our constitution.[70]

These texts highly recommended the 'discovery' of newer remedies through experiments with indigenous substances. Celebration of the 'indigenous' was indeed a compelling shared feature between discussions on homeopathy, family and nationalism. The proving of indigenous plants was upheld as an effective way to counter dependence on the west and to establish the self-sufficiency of Indians. The December 1928 editorial of the journal *Homeopathy Pracharak* proudly noted that the homeopathic drugs prepared from indigenous plants were selected for the exhibition marking the upcoming session of the Indian National Congress.[71]

These homeopathic texts also targeted the lay householders who were encouraged to actively participate in the experiments involving the productions of newer remedies with 'indigenous' vegetation. It was declared that such a

---

66 Anonymous (1925), p. 234.
67 'Swadeshi' literally meaning 'self-sufficiency' was a specific strand of nationalist ideology that emphasised confronting the colonial rule through the development of Indian economy. Strategies of the Swadeshi movement involved boycotting British products and the revival of domestic products and production processes. For a comprehensive history swadeshi see Sarkar (2010).
68 Anonymous: Deshiya Bheshaja (1899).
69 Pramada Prasanna Biswas: Materia Medica (1924), 'Note to Indian Physicians', page number not cited.
70 Ghose (1935), p. 79.
71 K.K. Ray (1928), p. 366.

'daunting task' would require the participation of 'thousands of amateurs, pa-
trons and practitioners of homeopathy.'[72] As an article in the *Calcutta Journal of Medicine* insisted,

> It is more than probable that the Indian flora contains specimens which would best be
> adapted to cure diseases peculiar to this country. Will there not be found, in that very
> same country, specimens of men, ready to subject themselves to proving the drugs of
> their own soil?[73]

Indeed, every individual, every householder in Bengal was encouraged to be
an 'active' and 'energetic' volunteer and participate in whatever capacity they
could.[74] It was pointed out that those who could not be involved in the direct
proving of drugs on their body could still contribute by consuming the drugs
once they had been proved.[75] They were encouraged to report their reactions
to the various doses of a proven drug. The participation of women was especially sought. Thus after proving the plant Atista Indica and publishing its result in the journal *Hahnemann*, physician Kalikumar Bhattacharya noted, 'before inserting this as an official remedy we need to get it tested in some other
humans. Especially in order to know how it works on the female constitution
and which organs it affects, we have to inspire some women to take up the
task.'[76] Participating as a family, involving many members of the same household, was highly recommended. The author of 'Bharat Bhaishajjya Tattwa:
Materia Medica of Indian Drugs' narrated that he and his family members
including other relatives were committed to the task of proving indigenous
drugs for malarial fever.[77] By way of preparing the 'ordinary', 'amateur' householders for such tests, the texts included elaborate instructions on reading 'relevant parts of the *Organon*'.[78]

These egalitarian invitations to 'ordinary' 'amateur' people were sometimes debated from within the ranks of the homeopaths themselves. Some
authors were doubtful of the viability of involving lay householders. To them,
it was dangerous for a lay person to test any plant and infer its medicinal values. They strongly felt that 'some specific knowledge and awareness was necessary for such mass participation in knowledge production.'[79] However, authors like Kalikumar Bhattacharya, contributing in the same journals, opposed
this view. In a letter to the editor of the journal *Hahnemann*, Bhattacharya took
a strong position against such advocacy of specialised knowledge.[80] In response to the attack by a younger colleague, he cited instances from his own
life where he had been guided in the discovery of new drugs by lay knowledge

72   Salzer (1869), pp. 177–178.
73   Salzer (1869), pp. 177–178.
74   Maity (1924), p. 174.
75   Pramada Prasanna Biswas (1923), p. 100.
76   Kalikumar Bhattacharya (1921), p. 323.
77   Pramada Prasanna Biswas: Materia Medica (1924), 'Note to Indian Physicians', page
     number not cited.
78   Pramada Prasanna Biswas (1923), pp. 463–466.
79   Maity (1924), p. 177.
80   Kalikumar Bhattacharya (1925), pp. 240–241.

among women.[81] To him, and many others, lay, familial participation was of utmost importance in not only the dissemination but also the production of homeopathic knowledge.[82] However, the texts admitted the importance of being extremely cautious in the attempts at proving. A pointed letter to the editors of the journal *Hahnemann,* written in 1925, initiated discussions on the precise methods of proving.[83] The writer noted that to eliminate any chances of error it was always advisable to test each plant with multiple groups of people of different age groups and constitutions.[84] To acquire fundamental knowledge of homeopathic drugs and their proving, Biswas advised his readers to read the relevant parts of Hahnemann's 'Organon' indicated in his article.[85] Those not conversant in English were referred to a particular Bengali translation published in an earlier edition of the journal *Hahnemann.*

Discussions on indigenous plants involved a range of species that were most easily available and 'often grown in the backyards of ones residence.'[86] Among those most extensively experimented with and written about were Ocimum (Tulsi), Kalmegh, Papaya, Neem and so on. The authors encouraged the ordinary householders to test these mundane, commonplace plants that one encountered daily. The article 'Talks about Homeopathy' in the journal *The Hahnemannian Gleanings* encouraged its readers to test 'Marigold (*Calendula officianialis*), known to you as the Gainder; sometimes you decorate your houses with it and make garlands from it.'[87] Deliberately diluting the possibility of any rigid professional/amateur divide, these texts upheld each Bengali household and its backyard as a potential laboratory of homeopathic drugs. Ordinary householders with no professional knowledge were shown to be capable of producing and positively contributing to the repertoire of homeopathic knowledge and pharmacopoeia.

Conclusion

Despite official bias against it, homoeopathy endured as a credible genre medicine among large sections of Bengali society since mid nineteenth century. This essay has reflected upon this intriguing fact. It has probed how homoeopathy could thrive as an intrinsic category of colonial modernity in Bengal, despite the evident lack of institutional state patronage. In so doing, it has studied the inherent tension in homeopathy's plural identity as the most appropriate 'indigenous' medical knowledge of India with distinct western roots. It shows the ways in which authors advocating homeopathy in Bengal crafted

---

81 Kalikumar Bhattacharya (1925), pp. 240–241.
82 Kalikumar Bhattacharya (1925), pp. 240–241.
83 Anonymous (1925), pp. 234–238.
84 Anonymous (1925), pp. 234–238.
85 Pramada Prasanna Biswas (1923), pp. 463–466.
86 Pramada Prasanna Biswas: Materia Medica (1924), p. 1.
87 Freebome (1932), p. 515.

it as a pragmatically hybrid science – one that was compatible with indigenous ways, yet also equipped with western scientific credentials. It complicates the existing revivalist narratives by elaborating on how such a hybrid category like homeopathy was celebrated as the ideal form of indigeneity in a colonial context.

The homeopathic writings of the late nineteenth and early twentieth century Bengal were entangled with the pervasive nationalist angst about the decline of Indian families due to unbridled westernization. Medical literature on homeopathy strategically intervened in the nationalist literature on family and quotidian health to uphold the practice of homeopathy as an ideal response to their anxiety. Consumption of homeopathy was written about as the most effective indigenous remedy for the corruptions induced by a colonial modernity in the pristine ways of Indian life. Homeopathy was shown to be in deep conversation with the larger nationalist ethos of self-reliance or swadeshi, with its emphasis on the consumption of things indigenous. In exploring this entanglement, this paper has studied how colonialism enabled an alternative institutionalization of homeopathy in Bengal primarily around the affective domain of the family. In so doing, it has delineated how understandings of 'family' and 'homeopathy' shaped one another in colonial Bengal.

Bibliography

Primary Sources

Anonymous: Advertisement of Improved Homeopathic Griha Chikitsha. In: Benimadhab Dey and Company Almanac. Calcutta 1896–97, page number not cited.

Anonymous: Atma Nirbharata. In: Swasthya 3 (1899), no. 7, pp. 204–205.

Anonymous: Deshiya Bheshaja. In: Swasthya 3 (1899), no. 2, pp. 35–37.

Anonymous: Letter to the Editor. In: Swasthya 4 (1900), no. 8, p. 238.

Anonymous: Preface. In: Homeopathy Mowt e Adorsho Griha Chikitsha. Calcutta 1914, page number not cited.

Anonymous: Letter to the Editor: Alochona. In: Hahnemann 8 (1925), no. 5, pp. 234–238.

Anonymous: Homeopathic Mowt e Saral Griha Chikitsha. 7th ed. Calcutta 1926.

Bandopadhyay, Raimohan: Homeopathic Griha Chikitshak. Calcutta 1926.

Bhattacharya, Benoytosh: Preface. In: Bhattacharya, Benoytosh: The Science of Tridosha. Calcutta [1951] 1975, page number not cited.

Bhattacharya, Kalikumar: Atista Indica Proving er Itibritta. In: Hahnemann 4 (1921), no. 9, p. 323.

Bhattacharya, Kalikumar: Ashar Alok. In: Hahnemann 7 (1924), no. 2, p. 80.

Bhattacharya, Kalikumar: Letter to the Editor: Alochonar Prattyuttor. In: Hahnemann 8 (1925), no. 5, pp. 239–248.

Biswas, Pramada Prasanna: Homeopathic Bhaishajya Tattwer Bisheshotto o Sustho Manob Dehe Oushadh er Porikkha. In: Hahnemann 6 (1923), no. 10, pp. 99–101, 463–466.

Biswas, Pramada Prasanna: Letter to the Editor. In: Hahnemann 7 (1924), no. 7, p. 332.

Biswas, Pramada Prasanna: Bharat Bhaishajya Tattwa: Materia Medica of Indian Drugs. Pabna 1924.

Chakrabarti, M.: Rog O Pashchatya Sabhyata. In: Hahnemann 3 (1920), no. 6, pp. 215–217.

Choudhury, Basanta Kumar: Baje Kharach. In: Grihasthamangal 5 (1931), no. 2–3, p. 35.

Dirghangi, G.: Bharatbarshe Homeopathy. In: Hahnemann 3 (1920), no. 11, pp. 401–407.

Dutta, Sarat Chandra: Primary Guide to Homeopathy or the Companion to the Family Medical Chest. Calcutta 1899.

Freebome, J. H.: Talks About Homeopathy. In: The Hahnemannian Gleanings 3 (Dec. 1932), p. 515.

Gangadin: European Guide and Medical Companion to India. Westminster 1895.

Ghose, Sarat Chandra: Life of Dr. Mahendralal Sircar. 2nd ed. Calcutta 1935.

Ghosh, Surendra Mohan: Susrut o Hyaniman. Calcutta 1906.

Kanjilal, Amaresh: Byaktigato arthoneeti. Calcutta 1921.

Laha, Satyacharan: Advertisement. In: Homeopathic Griha Chikitsha. Calcutta 1914, page number not cited.

Maity, H. P.: Deshiya Beshaja o Tahar Shakti. In: Hahnemann 7 (1924), no. 4, p. 174–177.

Mallika, Harikrishna: Sadrisa Byabostha Jwar Chikitsha, Berigny and Company's Bengali Homeopathic Series No II. Calcutta 1871.

Mukhati, H. N.: Pothyo Nirbachan. Dacca 1925.

Mukhopadhyay, Bhudeb: Paribarik Prabandha. 3rd ed. Hooghly 1889.

Mukhopadhyay, Shashibhushan: Baidya Chikitshak er Oshumpornota. In: Chikitsha Sammilani 8 (1891), pp. 269–272.

Ray, Haranath: Homeopathy Mowt e Jwar Chikitsha. In: Chikitsha Sammilani 3 (1886), pp. 217–222.

Ray, Haricharan: Kromo Nirnay ba Matra Bijnan. In: Hahnemann 1 (1918), no. 11, pp. 322–323.

Ray, K. K.: Editorial: Prodorshoni te Deshiya Homeo Oushadh. In: Homeopathy Pracharak 2 (Dec. 1928), no. 9, p. 366.

Raya, Jagachandra: Preface. In: Raya, Jagachandra: Garhasthya ebong Homeopathic Chikitsha Bigyan. Calcutta 1917, page number not cited.

Raya, Jagachandra: Garhasthya Swasthya ebong Homeopathic Chikitsha Bigyan. Calcutta 1917.

Roy, Madhusudan: Abadhoutik ba Sadrisa Chikitsha. In: Chikitsha Sammilani 2 (1885), pp. 146–161.

Salzer, Leopold: On the Necessity of Drug Proving in India. In: Calcutta Journal of Medicine 2 (May-June 1869), nos. 5 and 6, pp. 177–178.

Secondary Sources

Arnold, David; Sarkar, Sumit: In Search of Rational Remedies: Homeopathy in Nineteenth century Bengal. In: Ernst, Waltraud (ed.): Plural Medicine, Tradition and Modernity, 1800–2000. London; New York 2002, pp. 41–54.

Bakhle, Janaki: Two Men and Music: Nationalism in the Making of an Indian Classical Tradition. Delhi 2005.

Bean, Susan S.: Gandhi and Khadi: The Fabric of Indian Nationalism. In: Weiner, Annette B.; Schneider, Jane (eds.): Cloth and Human Experience. Washington 1989, pp. 355–376.

Bharadwaj, Surinder M.: Homeopathy in India. In: Gupta, Giri Raj (ed.): The Social and Cultural Context of Medicine in India. Delhi 1981, pp. 31–54.

Biswas, Arun Kumar: Collected Works of Mahendralal Sircar, Eugene Lafont and the Science Movement, 1860–1910. Kolkata 2003, pp. 231–247.

Chakrabarty, Dipesh: The Difference: Deferral of (A) Colonial Modernity: Public Debates on Domesticity in Colonial Bengal. In: History Workshop 36 (1993), pp. 1–36.

Chatterjee, Partha: The Nation and Its Fragments: Colonial and Postcolonial Histories. Princeton 1993.

Ernst, Waltraud: Colonial Psychiatry, Magic and Religion: The Case of Mesmerism in British India. In: History of Psychiatry 15 (2004), no. 1, pp. 57–68.

Hausman, Gary J.: Making Medicine Indigenous: Homeopathy in South India. In: Social History of Medicine 15 (2002), no. 2, pp. 303–322.

Hobsbawn, Eric J.; Ranger, Terence O. (eds.): The Invention of Tradition. Cambridge 1992.

Kishore, Jugal: About Entry of Homeopathy in India. In: Bulletin of the Institution of History of Medicine 2 (1973), no. 2, pp. 76–78.

Kumar, Anil: Introduction and Spread of Homeopathy in India. In: Medicine and the Raj: British Medical Policy in India 1935–1911. New Delhi 1998, pp. 62–68.

Mani, Lata: Contentious Traditions: the Debate on Sati in Colonial India. Berkeley 1998.

Mukherjee, S. N.: Calcutta: Essays in Urban History. Calcutta 1993.

Palit, Chittabrata: Dr. Mahendralal Sircar and Homeopathy. In: Indian Journal for the History of Science 33 (1998), no. 4, pp. 281–292.

Ramaswamy, Sumathy: Passions of the Tongue: Language Devotion in Tamil India 1891–1970. Berkeley 1997.

Sarkar, Sumit: Swadeshi Movement in Bengal, 1903–08. Delhi 2010.

Subramanian, Lakshmi: From Tanjore Court to the Madras Music Academy. Delhi 2006.

Warren, Donald: The Bengali Context. In: Bulletin of the Indian Institute of the History of Medicine 21 (1991), pp. 17–51.

Rethinking Asymmetries in the Marketplace: Medical Pluralism in Germany, 1869–1910

Avi Sharma

Introduction

When, in 1869, the Berlin Medical Association proposed a rider to pending trade legislation lifting all barriers to entry into the medical marketplace, medicine became one of the "Free Professions," open to all persons regardless of gender, confession, age, education, or accreditation.[1] Passage of this landmark legislation helped to create an extraordinarily unregulated market for medical care in Germany, one that was unique in the European world.[2] At first, doctors saw in the trade act welcome relief from the many and varied duties that, for almost six decades, had come with medical licensing.[3] Chief among these was the so-called "compulsion to cure" (*Kurierzwang*), which made the refusal to provide medical services a civil offense.[4] In calling for the incorporation of medicine as one of the free professions, then, the Berlin Medical Association was not knowingly advocating a more competitive medical marketplace. Instead, the rider was part of a more cynical effort to roll back obligations introduced in 1809 as part of efforts to modernize the Prussian civil services.[5]

The consequences of the deregulation of medical practice in Germany were not immediately clear. After all, doctors had long worked alongside surgeons, apothecaries, midwives, teachers, priests, and other non-licensed healers, with different practitioners offering services to different kinds of cure-seekers.[6] While the 1869 trade legislation changed the legal framework organizing the relationship between licensed doctors and non-licensed healers, the *de facto* division of labor did not immediately disappear.[7] This situation would change dramatically over the next three decades. As non-licensed healers targeted a more and more diverse audience, as they transgressed the informal rules governing the medical marketplace, they contributed to a breakdown of the medico-therapeutic division of labour. In the process, doctors were drawn, first slowly, then more rapidly, into a competitive relationship with "other healers." In part because of these new, more competitive dynamics, doctors'

---

1   Huerkamp (1985); Cocks/Jarausch (1990).
2   There was a brief interlude during the Jacobin phase of the revolution in which medicine in France was similarly freed of questions of accreditation. This period began with the law of 2 March, 1791, which abolished all trade associations and guilds, and persisted until 1803. Crosland (2004).
3   Huerkamp (1985), p. 242.
4   Huerkamp (1985), p. 255.
5   Huerkamp (1985), p. 255.
6   Robert Jütte offers a comprehensive discussion of medical pluralism. Jütte (1996).
7   Even in 1880, just 25 % of medical associations canvassed in a national survey expressed strong concerns about the activities of non-licensed healers. Huerkamp (1985), p. 259.

attitudes towards their non-licensed colleagues underwent a major reorientation.[8]

Faced with new and potentially threatening market forces, doctors began to call for the reinstatement of regulatory protections on the professional practice of medicine, and by the late 1890s, German medical associations were actively mobilizing to control the spread of what they called "quackery." They claimed that swindlers and charlatans were seducing the masses with potions and elixirs, and that uneducated lay-people were dangerously susceptible to their promises. In many cases, medical associations were joined in their crusade by bureaucrats, police superintendents, university professors and other educated elites, and these defensive alliances are important in understanding the asymmetries that organized the Wilhelmine medical landscape.

If a range of educated elites were concerned by the alleged spread of "quackery," though, this is only part of the story. Contrary to what contemporary critics of "quackery" would have us believe, attitudes towards non-licensed healers did not break down along class-lines, nor did an individual's level of education necessarily dictate his or her perception of a free medical marketplace. It was not, in other words, only "the masses" who were interested in "other" medicine, nor was it just the lower classes who defended the rights of "other" healers. Lawyers and parliamentarians, police superintendents and regional governors, workers and artisans, publicists and political activists, and even some doctors were active in their defense of right of lay-persons to practise medicine, and in their belief that "other" medicine should be considered one among many competing medical models.

These voices cast sometimes surprising light on popular attitudes towards scientific freedom, civil liberties, professional authority and the medical marketplace. They suggest that "other" healing traditions like *Naturheilkunde* were not a "survival" of an older medico-therapeutic worldview, as representatives of medical associations frequently claimed.[9] Nor should we assume that representatives of Wilhelmine state power were unified in their attitudes towards the practice of popular medicine. If it is relatively non-controversial to suggest that the 19th century European state increasingly considered the management of public health to be an important function of its responsibility, it does not follow that this growing concern with public health resulted in particular anxieties about practitioners of "other healing" traditions. As I try to show in this paper, bureaucrats and elected officials disagreed strongly about whether and to what extent the practice of popular medicine was actually a problem at all.[10] By focusing not just on the defensive alliances that pitted educated elites

---

8 For a systematic discussion of the German medical profession covering a far longer timespan than my present essay, see the excellent collection edited by Robert Jütte. Jütte (1997).

9 Uwe Heyll offers a rich portrait of *Naturheilkunde* over the *longue durée* in his monograph "Wasser, Fasten, Luft und Licht". Heyll (2006).

10 A piece by Florian Mildenberger suggests, for example, that the attempts to control the practices of non-licensed healers were a logical outcome of the growth of state power in

against "other healers," but on the range of actors who made their voices heard, I hope to show that healing traditions like *Naturheilkunde* occupied a less class specific, less discursively marginal place than we have sometimes assumed.[11]

Extra-Legal Measures in a *Rechtsstaat*

Calls for the increased regulation of the medical field appear to have stemmed, at least in part, from anxieties about the increased presence of non-licensed practitioners in the urban landscape. An October 1897 report on the consequences of de-regulation claimed that "the number of non-licensed practitioners [*Pfuscher*] had never been so great."[12] In Berlin, for example, the report cited the presence of 476 non-licensed practitioners, among them apothecaries, midwives, and orderlies.[13] If the increasingly shrill communications between local, state, and national officials are any indicator, the number of non-licensed practitioners had, in fact, grown dramatically during the 1890s. A 1911 report claimed that, between 1879 and 1898, the number of non-licensed healers active in Berlin had grown at a rate of 1,600%. Between 1901 and 1911, the numbers had grown by a further 300%, from 2,404 to 7,549.[14] While these numbers are surely exaggerated[15], they do point to the widespread belief that the practice of medicine by non-licensed healers had expanded in troubling ways.

If the desire to control the spread of "other" healing traditions like *Naturheilkunde* was the basis for expanding police power, though, the administration of justice varied dramatically. In Saxony, conviction carried with it a maximum penalty of 400 Marks or up to 40 days in jail[16], while in Schleswig, the same crime warranted a fine of just 60 marks or a "corresponding jail term"[17].

---

the late 19th and early 20th centuries. While his contribution is outstandingly researched, it will become clear in the course of this paper that I reject many of the assumptions on which it is based. Ultimately, my point here is that we should not easily assume that the practices of non-licensed healers were a "problem" that needed to be solved. Mildenberger (2012).

11   Martin Dinges gives a wonderful introduction to the range of movements critical of the medical establishment in his edited volume "Medizinkritische Bewegungen im Deutschen Reich". Dinges (1996).

12   GStA PK, I. HA Rep. 76 VIII B, 1328. "Sammlung auf M3658/97 betr. Ausscheidung der Ärzte aus der Gewerbeordnung. Zusammenstellung der auf den Erlaß vom 9. Oktober, 1897 eingegangenen Berichte der Regierungs – und Oberpräsidenten betr. die infolge der Kurierfreiheit auf gesundheitliche Gebiete gegenwärtig herrschenden Zustände."

13   GStA PK, I. HA Rep. 76 VIII B, 1328.

14   Alexander (1910), p. 258.

15   Anonymus (1914). See also the figures cited for Berlin in 1897 above.

16   GStA PK, I. HA Rep. 76 VIII B, 1329. Leipzig, October 23, 1900.

17   GStA PK, I. HA Rep. 76 VIII B, 1329. "Bekanntmachung, betreffend öffentliche Anzeigen von Heilmitteln und Heilmethoden," published in *Deutsche Medizinische Wochenschrift,*

Administrators were acting in improvised ways because elected officials were unwilling to legislate the practices of non-licensed healers. As the *Kölnische Zeitung* told its readers in 1902, members of the Prussian *Landtag* were divided over the question of new limits on the free medical marketplace.[18] In August of the same year, Minister of Ecclesiastical Affairs Konrad von Studt told Chancellor Bernhard von Bülow that the *Reichstag* was almost certain to reject revision of the 1869 legislation.[19] As a piece in *Deutsche Warte* explained, it was only because their demands for new rights and greater protections "found no echo with the people that doctors turned to the state authorities [...] This can be explained [by the fact that] doctors are represented in the state administrative apparatus in no small number."[20] These efforts, which found limited support from elected officials, got a better reception in ministerial audiences.

On June 28, 1902, despite the political and legal challenges certain to face efforts to regulate the professional practice of non-licensed healers, the Ministry of Ecclesiastical Affairs issued a series of decrees that would force non-licensed healers to register with local medical officers. Recognizing that print-media was an important vehicle for the spread of "other" therapies like *Naturheilkunde*, von Studt also tried to tighten the screws on the newspapers that carried advertisements for non-licensed healers, giving medical officers and police officials the broadly defined power to fine newspapers that failed to adequately oversee the content of advertisements from health and lifestyle entrepreneurs.[21] Non-licensed healers would now face oversight from the very group that most wanted to limit their access to the medical marketplace.

Given their own professional interests, it is unsurprising that natural healing associations responded to these measures with alarm, and this is where historians have typically focused their attention. The "Associations of Practising Natural Healers" (*Vereine Ausübender Vertreter der Naturheilkunde*), for example, claimed that state regulation of the medical marketplace amounted to a "Chinese Wall" on the road to scientific progress, inhibiting the competition between different medical models, and giving medical doctors what amounted

      June 5, 1902.
18   GStA PK, I. HA Rep. 76 VIII B, 1329. *Kölnische Zeitung*, July 11, 1902.
19   GStA PK, I. HA Rep. 76 VIII B, 1329. Minister of Ecclesiastical Affairs to the Chancellor, August 22, 1902.
20   GStA PK, I. HA Rep. 76 VIII B, 1330. "Die Aufhebung der Kurierfreiheit." *Deutsche Warte*, September 19, 1903. The text was highlighted in the archival copy, presumably in the Ministry of Ecclesiastical Affairs. This is a tension that Thomas Faltin explores extensively in his monograph "Heil und Heilung". He shows how elected officials and state administrators took very different positions on the issue of a more regulated medical marketplace. Faltin (2000), pp. 224–233. In that piece, Faltin also shows how the different agents? – lay-healers, medical associations, parliamentary, ministry and police officials – used data selectively to make arguments about the merits of legislative action. See, for example, Faltin (2000), p. 240. His piece offers a data-rich portrait of the Wilhelmine medical landscape. Faltin (2000), pp. 233–267.
21   GStA PK, I. HA Rep. 77 Tit. 719, 26. Minister of Ecclesiastical Affairs to District Governors and Police Chiefs, June 28, 1902.

to a professional monopoly.[22] A different group wanted to know how the measures would be applied. As members of the "Association for Healthcare and Natural Healing" (*Verein für Gesundheitspflege und Naturheilkunde – VGN*) pointed out, there was "no [legal] measure for physical unreliability, nor could there be, so long as lay certification boards, and lay healing institutes are not recognized by the state."[23] What, they asked, would be the grounds for declaring practitioners incompetent, and refusing them a concession to professionally practise medicine? Would it be applied to all non-licensed healers who treated a patient who later died? Would medical doctors consider dangerous all treatment that deviated from those accepted in the academy? As the *VGN* petition made clear, the proposed measures gave medical doctors, "who already see the absence of a medical license as evidence of [the lay-persons] unfitness for the healing trade," the tools to systematically persecute non-licensed practitioners. In the face of widespread disagreement over scientific best practices, the *VGN* argued that health-care decisions should be left to the patients themselves.[24] Copies of their petition were submitted to the Saxon Ministry of the Interior by 18 natural healing associations.[25]

It was not only natural healing associations that raised concerns about Minister Studt's June 28 directives, though. The national liberal newspaper *Kölnische Zeitung* noted, for example, that while the exclusion of swindlers and charlatans was generally desired, it was also generally recognized that the introduction of police measures opened the door to all manners of abuse. In particular, they pointed to problems related to the advertisement and distribution of controlled substances. While ministry officials may have been justified in their anxiety about the proliferation of advertisements showcasing the abilities of "other healers" and their products, editorial writers for the *Kölnische Zeitung* thought that only uniform regulatory steps would ensure the freedom of the press and the equal application of the law. The editorial staff was clear that their calls for caution should not be understood as "an endorsement of quackery [...]."[26] But how was the editorial staff supposed to judge the relative merits of one therapeutic regime in regards to another? Were they obliged to

22 GStA PK, I. HA Rep. 76 VIII B, 1327. "Denkschrift betreffend die Aufhebung der Kuri-erfreiheit und das Verbot der Kurpfuscherei". From the "Association of Practising Natural Healers" to the Ministry for Ecclesiastical Affairs.

23 GStA PK, I. HA Rep. 76 VIII B, 1330. *Verein für Gesundheitspflege und Naturheilkunde* (Freiberg) to the Prussian Ministry for Culture, September 30, 1903. The same petition can be found in the *Hauptstaatsarchiv* in Dresden. HstAD, 2te Abt.: 3.3.3, 15232. *Verein für Gesundheitspflege und Naturheilkunde* (Freiberg) to the [Saxon] State Minister of the Interior Metzsch. September 22, 1903.

24 GStA PK, I. HA Rep. 76 VIII B, 1327. "Denkschrift betreffend die Aufhebung der Kuri-erfreiheit und das Verbot der Kurpfuscherei". From the "Association of Practising Natural Healers" to the Ministry for Ecclesiastical Affairs. Undated though probably presented in 1896 or 1897.

25 GStA PK, I. HA Rep. 76 VIII B, 1330. *Verein für Gesundheitspflege und Naturheilkunde* (Freiberg) to the Prussian Ministry for Culture (sic), September 30, 1903.

26 GStA PK, I. HA Rep. 76 VIII B, 1329. *Kölnische Zeitung*, July 11, 1902.

conduct laboratory testing of controlled substances and evaluations of individual healers? Or did the spirit of the police directives really demand that the
medical qualifications of the advertiser be brought to bear on the decision
making process? While the commercial interests of the press should not be
ignored when evaluating their opposition to Studt's initiatives, their criticisms
highlight the complicated legal questions facing advocates of increased regulation.[27]

Opposition from a third party also suggests that critics of the June decrees
were motivated not just by economic interests. Just one day after the police
directives were circulated to German dailies for publication, the Chief of Berlin Police, von Windheim, wrote a letter to Minister Studt, arguing that there
were no legal grounds to compel non-licensed healers to register with their
local medical officer, and that directives covering the restriction of advertisement were completely outside the scope of police regulatory authority.[28] Von
Windheim's letter pointed to the constitutional limits to a policy of rule by
decree, writing that, in light of the "many police regulations stricken down by
the higher administrative courts and, in particular, the state superior courts[,]"
it was bad policy (and bad publicity) to put in place police directives that
would later be overturned.[29]

This case was made equally forcefully by chief of the Hanover police Graf
von Schwerin in a letter to the regional governor. Von Schwerin noted that
paragraph 29 of the North German Trade Federation Act made absolutely
clear its authors' intention to remove legal obstacles to the free practice of
healing by any and all persons. In his view, the attempt to regulate advertisements, as well as the obligation to register one's trade with the local medical
officer, were in direct conflict with both the spirit and the letter of the law.
While the dangers of quackery were real, von Schwerin thought that unlawful
rule by decree was ultimately more dangerous than strict adherence to the letter of the law.[30] Reactions to the June Decrees suggest that media elites and
police officials were as concerned with the uniform administration of justice as
they were with the specter of the swindler. Complaints about the "capricious-
ness" of the police directives and questions about the motives of medical doctors placed Minister Studt under considerable pressure, so much so that, by
December 1902 he felt compelled to revise the ministry's stance on advertisements. In a letter to regional governors dated December 31, 1902, Studt in-
structed police officials to warn editorial staff before fining them for running
advertisements that contained misleading or exaggerated claims.[31] Faced with

27   GStA PK, I. HA Rep. 76 VIII B, 1329. *Kölnische Zeitung,* July 11, 1902.
28   GStA PK, I. HA Rep. 76 VIII B, 1329. Chief of Police von Windheim to the Minister of
     Ecclesiastical Affairs, July 12, 1902.
29   GStA PK, I. HA Rep. 76 VIII B, 1329. Chief of Police von Windheim to the Minister of
     Ecclesiastical Affairs, July 12, 1902.
30   GStA PK, I. HA Rep. 76 VIII B, 1329. Graf von Schwerin to the Provincial Governor.
     September 25, 1902.
31   GStA PK, I. HA Rep. 76 VIII B, 1329. Minister of Ecclesiastical Affairs to the Provincial
     Governors, December 31, 1902.

widespread concerns over the implementation of police measures – concerns given voice not least by high-ranking police officials – ministry level officials seem to have recognized that the only way to resolve the problem of "quackery" was to draft national legislation.

Legislating the Medical Marketplace: Progress and Public Health in the *Reichstag*

After years of delay, draft legislation to regulate abuses in the healing trade was presented to the Royal Prussian Ministry of State on April 27th, 1910. The proposed law had its first hearing in the 90th Sitting of the Reichstag on November 30th, 1910, and the debate there crystallizes many of the issues raised so far. Dr. (Jur.) Martin Fassbender, representative of the Catholic Centre Party, was first to speak, and it quickly became clear that he was suspicious of the proposed legislation. That advocates of natural healing and those of allopathic medicine disagreed about the pathogenesis of illness was obvious to everyone. As Fassbender pointed out, though, this disagreement had no objective arbiter. Neither clinical study nor laboratory research had demonstrated the superiority of one medical model over the other. For all the many advances in biology and chemistry – advances that had important consequences for anatomy, physiology, and pathology – medical researchers simply did not understand the human body well enough to speak authoritatively about it. In fact, medical doctors often had just as much trouble explaining their therapeutic successes as they did their failures. As long as this was the case, as long as the medical sciences continued to evolve, Fassbender thought that researchers and practitioners should continue to test theory and practice in the marketplace of ideas. He also thought that participation in this marketplace of ideas should not be limited by one's educational, professional, or licensing background, but rather by one's ability to demonstrate the merits of ideas and practices in a competitive field.

Given the spaces of uncertainty that characterized the medical landscape, though, Fassbender wondered whether it was possible to target charlatans and swindlers without unduly affecting legitimate practitioners of other healing traditions.[32] Perhaps a law to control the fraudulent practice of healing was necessary. More important, though,

far more important than a law against quackery, is doubtless the better education [*Aufklärung*] of the public about the condition of the body, about questions of nutrition, about cleanliness, the dangers of alcohol, and also education about the dangers of quackery [...].[33]

32 GStA PK, I. HA Rep. 76 VIII B, 1332. "Auszug aus den Verhandlungen des Reichstags". 90th Sitting, 1910, 3278–3308. Dr. Fassbender.
33 GStA PK, I. HA Rep. 76 VIII B, 1332. "Auszug aus den Verhandlungen des Reichstags". 90th Sitting, 1910, 3278–3308. Dr. Fassbender.

In this regard and others, natural healing had contributed mightily to the ongoing evolution of medical theory and practice. His remarks were greeted by cheers of "quite right!" from the center.[34] Martin Fassbender was, himself, active in a range of reform initiatives, including land-reform, the Cooperative and life-reform movements.[35] Like millions of other Germans from across the class, confessional and party-political spectrum, Fassbender believed in a total reform of health and hygiene. But parliamentary testimony suggests that one did not have to be a follower of so-called 'Life-Reform' in order to question the merits of the law, and by the time the 32-year-old Social Democratic representative Fritz Zietsch took the floor, some themes were already becoming clear.

Zietsch, like Fassbender, was concerned that the draft legislation threatened "to affect not only the true charlatans, but to reach far beyond […]."[36] In a point that drew widespread calls of "Quite Right!", Zietsch asked "[b]ut what is a *Kurpfuscher?* If one wants to combat *Kurpfuschertum* on legal grounds, is it not then necessary to [first] define the term […]."[37] In Zietsch's view, a *Kurpfuscher* was someone who practised healing without being up to the job, a definition that, as he pointed out, had nothing to do with the question of licensing or education. "But one finds such people in all other trades, *without therefore having felt obliged to proceed against them legally.*"[38] Zietsch argued that doctors, anxious to secure for themselves new professional privileges, were trying to establish a different kind of monopoly, and to accomplish their goals, all they had to do was to convince the public "that anything learned on the basis of practical experience" rather than "through so-called academic training [*Schulweisheit*] […] is to be designated as suspect."[39] They were, in Zietsch's view, out to prove that anyone practising medicine without a medical degree was a "*Kurpfuscher.*" As the social democratic representative reminded the assembled audience, though, this definition was at odds with the spirit and the wording of the 1869 Trade legislation. In what amounted to a slander of the thousands "that practise healing with the utmost honesty"[40] – a characterization met with calls of "quite right!" from the social democrats – doctors were pushing a law based largely on professional self-interest.

34   GStA PK, I. HA Rep. 76 VIII B, 1332. "Auszug aus den Verhandlungen des Reichstags". 90th Sitting, 1910, 3278–3308. Dr. Fassbender.

35   Blessing (2011), p. 75. Blessing calls Fassbender a "conservative" politician, but my reading is rather different. See Sharma (2011) and Sharma (2012).

36   GStA PK, I. HA Rep. 76 VIII B, 1332. "Auszug aus den Verhandlungen des Reichstags". 90th Sitting, 1910, 3278–3308. Zietsch.

37   GStA PK, I. HA Rep. 76 VIII B, 1332. "Auszug aus den Verhandlungen des Reichstags". 90th Sitting, 1910, 3278–3308. Zietsch.

38   GStA PK, I. HA Rep. 76 VIII B, 1332. "Auszug aus den Verhandlungen des Reichstags". 90th Sitting, 1910, 3278–3308. Zietsch. Emphasis added.

39   GStA PK, I. HA Rep. 76 VIII B, 1332. "Auszug aus den Verhandlungen des Reichstags". 90th Sitting, 1910, 3278–3308. Zietsch.

40   GStA PK, I. HA Rep. 76 VIII B, 1332. "Auszug aus den Verhandlungen des Reichstags". 90th Sitting, 1910, 3278–3308. Zietsch.

It was clear, at least to Zietsch and those who cheered him on in his remarks, that in "untold thousands of cases, *Naturheilkunde* had demonstrated its value."[41] The law, said Zietsch, "will not find the approval of parliament, because [...] *Naturheilkunde* might in this way be destroyed [*totgeschlagen*] with a single blow."[42] In the end, the Reichstag was not the place to adjudicate the relative merits of *Naturheilkunde* and academic medicine. Critics of the law understandably focused their attacks on legal and administrative questions, but their general orientation towards regulation rested on deeper assumptions. On the floor and in committee, critics from across the party-political spectrum defended the free medical marketplace because they believed that citizens had the federally guaranteed right to choose between competing therapeutic traditions. Whether they themselves subscribed to *Naturheilkunde*, homeopathy, allopathy, or some hybrid version of the three, they all (at least implicitly) accepted the legitimacy of these diverse medical epistemologies. While doctors and doctors' associations wanted to convince the decision-making classes that other healing appealed primarily to the gullible masses, this was more a professional fantasy than it was an objective representation of the Wilhelmine landscape. As the parliamentary record shows, the defense of medical pluralism was by no means confined to the socio-cultural margins, it was not intrinsically tied to questions of professional interest, nor was it the pet-issue of one political party. Medical Pluralism was a shared commitment that cut across class, party, and even confessional lines.[43]

There were, of course, supporters of the proposed legislation. Expressing surprise at the vigorous attacks on the proposed law, the eye doctor and National Liberal from Hanover, Wilhelm Arning, departed from his planned comments almost immediately. Instead of focusing on the wording of the law, Arning used his time to defend his profession from perceived attacks, and to speak of the pressing need for legislative initiative on the part of his colleagues. While acknowledging that medicine was indeed an art, and that there were, in some rare cases, individuals gifted with a natural ability that had nothing to do with training or education (!), he also argued that the law was designed to deal with the general rule, and not its exception. The general rule was, in his view, one in which swindlers and confidence men worked to defraud the sick and the gullible of their hard-won wages.[44] Raising the spectre of unregulated swindlers and criminally insane confidence men populating the ranks of the non-licensed healers, Arning thought that it was obvious that strong legislation was required to control the situation. The problem, of course, was that not

---

41 GStA PK, I. HA Rep. 76 VIII B, 1332. "Auszug aus den Verhandlungen des Reichstags". 90th Sitting, 1910, 3278–3308. Zietsch.

42 GStA PK, I. HA Rep. 76 VIII B, 1332. "Auszug aus den Verhandlungen des Reichstags". 90th Sitting, 1910, 3278–3308. Zietsch.

43 On the organizational structure of the natural healing movement, see Regin (1995), pp. 45–90. See also Florentine Fritzen's wonderful monograph "Gesünder leben" (2006). Taken as a whole, Fritzen's work suggests just how impactful the so-called Life-reform movement was.

44 Regin (1995), pp. 426ff. Dr Arning, MD.

everyone agreed with him. No small number of those skeptics happened to be sitting in parliamentary chambers.

The weeks following the first parliamentary hearing saw widespread press coverage of the proposed legislation, and debates in the press bear striking similarity to the parliamentary debate. On December 1st, under the banner "The Quackery Law in the Parliament," the *Deutsche Tageszeitung* editorialized that efforts to address abuses in the field of health failed to draw distinctions between "other healers" who rejected the principles of orthodox medicine, and the quacks and charlatans who put public health at risk. As the author pointed out, "[n]ot every natural healer is a swindler, or even a *Kurpfuscher* in the typical sense of the word."[45] He cited widespread concerns that the proposed legislation would indiscriminately affect all non-licensed healers without significantly improving public health.

In their report one week later on a public meeting at the Germania hall on Berlin's Chaussee Strasse, the *Berliner Tageblatt* echoed many of the concerns raised in the *Deutsche Tageszeitung* piece cited above. Describing a crowd of some 2000 people, and the flurry of 300 telegrams posted from all over Germany, the author claimed that, while the crowd appeared unified in their desire to exclude charlatans and swindlers from the medical marketplace, they were also convinced that the present law would open "[g]ate and door to hateful denunciations."[46] The very vocal crowd "sees in the draft law a thoroughly unsuitable measure for pulling the floor out from under the true quacks, because these can only be destroyed through [...] the education of the people [...]."[47] Reports in the press struck a relatively even balance between practical concerns about the implementation of the law, and more philosophical concerns about freedom of choice and the rights of "other healers."

Opposition to the law came from a number of different directions, but medical associations did little to counter their critics. In fact, medical associations themselves attacked provisions in the law, in particular, the "compulsion to cure" (*Kurierzwang*) that made it obligatory for doctors to treat patients in need of immediate medical attention. Hostility to the so-called *Kurierzwang* had been an important part of medical association platforms for more than four decades, and played a catalyzing role in the creation of the free medical marketplace in 1869. At that time, the Berlin Medical Association pushed the "North German Free Trade Act", in part to free medical doctors from a whole range of professional responsibilities, chief among them, the "compulsion to cure." Freedom came at a price, though. If doctors were unwilling to provide medical attention on demand, then patients must have the freedom to seek care from a willing provider. As an editorial in the *Nationale Zeitung* put it in

45   BA, R/8034II, 1808. "Das Kurpfuschereigesetz im Reichstage," *Deutsche Tageszeitung*, December 1, 1910.

46   BA, R/8034II, 1808. "Protestversammlung gegen den Entwurf des Kurpfuschereigesetzes," *Berliner Tageblatt*, December 8, 1910.

47   BA, R/8034II, 1808. "Protestversammlung gegen den Entwurf des Kurpfuschereigesetzes," *Berliner Tageblatt*, December 8, 1910.

1900, if "the state fails to ensure [medical] care for all, it cannot deny the right to seek assistance" from non-licensed persons.[48]

Parliamentary hearings echoed these points, now almost a decade old. As committee members Stadthagen, Stücklen, and Zietsch made clear in riders to the legislation, a return to the 1869 *status quo ante* was only possible if doctors submitted to the "compulsion to cure." Why was this such a sticking point for both sides? Because the *Kurierzwang* acted as a potential check on a medical monopoly, a check ensuring that patients would receive adequate care even if doctors tried to use their control over the medical marketplace to extort wage concessions or other professional advantages. This was not just an academic point. Physicians had, in fact, repeatedly withheld care in exactly this way. *Kurierzwang* was, then, an important condition for doctors as they tried to assert control over the medical marketplace. For some elected officials, the "compulsion to cure" clause was a way to ensure that doctors' associations could not use their monopoly to manipulate the marketplace by choking off access to an essential service. Ultimately, it was this unwillingness of medical associations to accept the reintroduction of the "compulsion to cure" as the price for increased regulation that led to the failure of the law.

The proposed law had a number of factors in its favour: anxiety about unlicensed and unregulated healers, fears of a population crisis, and suspicions that charlatans and confidence men were using the absence of regulation to defraud the German public. But doctors had done little to leverage this support to ensure passage of the law, antagonizing important officials, the popular press, and public opinion with their aggressive defense of largely material interests. And this ultimately helps us to understand why the defense of medical pluralism was so effective. Medical pluralism was not just a matter of medico-scientific progress. It was implied in debates about individual rights and personal choice, in conflicts over state power and freedom of the press. The defense of medical pluralism also occurred in a particular moment in German history. It was shaped by new media and publicity outlets, it evolved in an age of mass political mobilization.

For almost five decades, the free medical marketplace was an important index of Germany's remarkably exuberant public sphere, and the end of one signaled the decline of the other. During World War I, centralizing forces were increasingly able to silence both the defenders of the free medical marketplace and to short-circuit civil and political dissent. The war, then, accomplished what decades of agitation by doctors' associations had failed in peacetime to do. On the prerogative of some military governors general, and at the urging of the Ministry of War, natural healers were forbidden to treat sexually transmissible and infectious diseases in combat zones – a decree that would have essentially excluded natural healers from practising in those areas.[49] 1914/1915 were very bad years for medical pluralism in Germany.

48 GStA PK, I. HA Rep. 76 VIII B, 1329. "Die Bekämpfung der Kurpfuscherei," *Nationale Zeitung,* July 11, 1902.
49 Regin (1995), p. 445.

Conclusion

It is not often that one finds historians trying to "recover" elite discourses these days, but that is precisely what I try to do in this paper. In writing about "other healing" traditions, historians too often suggest that these traditions were somehow insurgent, or that they expressed a more authentic popular culture. In some instances, this may be true. In the German case, though, I think this reading has the potential to marginalize what were in fact very widespread practices. To ignore the place of elites in writing the histories of medical pluralism is to wrongly imply that "other healing" traditions appealed mostly to the popular classes. This has the effect of undermining the authority of these medical alternatives, because – rightly or wrongly – elite knowledge / expert knowledge / bourgeois knowledge / colonial knowledge are powerfully normative. In Wilhelmine Germany, medical pluralism was a widely shared value. For some of its defenders, this was a question of individual rights and personal choice. For others, it was about scientific progress and the marketplace of ideas. For others still, it was an expression of Germany's national self. Whatever the reasons were that people came together in defense of the free medical marketplace, it is clear that they came from diverse social, economic and cultural backgrounds. By focusing not just on the defensive alliances that pitted educated elites against "other healers," but on the range of actors who made their voices heard, I hope to have shown that healing traditions like *Naturheilkunde* occupied a less class-specific, less discursively marginal place than we have sometimes assumed.

These conclusions resonate in interesting ways with some of the other papers presented in this volume, in particular, those by Nupur Barua and Harish Naraindas. These papers, in particular, illustrate ways in which conventional medicine has achieved a kind of hegemonic status, shaping the therapeutic, rhetorical and administrative practices even of those who claim, at first, to be offering medical alternatives. Barua, for example, describes a "global medicine" in "local garb," where the delivery mechanism – the "pill" – is thought to be a panacea for reasons both of political economy and of ideology. Naraindas shows how even the practices of those trying to differentiate themselves from conventional medicine are forced to conform to established norms that promise consumers a quick fix to all of their complaints. Whether it is the local healer who treats slum-dwellers, or practitioners of Ayurveda catering to a global audience, even "alternatives" to conventional medicine are over-determined by their relationship to its authority. And as Harald Walach and William Sax noted in the closing discussion, this profoundly asymmetrical relationship has structural consequences. It determines where research funds are allocated, which therapies are reimbursed by insurance schemes, and what is taught in medical schools.

All of this helps to explain why the histories of "other medicine" in the 19th and early 20th centuries are written in the ways that they are, with healing traditions like homeopathy and *Naturheilkunde* identified as local rather than universal, folkloric as opposed to scientific, superstitious instead of rational. Historical writing about "other medicine" is itself defined by the post-war hegemony of conventional medicine, which has made it remarkably difficult to recognize other forms of medical knowledge as legitimate. For decades, now, the medical marketplace has been defined by asymmetry. And this has defined the way that historians have written and thought about medicine – conventional and otherwise.[50]

There were, of course, asymmetries in the Wilhelmine medical marketplace, too. But my paper suggests that the hegemony of conventional medicine had not yet been achieved, nor was it normative in the way that Barua's and Naraindas' papers show that it has become. The hegemony of conventional medicine, then, is a development of relatively recent provenance, and it remains to be seen whether and to what extent this global dominance will persist in the future. The Wilhelmine story that I tell also offers hope for a more plural marketplace in our own time, precisely because it shows that the dominance of a "university medicine" that has become "conventional" was never quite as complete as it seemed to be. Taken together, the papers in this collection suggest that a more plural, more inclusive, more accessible medicine is not just a thing of the past.

Bibliography

Archival Sources

Bundesarchiv, Berlin (BA)
R/8034II
Hauptstaatsarchiv Dresden (HStAD)
2te Abt.: 3.3.3
Geheimes Staatsarchiv Preußischer Kulturbesitz, Berlin (GStA PK)
I. HA Rep. 76 VIII B
I. HA Rep. 77 Tit. 719

50 This is particularly glaring in the work of historians who claim to be working to recover plural knowledge. Michael Hau, for example, tells us at one point that medical cosmologies like *Naturheilkunde* were really just an attempt to simplify medicine so that the simple people could understand it. Hau writes "I argue that the holism of most of the etiologic concepts of life reformers were simply a way to avoid the necessity of complex analysis by reducing pathological symptoms to a single cause that could easily be understood by lay people." Hau (2003), p. 113. Earlier, though, he tells us that the *Lebensreform* movement should not be understood primarily as a "protest against modernization [...] [but as] an expression of the contradictions and tensions of the period of classical modernity." Hau (2003), p. 3.

Printed Sources and Literature

Alexander, Carl: Das Kurpfuschertum und seine Gegner. In: Gesundheitslehrer 13 (1910), pp. 258–261.

Anonymus: Eine Erklärung des Reichsamtes des Innern über die Zahl der Kurpfuscher. In: Gesundheitslehrer 17 (1914), p. 28.

Blessing, Bettina: Pathways of Homeopathic Medicine. Heidelberg 2011.

Cocks, Geoffrey; Jarausch, Konrad (eds.): German Professions, 1800–1950. New York 1990.

Crosland, Maurice: The *Officiers de Santé* of the French Revolution: A Case Study in the Changing Language of Medicine. In: Medical History 48 (2004), pp. 229–244.

Dinges, Martin (ed.): Medizinkritische Bewegungen im Deutschen Reich (ca. 1870-ca. 1933). Stuttgart 1996.

Dinges, Martin (ed.): Patients in the History of Homeopathy. Sheffield 2002.

Dirlik, Arif: The Post-Colonial Aura: Third World Criticism in the Age of Global Capitalism. Boulder, CO 1998.

Fabian, Johannes: Out of Our Minds: Reason and Madness in the Exploration of Central Africa. Berkeley 2000.

Faltin, Thomas: Heil und Heilung. Geschichte der Laienheilkundigen und Struktur antimodernistischer Weltanschauungen in Kaiserreich und Weimarer Republik am Beispiel von Eugen Wenz (1856–1945). Stuttgart 2000.

Foucault, Michel: Discipline and Punish: The Birth of the Prison [Trans. Allan Sheridan]. New York 1977.

Fritzen, Florentine: Gesünder leben: Die Lebensreformbewegung im 20. Jahrhundert. Stuttgart 2006.

Hau, Michael: The Cult of Health and Beauty in Germany: A Social History, 1890–1930. Chicago 2003.

Heyll, Uwe: Wasser, Fasten, Licht und Luft. Die Geschichte der Naturheilkunde in Deutschland. Frankfurt/Main 2006.

Huerkamp, Claudia: Der Aufstieg der Ärzte im 19. Jahrhundert. Vom gelehrten Stand zum professionellen Experten. Das Beispiel Preußens. Göttingen 1985.

Jütte, Robert: Die Geschichte der alternativen Medizin: von der Volksmedizin zu den unkonventionellen Therapien von heute. München 1996.

Jütte, Robert (ed.): Geschichte der deutschen Ärzteschaft: organisierte Berufs- und Gesundheitspolitik im 19. und 20. Jahrhundert. Köln 1997.

Mildenberger, Florian: Sanatorien für Touristen – Medikamente für zu Hause – Heilkundige nach Bedarf: Heilkulturen im Herzogtum Gotha (ca. 1850-ca. 1950). In: Medizin, Gesellschaft und Geschichte 30 (2011), pp. 171–205.

Regin, Cornelia: Selbsthilfe und Gesundheitspolitik: die Naturheilbewegung im Kaiserreich, 1889 bis 1914. Stuttgart 1995.

Sharma, Avi: Medicine From the Margins? From Medical Heterodoxy to the University of Berlin. In: Social History of Medicine 24 (2011), pp. 334–351.

Sharma, Avi: Wilhelmine Nature: Natural Lifestyle and Practical Politics in the German Life-Reform Movement. In: Social History 37 (2012), pp. 36–54.

A Homeopathic Clinic in a Multispeciality Hospital. Reflections from Practice

Ameeta R. Manchanda

Introduction

Traditions and culture play a vital role in the practice of health services where people adopt and utilize them in synchrony with their beliefs, values, accessibility and socioeconomic status. The level of acceptance of a medical therapy by society is of utmost importance for the relevant practitioners and the consumers. Medical pluralism is more than a phenomenon of the mix of traditional and modern medicine; it is rather a function of political economy and cultural hegemony[1] and a result of complex factors within medical and other systems which are intertwined. Medical pluralism in health care signifies the provision of multiple systems of therapies for the promotion of health and prevention/cure of diseases. Pluralism has been conspicuous in healthcare amid various medical therapies, with their salient healing effects. The Integration of diverse philosophies in the delivery of health services is indeed challenging. Medical pluralism is more readily observed in societies where the role of the state is considered significant to the phenomenon of its application.

The Government of India has granted official recognition to traditional systems known as Ayurveda, Yoga & Naturopathy, Unani, Siddha and Homeopathy (AYUSH) systems and it is legal for any allopathic hospital to provide these services; the Government even encourages and provides financial grants to establish departments of AYUSH systems.[2] In India out of pocket expenditure on health services is to the tune of 85%, which is the highest in the world.[3] The patients' decision is often driven by factors like accessibility, affordability and personal preference rather than the hegemony of insurance sector and pharmaceutical industry.

Homeopathy received recognition and patronage from the Government of India immediately after independence along with the other Indian systems. Statutory provisions for university level education in homeopathy were approved by the Indian Parliament, when Central Council of Homeopathy Act was passed in the year 1973.[4] The impact was evident from the proliferation of homeopathic infrastructure at all levels, including the number of colleges, dispensaries supported by the charitable institutions, and advancements in the state and private sectors. Masses were seen seeking this therapy with renewed faith and confidence. The majority of the clinics were established either as standalone clinics or at the level of primary health care. However, the last two

---

1 Elling (1981); Myntti (1988).
2 http://www.indianmedicine.nic.in (last accessed on May 5, 2013).
3 Mudur (2011).
4 http://www.cchindia.com/hcc-act.htm (last accessed on May 8, 2013).

decades witnessed the emergence of these clinics at secondary level multispe-
cialty hospitals, signifying their enhanced popularity.

The health sector in India is in an ever-evolving phase, wherein AYUSH
systems play an important role. This paper is a humble endeavor to illustrate
the dynamics of establishing and running a homeopathic clinic in a reputed
multispeciality hospital of Delhi using case study methodology.

The Homeopathic Clinic in Holy Family Hospital (1990–96)

The Holy Family Hospital is a general multi-speciality hospital established in
the year 1958 run by the Delhi catholic Arch-Diocese and registered as a charitable non-profit organization under the Societies Act XXI of 1860 and has the
Archbishop of Delhi as its Chairperson.[5] The homeopathic and ayurvedic
clinics started in the year 1988. The Homeopathic consultation was initially
provided by a clergyman who treated patients with bio-chemic tissue salts and
combinations of homeopathic drugs, known as Father Muller Combinations.
During 1988–90, the clinic was managed by a part time homeopathic doctor
after which the authorities decided to recruit graduate doctors by advertising
in the newspapers. Two graduate homeopathic physicians were recruited by a
panel committee of medical superintendent, medical director, and one senior
homeopathic doctor.

The homeopathic clinic was given separate identity as a department with
one consultation room, an examination table, sphygmomanometer, ENT set,
thermometer, tongue depressor, torch etc. There was an attached pharmacy
chamber with a support staff to dispense the medicines.

The author, along with one male homeopathic physician, joined the department on 1st May 1990 and was given the morning shift (9am-12noon) at a
salary of Rs 2,000/per month (35 Euro) during the first year of probation,
which was subsequently raised to Rs 3,000/pm (50 Euro). During the formal
induction session, the mission, vision and activities of the hospital were detailed with a tour to various departments i.e. emergency, intensive care unit,
intensive coronary care unit, efficient laboratories, X rays, ultrasound and CT
scan, blood bank, physiotherapy etc. The hospital also undertook public
health projects and activities in the form of mobile health clinics, well baby
clinic, social counselling for the patients and free homeopathic consultation
for poor patients once every week. We were advised to develop rapport with
allopathic specialists and refrain from modifying or revoking prescriptions of
other therapists without their consent. We had autonomy to admit patients to
the in-patient department (IPD) under our care and also utilize state of art diagnostic facilities at par with other consultants. Attending the monthly clinical
meeting was mandatory, so as to keep abreast with new activities and ensure
healthy discussion among the different health systems. The patients visiting

---

5   http://www.hfhdelhi.org/ (last accessed on May 8, 2013).

the hospital were issued a consultation booklet at a registration fee of Rs 50/- (0.75 Euro) & Rs 270/- (4.1 Euro) for general and private patients respectively. The same booklet was being utilized by all the departments where the doctor would write the short history, diagnosis and prescription for each patient. Subsequent consultations were also recorded in the same booklet with a nominal fee for each visit. A carbon copy of each prescription was kept in the respective department as a record.

The initial patients were the hospital staff, resident doctors and a few referrals from the allopathic specialists; gradually patients from the general pool of the outpatient department (OPD) also started to visit the clinic. Patients were from diverse religious backgrounds that included Muslims, Hindus and Christians. Those from the middle and lower middle classes were seen as general patients and the affluent ones as private patients. A major patient percentage (about 75%) included women, children and old people. The overall response was encouraging, as awareness of the clinic gained momentum. This was evident from the consistent increase of patient numbers. At first the clinic was visited by 15–20 patients/day, a number that rose to about 40–50 a day, with Saturdays witnessing numbers of about 75–90 within one year of its establishment. The total patient turnover at the hospital's OPD was about 1,400–1,500 patients a day, of which about 5–8% were catered for by the homeopathic clinic. The hospital staff who had benefitted from homeopathic treatment were the brand ambassadors who promote the clinic.

The clinic primarily provided consultation in both acute and chronic cases. At times, at the behest of either the patient or the attending physician, IPD consultations were sent for. We were required to advice treatment after discussion with the unit in-charge about the possibility of recovery with homeopathy. The common clinical conditions treated in this clinic are given in Table 1.

About 7–10% patients were referred by allopathic consultants. These were primarily the patients suffering from respiratory allergies, anxiety neurosis, chronic arthritis, recurrent infections, warts, callosities, migraine, dentition complaints etc. For medical and surgical conditions where little could be achieved through homeopathy (e.g. tuberculosis, leprosy, large benign tumours, acute asthma, high fevers, acute abdomen, very high blood pressure, blood sugar levels etc.) patients were referred back for allopathic treatment, but often continued homeopathic treatment as well. It was indeed heartening to see the integration of different systems in one prescription booklet. The referrals depended on the conviction of the other consultants, as some allopathic doctors consulted us for themselves and their family members too.

The clinic achieved breakeven point in the first few weeks and thereafter continued to yield good revenue though the profit margins were comparatively low in contrast to other specialities owing to the cost effectiveness of homeopathic medicines. This was often a point of concern for the hospital administration.

Table 1: Common clinical conditions treated in the Homeopathic clinic

Allergic asthma	Adenoids	Anal fissure	Ankle sprain
Addictions	Behavioural problems in children	Bed wetting	Bronchitis
Childhood diarrhoea	Childhood fever	Chronic fatigue syndrome	Common cold
Cough	Dysmenorrhoea	Fibromyalgia	Gastrointestinal cramps
Hay fever	Headache	Infertility (female)	Influenza
Insomnia	Irritable bowel syndrome	Kidney failure	Low back pain
Migraine	Nervousness	Obesity	Osteoarthritis
Otitis media	Plantar fasciitis	Post-operative pain	Psychosomatic disease
Premenstrual syndrome	Pruritus	Psoriasis	Respiratory tract infection
Seborrhoea	Sepsis	Sinusitis	Stomatitis
Tonsillitis	Vertigo	Viral infections	Varicose veins

The clinics functioned as per the expectation of the administration with no financial burden. Many patients visited the hospital only for homeopathic consultation and for others it was an added facility. It is general practice in India that homeopaths seldom reveal their prescriptions but in the hospital, all prescriptions were open and this fact was often appreciated by patients.

This is a brief summary of the functioning of a homeopathic clinic in a multispeciality setup. Similarly an ayurvedic clinic is also functioning successfully in the hospital with a better infrastructure in terms of manpower and space allocated. The clinic, besides consultation, is providing panchkarma treatment, which includes famous ayurvedic massages with special focus on chronic diseases such as low back pain, arthritis, spondylitis etc.

Reflections

The success of homeopathic and ayurvedic clinics in a multispeciality hospital indicates that an integrated medical approach is definitely way ahead in imparting astute and rational treatment to the patients. The objective of these clinics was to provide holistic care to the patients in line with the mission of the hospital i.e. to provide multidimensional comprehensive medical care to strengthen the preventive, promotive, curative, emergency and rehabilitative services including education and training in medical, paramedical and support facility.

One of the advantages of this clinic was to keep patients from migrating to other private clinics or hospitals for homeopathic treatment. The transparency in prescriptions generates additional confidence in the patient and helps in mainstreaming traditional systems. The scope of the traditional system in providing treatment to patients with chronic recurrent infection, neurosis, allergies, arthritis and dyspepsia is well appreciated by allopathic physicians. The clinic could also treat cases of alcohol and smoke addiction, apart from helping patients with various psychosomatic diseases. Homeopathy was also preferred by sportspersons of repute for minor injuries when it was not possible to use allopathic drugs due to their doping effect before the tournaments. These situations often presented homeopathy as a great alternative for patients. Although this clinic offers the opportunity to work in collaboration with the allopathic specialists, with full support of state-of-the-art diagnostic facilities, it is rather disconcerting to see that due research is not being undertaken. As a consequence data pertaining to the homeopathic practice in an integrated set up is often lacking.

Overall, the author's experience reflected that the knowledge, attitude and behaviour of the homeopathic doctor, the ability to diagnose and treat patients logically goes a long way in making the clinic a success in an integrated medical set up. The doctor must understand the limitations and scope of homeopathy. Their clinical acumen should be in line with hospital protocol and, where it is not possible to cure the patients completely, one should be open to providing only symptomatic support and must allow/refer the patient to seek help from allopathic doctors.

The number of minor surgical procedures was marginally reduced in the hospital as patients with enlarged adenoids, tonsils, simple cyst, callosities, warts etc. preferred and were cured with homeopathy. The feedback of such patients often revealed very high satisfaction levels. Although we do not have any specific data, this fact was often stated by the specialists concerned in clinical meetings.

Homeopaths should also advocate the general measures of good nutrition, general hygienic measures, supportive life style therapies, healthy social relationship and counselling. The controversial issues related to vaccination, use of two therapies simultaneously etc. should not be debated unnecessarily. The approach towards the patients should be practical and credible. It is also important to discuss and share one's experiences with the allopathic colleagues on scientific lines. After witnessing the benefits of homeopathy, few specialists showed interest in doing a short course in homeopathy, but were content with referring the patients.

The clinic still continues to function successfully today and is generating goodwill and revenue. Presently the hospital has employed a full time homeopathic post graduate doctor. There is a need to further develop facilities for undertaking research activities for the development of this science. The main reason for their absence is the focus of the administration on patient care rather than research. Even the allopathic doctors working there do not have much research orientation or training, which makes it all the more challenging, but equally important, to create an opportunity for undertaking organized research in the hospital.

The popularity of the integrated approach at Holy Family Hospital encouraged many multispeciality hospitals to establish such departments during the last two decades. Currently, many major allopathic hospitals in Delhi, such as Sir Ganga Ram Hospital (http://www.sgrh.com/, last accessed on May 8, 2013), Vidyasagar Institute for Mental Health, Neuro & Allied Sciences (http://www.vimhans.com/, last accessed on May 8, 2013), Indian Spinal Injuries Centre (http://www.isiconline.org/, last accessed on May 8, 2013) and Pushpanjali Crosslay Hospital (http://www.pushpanjalicrosslayhospital.com/Homeopathy-Overview, last accessed on May 8, 2013) have started homeopathic clinics, while several others have a homeopathic consultant on their list of specialists.

There are many such success stories of homeopathic clinics in India. It has been observed that formal recognition and political support of the management is vital to sustain these clinics in the beginning and later on these clinics fend for themselves adding value to the hospital services. During the last decade, the Government of Delhi has also opened 15 homeopathic clinics at secondary level allopathic hospitals (http://www.homeo.delhigovt.nic.in, last accessed on May 8, 2013), whereas earlier the services were limited only to primary health centres/dispensaries. This could be attributed primarily to the cumulative impact of the success of several such clinics in the private sector.

Bibliography

Internet Links

http://www.indianmedicine.nic.in (last accessed on May 8, 2013)
http://www.cchindia.com/hcc-act.htm (last accessed on May 8, 2013)
http://www.hfhdelhi.org/ (last accessed on May 8, 2013)

Literature

Elling, R. H.: Political economy, cultural hegemony and mixes of traditional and modern medicine. In: Social Science & Medicine Part A, Medical Psychology and Medical Sociology 15 (March 1981), no. 2, pp. 89–99.
Mudur, G. S.: Tax cry for wider health net. In: The Telegraph (January 13, 2011), URL: http://www.telegraphindia.com/1110113/jsp/frontpage/story_13432596.jsp (last accessed on May 8, 2013).
Myntti, C.: Hegemony and healing in rural North Yemen. In: Social Science & Medicine 27 (1988), no. 5, pp. 515–520.

Homeopathy in Urban Primary Healthcare Units of the Delhi Government: An Assessment

Raj Kumar Manchanda, Surender Kumar Verma, Leena V. Chhatre, Harleen Kaur

Introduction

Homeopathy was officially introduced in Delhi when the Delhi Homeopathic Act was passed by the State Legislative Assembly on 1st October 1956 to provide for the registration of medical practitioners and to undertake education and research activities of homeopathy.[1] Subsequently, Nehru Homeopathic Medical College was established in 1964 by a Non-Governmental Organization (NGO), the Dr Yudhvir Singh Charitable Trust, which was later handed over to Delhi Administration. In 1978, twenty eight homeopathic units were established in the allopathic primary health centres. In the year 1996, on the recommendations of the Homeopathic Advisory Committee, a scheme providing for the opening of 5 new homeopathic units every year in the existing or upcoming allopathic primary health centres was approved. To give further impetus to the development of Indian Systems of Medicine and Homeopathy, the Directorate of Indian Systems of Medicine and Homeopathy (ISM&H) was established on 1st August 1996, with an independent wing of homeopathy.[2] Presently the homeopathic infrastructure comprises of 92 homeopathic units in primary health centres, a Research and Development Centre (*Dilli Homeopathic Anusandhan Parishad*), a Statutory Body (Board of Homeopathic System of Medicine) and two medical colleges.[3] There are currently about 5,000 registered homeopathic doctors in Delhi.

A study by Manchanda & Kulashreshtha[4] (2005) analyzed the importance of homeopathy in the delivery of healthcare in Delhi. During the year 1999–2000, out of 139 allopathic health centres, 48 centres had homeopathic units. Analysis of a total of 1.2 million patients who sought consultation during that period made the base of the study. This study revealed that the expenditure per patient of homeopathic units was one-fifth of that of allopathic primary healthcare units. The morbidity profile of both, the allopathic and homeopathic units, largely consisted of the diseases of the respiratory tract, skin, infections, gastrointestinal and female disorders. However, it was observed that allopathy was preferred by patients with acute symptoms and homeopathy for

1   Official Website of Board of Homeopathic System of Medicine, Delhi: http://www.delhihomeoboard.com (last accessed on May 15, 2013).
2   Official Website of Government of Delhi: http://delhi.gov.in (last accessed on May 15, 2013).
3   Official website of Department of Homeopathy, Government of Delhi: http://www.delhihomeo.com (last accessed on May 15, 2013).
4   Manchanda/Kulashreshtha (2005), URL: http://www.delhihomeo.com/paperberlin.html (last accessed on May 15, 2013).

sub-acute and chronic symptoms. The study suggested that under one roof, these primary healthcare units complemented each other and the patients sometimes sought treatment from both the units concurrently for certain diseases. These included rheumatoid arthritis, asthma, hypertensive heart disease, conjunctivitis, endocrinal and metabolic diseases. The reason behind this trend could be the growing awareness of the fact that homeopathic therapy can act as an adjuvant to allopathy and that the summative effect of the two may be better than the action of either, when taken individually.

The study also informed about a field survey undertaken by the Planning & Evaluation Cell of the Delhi Government in 2001, which covered 57 homeopathic healthcare units and 840 patients. 10 to 15 patients from each unit and the staff working in homeopathic and allopathic units were interviewed during the field visit. Separate structured questionnaires were used for both types of interviews. This survey revealed that allopathic and homeopathic units were working symbiotically under one roof and 46 out of 53 (87%) allopathic doctors believed that such a model was beneficial for the overall healthcare delivery. 41 doctors (78%) confirmed to the fact that working in the same premises did not create any functioning problem for either of the units. These questions revealed the changing mindset of the allopathic doctors towards the homeopathic system. The positive change can be attributed to the enhanced interaction of allopathic doctors with their homeopathic colleagues, who share the same workplace, which, in turn, gives them a fair chance to have a closer look at the efficacy of homeopathic medicines in treating various conditions. Incidents of the allopathic physicians getting not only their patients, but also their family members treated by their homeopathic counterparts and vice versa are not uncommon. Furthermore it was observed that a large number of patients (47%) based their opinion about homeopathy on their own experiences, while those who resorted to it upon somebody else's advice were a close second (45%). Nevertheless the study was reflective of only a low-income group of people. The trend among the middle or rich classes, who, as per common knowledge, prefer to see a private practitioner for their treatment, could not be explored in the study. Another nationwide survey[5] conducted in 2001–2002, however, covered this aspect. The survey, which involved 35 districts spread over 19 states of India, included a fair distribution of urban and rural groups and of income as per salary structure, and found that the percentage of households preferring ISM&H increased with increased level of income and literacy. It also predicted that with an increase in income and literacy, the preference for ISM&H might go up over time.

In order to further the outreach of homeopathic services, the Government of Delhi launched a pilot scheme in 2003 to provide financial grants to NGOs for running homeopathic healthcare units. To evaluate the outcome of this scheme under Public Private Partnership (PPP), an in-depth case study of the six NGOs that participated in the scheme was undertaken.[6] The study sug-

---

5   Singh/Yadav/Pandey (2005).
6   Venkat Raman/Manchanda (2011).

gested that out of the estimated 5,000 homeopathic practitioners in the city of Delhi, 90% were considered to work in the private sector. Apart from that, the study also mentioned that there were 149 government primary healthcare units and about 600 charity units in the city and anecdotal evidence suggested that most dispensaries were run by single practitioners who charge nominal fees. It is alleged that the private sector tends to employ self-taught, unqualified, unregistered practitioners. The study argued that the involvement of private providers will improve the quality of homeopathy services by ensuring the employment of only qualified and skilled homeopathic doctors, strengthen the public health system, wean away people from quacks, improve access to healthcare at relatively low cost, help mainstream the homeopathy system, and avoid malpractice. As per the study, the budget required to run a primary healthcare unit through private partnership was only about 30% of the budget needed to run a government unit. It also suggested that there was a possibility of making these health services self-sustainable provided the government innovated and modified the scheme to better suit the needs of the NGOs, such as redesigning the model from grant-in-aid to a contract-based partnership model. This, in turn, would motivate the NGOs to perform better. The study also emphasized the need to develop the managerial capacity of both NGO and government officers engaged in the scheme. Homeopathic units are known to be cost-effective and safe, requiring minimal space and low technological input. These, therefore, seem to be a more practical option for several religious organizations and resident welfare societies, and would therefore ensure the success of such a PPP model.

Delhi is fast becoming a hub of medical tourism with patients pouring in from across the borders to receive quality treatment at costs less than those prevalent in the more developed nations. Ironically, the same state is finding it hard to provide a reasonably sound and responsive Primary and Secondary healthcare system for those of its habitants who cannot afford to pay. The 'Tale of two cities' phenomenon is especially pronounced in Delhi.[7] Homeopathy can be an answer to this irony by providing economical treatment to all. During the last decade (2001–2011), the Government of Delhi has established 40 new homeopathic units in the city. This paper analyzes whether this number is sufficient in comparison to the population explosion. An attempt also has been made to assess whether, as observed in the 2001 study, these units are as popular and cost-effective. An analysis of the shift in the overall scenario from the last decade in terms of utility of the homeopathic services, the morbidity profile of the patients and infrastructure has also been made. The paper also suggests the economically viable options and policy initiatives the government could consider to provide impetus to the growth of homeopathy in Delhi.

---

7   Link to the official Website of the Government of Delhi: http://delhi.gov.in/wps/wcm/connect/bd5a8c80405403b0ababaf34262e20fd/State%20PIP%202009–10.pdf?MOD=AJPERES (last accessed on May 15, 2013).

The data of previous studies, secondary data sourced from the official records of the homeopathic and allopathic primary healthcare units of the Government of Delhi and the data of the population survey conducted in Delhi as part of the national census in 2011 have been used in this study.

Findings

During the last decade, the population of Delhi[8] has increased from 14 million to 17 million (21 %) (Fig. 1). The number of homeopathic primary healthcare units has risen from 51 in 2001 to 92 in 2011 (Fig. 2), which is approximately 4 units per year against the target of five units, as mentioned in the 9th & 10th Five Year Plans of the Indian Government.[9] Consequentially, the outreach of the primary healthcare units to the Delhi population has marginally increased from about 4 units per million people in 2001 to 5 in 2011 (Fig. 3), but it is still far less than the desired limit of one public health facility per 50,000 people.[10]

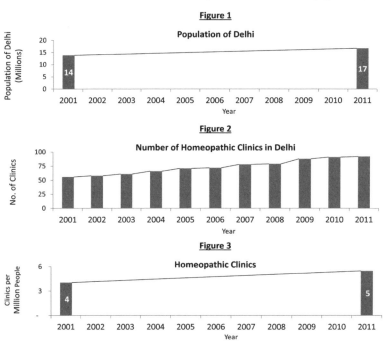

The patient inflow data of 2001 to 2011 reveals that after a plateau of four years, the rise has been relatively sharp from 2005 until 2008. The overall in-

8   Directorate (2011), pp. 2–3.
9   The link to the official website of the Government of Delhi is: http://delhiplanning.nic.in/write-up/2002–03/volume-ii/medical.pdf (last accessed on May 15, 2013).
10   http://delhi.gov.in/wps/wcm/connect/bd5a8c80405403b0ababaf34262e20fd/State%20PIP%202009–10.pdf?MOD=AJPERES (last accessed on May 15, 2013).

crease in the total number of patient visits was from 1.13 million in 2001 to 1.8 million in 2011. There has been a consistent rise in the number of patients in homeopathic primary healthcare units and the patient inflow has increased by 58% over the last decade (Fig. 4), as opposed to a 21% rise in the Delhi population (Fig. 1). This suggests a growing public demand and popularity for homeopathy among people.

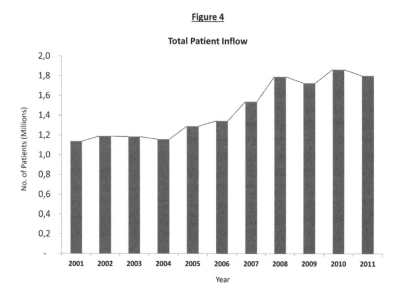

Figure 4

Total Patient Inflow

The average patient load in homeopathic units reflected in Fig. 5 reveals that each homeopathic unit is attending to about 20,000 patients annually. It is also evident from Fig. 6 that an allopathic doctor attended 15,512 patients in 2011, as compared to 19,580 attended by a homeopathic doctor. This could be attributable to a lower number of homeopathic doctors per primary healthcare unit. As opposed to 3 doctors in an allopathic health centre, only 1 doctor is posted in a homeopathic primary healthcare unit, thus increasing the burden on a homeopathic doctor. As a consequence, in 2011, an allopathic doctor had 12.9 minutes to attend to a patient, while a homeopathic doctor could spare only about 5.2 minutes per patient.

Figure 5

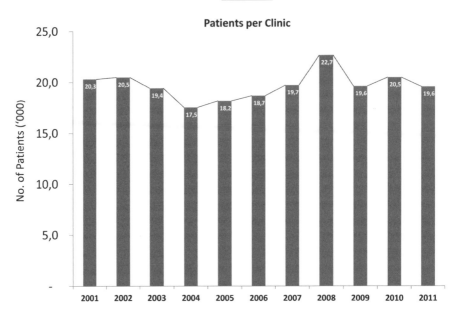

Patients per Clinic

Figure 6

Patients attended Per Physician

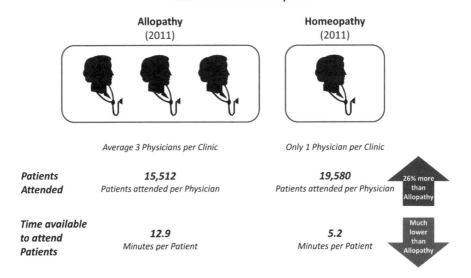

The gender break up of patients in Fig. 7 reveals that in 2001 there were 479,738 females and 344,566 children among 1.13 million patients, whereas in 2011 the number of female patients rose to 860,505 and that of children reached 388,869 among the total of 1.8 million patients (Table 1). There has also been a distinct push (5%) towards the utilization of services by males in 2011. Popularity among females has remained fairly constant (46–47%).

Figure 7

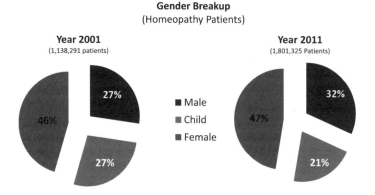

Gender Breakup
(Homeopathy Patients)

Table 1

Gender Breakup of Patients

Year	Male	Female	Child	Total
2001	313,987	479,738	344,566	1,138,291
2011	551,951	860,505	388,869	1801,325

The morbidity profile of patients attending homeopathic primary healthcare units reveals that the top five diseases treated in homeopathic primary healthcare units continue to remain the same even after a decade (Fig. 8). Among the patients who reported, the majority was suffering from either chronic or sub-acute problems related to skin, respiratory, infectious, female and digestive disorders. In 2011, patients with skin diseases topped the list leaving those with respiratory diseases a close second. It seems that awareness for efficacy of homeopathy in treating skin disorders has increased, and the fraction of patients seeking consultation for the skin problems has increased from 10.8% in 1999 to 18.8% in 2011, the highest in the profile chart.

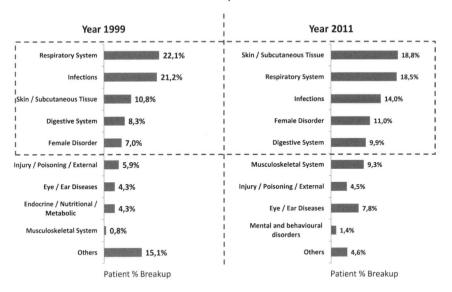

Figure 8

Morbidity Profile

Patient % Breakup

Table 2 shows a comparison of the total expenditure of allopathic and homeopathic primary healthcare units in 1999 and 2011. The Government is spending between 5–6% of budget on homeopathic units in comparison to the allopathic primary healthcare units (Fig. 9). Even after 10 years, homeopathy continues to be less expensive. Fig. 10 reveals that the cost per patient in allopathic primary healthcare units has risen from INR 77 in 1999 to INR 104.2 and in homeopathy from INR 15 to INR 27.7. Even now the cost per patient in homeopathic units is four times lower than that in allopathic primary healthcare units but it has increased by 1% due to the increased expenditure on staff salaries in homeopathic units. The Delhi government by order has granted to homeopathic doctors a status on a par with their allopathic counterparts.

Table 2

Expenditure Breakup

Total Expenditure	1999	2011
Allopathic Health Centers	INR 2,939 Lacs (EUR 4.3 Million)	INR 10,355 Lacs (EUR 15 Million)
Homeopathic Clinics	INR 188 Lacs (EUR 0.3 Million)	545 Lacs (EUR 0.8 Million)

Note: Exchange rates have been taken as on August 22, 2012

Figure 9

Expenditure Breakup

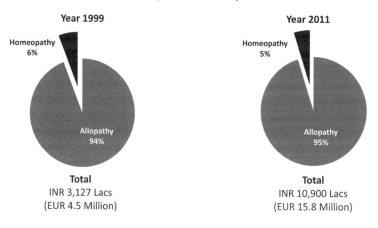

Year 1999

Homeopathy 6%
Allopathy 94%

Total
INR 3,127 Lacs
(EUR 4.5 Million)

Year 2011

Homeopathy 5%
Allopathy 95%

Total
INR 10,900 Lacs
(EUR 15.8 Million)

Note: Exchange rates have been taken as on August 22, 2012

Figure 10

Expenditure per Patient

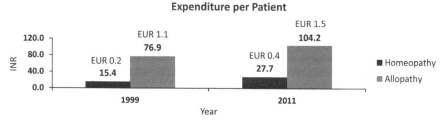

Note: Allopathy bears the cost of investigations and other supportive care advised by doctors in homeopathic clinics.

In another analysis, shown in Fig. 11, it is revealed that homeopathic units are available in 30% of the total allopathic health centres but expenditure for these primary healthcare units is only 5% of the total budget.

Figure 11

No. of Clinics vs. Expenditure

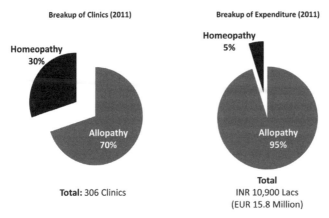

Breakup of Clinics (2011)   Breakup of Expenditure (2011)

Homeopathy
30%

Homeopathy
5%

Allopathy
70%

Allopathy
95%

Total: 306 Clinics

Total
INR 10,900 Lacs
(EUR 15.8 Million)

Note: Exchange rates have been taken as on August 22, 2012

Discussion

Homeopathic outreach to the Delhi population

A policy document of the Delhi Government estimates that 29% of the population in Delhi depends on public medical facilities out of which 39% are households with poor living standards. It also mentions that a good 53% of the population seeks private medical care. 44% of the population seeking private care are satisfied with the services received, as opposed to only 21% of those seeking care in government facilities.[11] In order to overcome these challenges in the health sector of the government, the healthcare delivery system needs to be improved further, both in quality and quantity. It is obvious from the trends shown above that homeopathy is gaining popularity in Delhi. The Government of Delhi is trying to widen the outreach of homeopathic facilities to the Delhi population, which has increased by 21% over the last decade, by opening new homeopathic units. So far, there are 92 homeopathic primary healthcare units catering to this population, with a presence of 5 units per one million people. However, the pace of opening these primary healthcare units is not fast enough to meet the increasing demand for homeopathic services. This rise in popularity for homeopathy concurs with a recent national survey that also reflects an increasing popularity of AYUSH systems.[12] The homeo-

11 http://delhi.gov.in/wps/wcm/connect/bd5a8c80405403b0ababaf34262e20fd/State%20
PIP%202009–10.pdf?MOD=AJPERES (last accessed on May 15, 2013).
12 Priya/Shweta (2010), pp. xxii–xxiii.

pathic services are being used optimally and the units are running to their full capacity with every unit seeing about 20,000 patients annually. Despite the rising demand, these primary healthcare units cannot accommodate more patients under their present staffing arrangement. Homeopathic services have, thus, reached a bottleneck where each unit is serving to its full capacity and the doctors are not able to spare more than 5–6 minutes for a patient. This could mean that a big portion of the patients willing to receive homeopathic treatment is perhaps being left untreated because there are not enough primary healthcare units. The unattended patients are then pushed towards the private doctors or to allopathy as there are fewer patients per doctor in allopathic health centers. Therefore, there is an urgent need to strengthen the homeopathic units by employing one more homeopathic doctor in the units already attending to more than 60 patients a day. Also, more homeopathic units need to be opened to overcome the saturation point these units seem to have reached.

Furthermore, as was suggested in a previous study[13], the private sector needs to be involved so that the rising public demand for homeopathic services can be met. To achieve this, the PPP model should be adopted in a more evolved way, with the NGOs running charitable and low-cost homeopathic care being allowed to retain the surplus funds generated through PPP units or donations for further development as a corpus fund. This would, over a period of time, make these PP units self-sustaining. Currently, due to the opening of new homeopathic clinics by the government, the share of patients visiting these charitable clinics has declined. An average patient prefers to visit a nearby government homeopathy health unit in hope of being attended by a better qualified doctor and of receiving superior services, thereby adding further to the patient load in government units. With adequate funds, these charitable clinics can aim to hire qualified homeopathic doctors with comparable wages and also offer better services. Therefore, successful implementation of the PPP concept would not only promote homeopathy among the masses, but also revive the dying concept of charitable homeopathic healthcare units in Delhi. Currently, most of these charitable units are in a poor condition owing to lack of funds and infrastructure.

This proposal of involving the private sector is also reiterated by the Planning Commission of Government of India in its 12th Five Year Plan (2012–17).[14] The health chapter of the plan calls for the introduction of a 'managed network approach' where health services will be largely privatized and payments for health services will be made to a network of private service providers on a per-patient basis. The government's role will in effect be reduced from providing health services to managing the network. The implementation of this plan is, however, subject to its acceptance by the health authorities at various levels.

13   Venkat Raman/Manchanda (2011).
14   http://www.livemint.com/2012/08/06222127/Ministry-opposes-plan-to-overh.html?h=B
      (last accessed on May 15, 2013).

The patient profile in homeopathic primary healthcare units

The types of diseases being reported in the homeopathic units have largely remained similar for almost a decade. This seems to suggest that a sound understanding is developing among the patients for the range of illnesses that are well treated with homeopathy. The study also reveals that the patients suffering from other conditions that are usually recommended for surgery by the allopathic doctors, like benign tumours, haemorrhoids, chronic diseases of the tonsils and adenoids, urinary calculi or uterine fibroids continue to report to homeopathic units, in the hope of avoiding going under the knife, thereby making the general perception of homeopathy being capable of averting surgery evident in the statistics. On the other hand, patients with conditions that call for urgent surgical care, or with infections included in the public health programs, like STDs, tuberculosis, leprosy, HIV/AIDS, malaria, filariasis, malignant tumours, abdominal hernia, appendicitis, cholecystitis and open wounds or injuries to blood vessels do not generally report to the homeopathic units or are referred to allopathic primary health care units for specific intervention, perhaps due to the serious nature of the ailment. This correlates with another similar study that reveals that 33 % of the patients preferred ISM&H for common ailments, while only 18 % preferred it for a serious ailment. Among those who opted for these therapies for serious ailments, a good 11.4 % preferred homeopathy over other ISM&H systems.[15] Apart from that, most chronic problems, such as chronic bronchitis, chronic dyspepsia, osteoarthritis, chronic otitis media, chronic liver diseases and menopausal problems continue to be reported to homeopathic units. Furthermore, respiratory problems still form the second most common group of illnesses, largely including chronic bronchitis, emphysema, asthma, bronochiolitis, chronic diseases of the tonsils and adenoids, influenza etc.

However, over this period, the primary focus seems to have shifted from respiratory problems to skin. The skin problems reported at the units largely included scabies, fungal infections, pyoderma, molluscum contagiosum, impetigo, furuncles, exfoliative eczema/atopic dermatitis, seborrhoeic dermatitis, warts; pruritis; psoriasis, pityriasis rosea; lichen planus; urticaria; sunburn; alopecia areata; acne; vitiligo etc. This is an interesting finding as skin disorders are known to affect 20–30 % of the general population at any one time.[16] In India, skin problems are extremely common and approximately 6 % of visits to all physicians are due to skin, hair or nail problems.[17] In addition, skin problems like psoriasis and vitiligo cause social embarrassment and the scope of their treatment with allopathy is very limited. Considering the large fraction of the population suffering from skin diseases, the direct effect of these diseases on the quality of life of patients and the established efficacy of homeopathy in their treatment, it is desirable that the Indian Government should launch a

15 Singh/Yadav/Pandey (2005).
16 Rea/Newhouse/Halil (1976).
17 Thappa (2002).

nationwide campaign to raise awareness of the role of homeopathy in the treatment of skin diseases. This will also result in the decreased reliability of these patients on steroid-based local applications or on surgery for minor skin conditions like warts or lipomas which can easily be treated with homeopathy.

Females continue to make up the biggest section of visitors to the homeopathic primary healthcare units. This can be interpreted in more ways than one. The general perception in India that homeopathy works better in female disorders seems to be playing its role in driving more females to the units. As indicated in a survey, most of these females happen to be housewives.[18] This suggests a probable added convenience of these women to report to the units within the opening hours of 8 am to 2 pm or 9 am to 4 pm on workdays. However, neither that study nor this one was able to include the weekend data separately to observe any change in the trend, such as a comparative increase in the number of working females or males on weekends. This would be an advisable topic for future research or surveys of this kind.

Economic viability and cost effectiveness

Another interesting finding is that despite the fact that the cost per patient for homeopathic treatment has gone up over the last decade, homeopathy continues to be four times cheaper than allopathy. Of the total expenditure incurred by allopathic and homeopathic primary healthcare units, only 5% is used to run 92 homeopathic units, which, in turn, is 30% of the total primary healthcare units. It is quite probable that, with the advances in medicine, the cost per patient will go up for all the therapies. However, it is clearly evident that the running costs of a homeopathic unit will continue to be a more economical option than an allopathic one. So, more policy initiatives to make homeopathy more accessible would be the right step in providing maximum health benefits to the common man with a minimum budget.

Conclusion

Over the last decade, homeopathy has gained more popularity and proven to be an economically viable part of the healthcare delivery system of Delhi. The preference for homeopathy for subacute and chronic diseases has remained unaltered over the decade and homeopathy is now the preferred approach for skin diseases. There is a need to launch a public campaign to raise awareness of the efficacy of homeopathy in the treatment of skin diseases among the patients. It is also evident that the homeopathic primary healthcare units run by the government are currently working to their full capacity. To meet the rising demand, it is imperative that homeopathy is made more accessible by open-

---

18 Manchanda/Kulashreshtha (2005), URL: http://www.delhihomeo.com/paperberlin. html (last accessed on May 15, 2013).

ing more homeopathic units and appointing more homeopathic doctors. The government also needs to create policies to provide adequate homeopathic services. As homeopathy is a cost-effective therapy, a larger homeopathic infrastructure will ensure the optimal usage of the national health budget. The abundant potential existing in the homeopathic private sector also needs to be tapped through the PPP model to further bring down the cost of homeopathic treatment and to increase the outreach of homeopathy to the population of Delhi.

Bibliography

Internet Links

http://www.delhihomeoboard.com (last accessed on May 15, 2013)
http://delhi.gov.in (last accessed on May 15, 2013)
http://www.delhihomeo.com (last accessed on May 15, 2013)
http://delhi.gov.in/wps/wcm/connect/bd5a8c80405403b0ababaf34262e20fd/State%20PIP %202009–10.pdf?MOD=AJPERES (last accessed on May 15, 2013)
http://delhiplanning.nic.in/write-up/2002–03/volume-ii/medical.pdf (last accessed on May 15, 2013)
http://www.livemint.com/2012/08/06222127/Ministry-opposes-plan-to-overh.html?h=B (last accessed on May 15, 2013)

Literature

Directorate of Economics & Statistics, Government of Delhi: Delhi Statistical Handbook 2011. Delhi 2011.

Manchanda, Raj Kumar; Kulashreshtha, Mukul: Cost Effectiveness and Efficacy of Homeopathy in Primary Health Care Units of Government of Delhi – A study. Paper presented at 60th International Homeopathic Congress organized by LIGA at Berlin, Germany, 2005, URL: http://www.delhihomeo.com/paperberlin.html (last accessed on May 15, 2013).

Priya, Ritu; Shweta, A. S.: Status and Role of AYUSH & Local Health Traditions under the National Rural Health Mission. New Delhi 2010, URL: http://nhsrcindia.org/pdf_files/ resources_thematic/Public_Health_Planning/NHSRC_Contribution/Status%20and%20 Role%20of%20AYUSH%20_451.pdf (last accessed on May 15, 2013).

Rea, J. N.; Newhouse, M. L.; Halil, T.: Skin disease in Lambeth: a community study of prevalence and use of medical care. In: British Journal of Preventive & Social Medicine 30 (1976), pp. 107–114.

Singh, Padam; Yadav, R. J.; Pandey, Arvind: Utilization of indigenous systems of medicine & homeopathy in India. In: Indian Journal of Medical Research 122 (August 2005), pp. 137–142.

Thappa, Devinder Mohan: Common skin problems in children. In: Indian Journal of Pediatrics 69 (2002), no. 8, pp. 701–706.

Venkat Raman, A.; Manchanda, Raj Kumar: Public-private partnerships in the provision of homeopathic services in the city of Delhi. In: India International Journal of High Dilution Research 10 (2011), no. 37, pp. 353–361.

Nosopolitics.
Epistemic Mangling and the Creolization of Contemporary Ayurveda[1]

Harish Naraindas

The Therapeutic Landscape in India

If one were ambitious enough to produce a mere list of therapeutic possibilities in South Asia, or in any part of the world, and especially Germany, one would soon give it up as a hopeless task. But I shall nevertheless attempt it by saying that unlike anywhere else in the world, perhaps with Germany as a part exception, India possibly represents one extreme and exemplary variant of a nation-state that formally recognises a number of therapeutic "systems". By formal recognition it is meant that one is legally allowed to practise these systems, which is made possible by legally granted degrees with full courses of studies and training. Moreover, all these systems are actively promoted by the state, in so far as the state health system has departments and dispensaries of all these systems to varying degrees, marked by severe asymmetries and regional variations. Interestingly enough, many of these systems are not native to what is now called India. Apart from the most obvious case of biomedicine, or to use the more familiar term "allopathy", whose origin is quite clear from epithets such as "English medicine", "English *marundu*" in Tamil, or *angrezi davā* in Hindi/Urdu, and which is now almost universal as "state medicine" the world over, the Indian state also formally recognises Homeopathy and Naturopathy. Both these medical systems have German roots, although "modern Naturopathy", depending on how one writes its history, is seen to begin around 1826 with Priessnitz in Silesia (now largely in Poland and the Czech Republic).

The Department of AYUSH in India, which is under the Ministry of Health, is an acronym that stands for Ayurveda, Yoga & Naturopathy, Unani, Siddha, and Homeopathy. If we add allopathy to this pentad, we get Sanskrit, Sanskrit and German, Arabic/Persian, Tamil, German and English as nominal root languages for these systems, a claim that I am aware is contentious.[2] Of

---

1 It is imperative that the reader reads all the appended notes diligently. They are an intrinsic part of the essay and the argument is unlikely to make sense without them.

2 There are Unani texts in Tamil (apart from several other languages), Ayurvedic texts in Persian, Arabic or Urdu, etc. Contemporary linguistic politics, as a sub-species of postcolonial nationalism and sub-nationalism has, to merely illustrate, identified Unani with Persian/Arabic/Urdu/Muslim; Ayurveda with Sanskrit/Hindu/Brahmin; and Siddha with Tamil/Hindu/non-Brahmin. This not only provides grist to the mill for contemporary electoral politics, but is also symptomatic of how scholarship is practised by Indians in India: where there is an Ancient India where the sources are largely seen to be in Sanskrit and is hence practised by (Brahmin?) Hindus; Medieval India, which is primarily seen as being Persian and Muslim, and practised largely by (Ashrafi?) Muslims; and

these six systems, the German ones (not that allopathy is any less German) did not come piggyback on the colonial state. Homeopathy purportedly arrived in 1835 in Maharaja Ranjit Singh's court;[3] and Naturopathy, or hydrotherapy as it was called in the nineteenth century, or what the Germans popularly call "Kneippkur", may have at least two lineages. One of them is the prestigious lineage of Mahatma Gandhi, whose first public performance with Naturopathy/hydrotherapy appears to have been during a plague outbreak in South Africa, where two of the three patients with pneumonic plague who volunteered to try his treatment survived, while the remaining 21 who did not volunteer died.[4] But this was not the way many students, who were doing a formal five-and-a-half year course in what is now called a Bachelor's degree in Yoga & Naturopathy (BYNS) in South India, saw their own history. The first batch of students from Udupi that I spoke to in the mid-1990s were certainly not aware that Gandhi was part of their lineage, and most of them were not only not aware of Naturopathy's German roots (unlike homeopathy), but insisted that this system was a wholly Indian invention and all the remedies could be found in some canonical Indian text or other. Instead of seeing Vincenz Priessnitz, or Gräfenberg (now *Lázně Jeseník*), as either a Guru or *prārambha-sthāna* (place of origin), most of these students traced Naturopathy

modern India with its "colonial archive", which to caricature further, is (largely?) practised by Bengalis – the Bhadralok of Brahmins, *Vaidyas* and *Kayasthas* to be more precise – who may be seen, and often see themselves, as the first citizens of the new language of rule, namely English. Then there are "regional histories" (which largely means South India) practised by "regional scholars". In the rare instance a Hindu writes the history of medieval (North) India, the language of choice for training to look at the sources would still be Persian/Urdu, as Medieval India and Persian (or Early Modern and Mughal) have by convention become coeval. Since university careers have to be made, it might not pay in the long run to learn Avadhī (there might not be anyone to teach it; one confines oneself to a smaller region rather than a large swath of territory and time, etc.). I say this, and more below, to indicate that university disciplines and their conceptual underpinnings are not merely not exempt from the populism they often decry, but are deeply implicated in creating the very categories that are mobilised by politics. In the same vein, this article attempts to demonstrate a similar argument with respect to "medical disciplines", their curricula, and the effect of these curricula on clinical practice, especially insofar as prescribing practices go. I attempt to address, in a forthcoming article, called "From shastric yogams to poly herbals", the effect of disciplines and curricula on pharmaceutical practices. This is a companion piece that attempts to see what underpins "pharmacy in the clinic", and what is mobilised (or not mobilised) by practitioners when they diagnose and prescribe.

3   Kumar (1998).

4   Albert West, Gandhi's collaborator in South Africa, who because of the plague outbreak took over the *Indian Opinion* at Gandhi's request and ran it for 14 years, writes of the outbreak of plague in March 1904 in the *Indian Location* of Johannesburg: "Instructions were issued that frequent doses of brandy had to be given to the patients. Gandhi had no faith in this. With the permission of Dr. Godfrey he put three patients, who were prepared to do without brandy, under earth treatment, applying wet-earth poultices to their heads and chests. Two of these were saved. The other twenty-one died." West (2013), URL: http://www.mkgandhi-sarvodaya.org/articles/earlydays.htm (last accessed on May 15, 2013). For more on this aspect of Gandhi see Alter (2000).

to the *Caraka Saṃhitā*, which is now one of the three canonical texts of contemporary Ayurveda. While I could not clearly determine if this was partly or wholly due to the way Naturopathy's lineage was constructed for them in the classroom, what it did indicate was that it was possible for them, their teachers and their textbooks to construct this lineage in a way that did not merely conceal their German roots, but allowed them to either replace these roots or trace them it further back to ancient Indian roots.[5] This construction of an alternative genealogy is possible only because there exists, or more precisely there has come to exist, an alternative canon.[6] This may not be possible in Europe, or at least not legally.

If one walks into Middlesex University[7], for example, and examines their curriculum for a BSc degree in Herbal Medicine, which also began in the 1990s, one will find that the curriculum is broadly divided into two cognitive universes: a therapeutic universe that is "Herbal" and, for the lack of a better word and because I do not wish to prejudge the issue, a non-herbal world of what in the syllabus is called "Herbal sciences," and thereafter simply "Clinical sciences" and "Diagnostic skills." None of these terms draw upon any kind of alternative canon to either understand or elucidate an alternative anatomy, physiology, or most importantly an alternative nosology. To put this shortly at the expense of some simplification, what is called Complementary and Alternative Medicine (CAM) in Europe does not seem to possess, *in toto*, an alternative science of "anatomy," "physiology," or any of the "sciences" that underlie or inform the herbal therapeutics, except the "herbal" pharmacopeia, which is also sometimes called Galenic. They certainly seem to have no alternative

---

5 For a similar Indian "scholarly" rendering that fully acknowledges the "modern founding" of the water cure by Priessnitz and at the same time says that all the principles were known before in India and among the Greeks and the Romans, see S. N. Pandey, who offers his own interesting "history" of naturopathy, and locates both Caraka and Priessnitz in it: http://www.drsnpandey.com/Origin%20of%20naturopathy.html (last accessed on May 15, 2013) (same remark about citing as in previous note).

6 A canon that was first shaped, or started to take shape, in the early twentieth century and one that has continued to "evolve" ever since and whose comprehensive history is yet to be written.

7 I discovered this when I was invited by the very first graduating class of Middlesex University to deliver a lecture organised by their "Herb Society." At that time, I was also doing fieldwork at the College of Naturopathy and Osteopathy in Hampstead, whose syllabus was similar in structure to the syllabus for Herbal Medicine at Middlesex University. But Naturopathy at that particular historical juncture, at least in Hampstead, seemed to be piggybacking on Osteopathy, which was far more established at that moment and had received a Royal Charter in 1993. This is to indicate that curricula are often the product of several "regimes": there is nothing intrinsic about their form and neither are they necessarily a simple reflection of a "system" bounded by either a body of theory or a therapeutic modality. They are best seen as historically contingent rhetorical frames that make claims on the world (Burke (1969)) through an act of framing in both senses of the term. But once these frames are stabilised they may endure for surprisingly long periods. For an extended demonstration of such an enduring frame, where the discipline called Tropical Medicine is brought into being in the late nineteenth century through rhetorical claims, and survives splendidly until today, see Naraindas (1996).

nosology either. Even if they do (which is unlikely, as no other nosology is available as a possible *lingua franca* to either practitioners or patients), they are invariably led to use a biomedical nosology, at least for legal and conventional reasons. Similarly, their concepts of "the body" and its workings, or the dynamics of drug action, or the aetiology of diseases, are all informed by biomedicine and conventional science in rather important ways.[8] While it would be interesting to see how this conventional science is inflected and possibly transformed and negated, if at all, in both herbal pedagogy and herbal practice (diagnostic and therapeutic), the fact remains that they have to formally contend with it and partly, I suspect, for legal reasons.[9]

This is not nominally the case in India, where Ayurveda, Unani and Siddha provide pedagogues and practitioners with another possible canon: a

8   Here is a description of three of their modules from their website: http://www.mdx.ac.
     uk/courses/undergraduate/complementary_health/herbal_medicine_bsc.aspx (last ac-
     cessed on May 15, 2013):
     "-   Herbal Sciences (30 Credits) – Compulsory
     This module provides an introduction to the study of herbal medicine through considera-
     tion of a number of aspects of herbs as medicines. Students will encounter plants in the-
     ory and in practice from the microscopic to the whole plant level. Overall this module
     aims to deliver the basic knowledge needed for the understanding of plant biology and
     chemistry and includes elements of phytochemistry, botany, horticulture, biodiversity as
     well as, regulation of plant medicines and introductory Materia Medica. These aspects of
     herbal sciences will be the foundation of training as a professional in herbal medicine.
     Human Sciences (30 Credits) – Compulsory
     This module aims to provide students with the knowledge and understanding of human
     anatomy and physiology required to underpin their future learning. The unifying theme
     of homeostasis is used to show how a healthy structure and function are maintained and
     how failures of homeostasis can result in disease.
     [...]
     Clinical Sciences (30 Credits) – Compulsory
     A thorough knowledge and understanding of the normal and abnormal structure and
     functions of the tissues, organs and systems of body and the general principles of ortho-
     dox medical treatment are essential for safe and effective complementary medicine prac-
     tice. This module offers students an opportunity to study the causes, mechanisms and
     general pathological changes underpinning disease and to integrate this knowledge with
     that of normal form and function learnt in the study of human sciences. Also included is
     an overview of the general mechanisms of drug action, drug categories and principles of
     infection control that need to be taken into account by the CAM practitioner. This mod-
     ule emphasises causes and mechanisms of systemic diseases and the pharmacological
     basis of management, rather than the details of clinical presentation and diagnosis, both
     of which are comprehensively covered in the Diagnostic Skills module."
9   A good example is the anthroposophist, who "builds on" a biomedical anatomy and
     comes up with other kinds of "bodies." He or she may certainly inflect and transform its
     nosology to offer other therapeutic possibilities. For an example, see Spiegel/Sponheuer
     (2011). But anthroposophists do not fully negate the biomedical canon and appear to be
     anthroposophists along with (and after) becoming allopaths. This is also the case with
     homeopathy in Germany, unlike in India, where one could become a homeopath, quite
     like an Ayurvedic, Unani, or Siddha doctor, without first becoming an allopath. It is for
     this reason one is awarded, I suspect, a BSc (and I presume an MSc after that) and not an
     MD in Herbal Medicine in the UK.

canon that, quite like the ancient Greek and Roman medicine, does indeed marshal water and the "natural elements" as therapeutic resources. It is this that probably allowed the students, and possibly their teachers and textbooks, to construct a genealogy for Naturopathy, for better or for worse, which is Indian (and specifically Ayurvedic) rather than German. Given this possibility for an "imported" system, one could easily be led to imagine that as far as Ayurveda, Unani and Siddha are concerned, teachers, students and practitioners would subscribe, if one takes Ayurveda as an example, to a wholly Ayurvedic aetiology, nosology, etc. But it transpires they do not, even when, unlike in the European world, such a nosology and aetiology are clearly and self-evidently available to them. I will not here go into why this is the case as I have done so elsewhere[10], except to state that all the Indian systems of medicine, much like CAM in Europe (with the BSc in Herbal Medicine that I have alluded to above as a good example), when they are taught in a formal university setting, invariably socialise students also into a biomedical nosology, anatomy, physiology, and so forth, apart from what passes for Ayurvedic "equivalents" of these disciplines. This results in the students, and future practitioners, having to straddle at least two different cognitive universes, which is reflected not only in their examinations, but also in their future clinical practice.

The formal proof of this comes from the fact that the degree that is awarded, namely BAMS, is often interpreted as meaning a bachelor's degree in Ayurveda, which is seen as a category *sui generis,* and which is what the A in BAMS stands for, with the M and S in the degree standing for medicine and surgery, that is medicine as in "universal" biomedicine and "universal" surgery. This acronym came into being in the late 1960s as a result of a bitter political struggle over the curriculum between what may be called "purists" and "integrationists".[11] It was established as a general acronym across India much later, following on from one dominant strand in the continuous framing of the curriculum and its meaning in post-independent India and other parts of South Asia, such as Bangladesh and Sri Lanka where Ayurveda is taught. This dominant strand is what is called "integrated medicine and surgery", where the attempt is to integrate Ayurveda (or Unani or Siddha) with allopathy, or to integrate allopathy into Ayurveda.[12] These acronyms are part of an ongoing dialogue and are best seen as being symptomatic of attempts to make allopathy and Ayurveda cohabit with each other, quite like Herbal Medicine and allopathy at Middlesex, or Osteopathy, Naturopathy and allopathy at Hampstead, or the cohabitation of Yoga, Naturopathy and allopathy in India, with allopathy being a given. This clearly and evidently produces at least two cognitive universes, with allopathy being one of them, which both pedagogues and students are called upon to straddle and negotiate.

This paper deals with one such practitioner who happily straddles these two universes, partly by pedagogic training, partly by conscious choice, and

10   Naraindas (2006; 2014).
11   Brass (1972).
12   Brass (1972).

partly by his employment or contractual obligations. Such practitioners, whom I refer to as "modern doctors of traditional medicine" (hereafter MDTM), are not only ubiquitous, but indicate where Ayurveda (and Unani and Siddha) is possibly headed. They are, in other words, if not the future, then certainly the present reality (of the mid 1990s and I believe even today) for university trained doctors of Ayurveda, Unani and Siddha.

Excising *Bhūta* and rescuing rationality

Before one proceeds through the portals of this practitioner to see what transpires in his clinic when he straddles these two cognitive, epistemic and, as I will presently show, ontological universes, it is important to survey the therapeutic landscape thoroughly to see what has been excluded from the training of this MDTM. In fact, it is through these acts of exclusion and inclusion, and more importantly translation and transmutation, that Ayurveda as a canonical form takes shape in the early twentieth century. This canon, which is not fixed but is constantly shifting, articulates the pedagogy and in turn the clinical practice of practitioners, one of whom we intend to examine. This is not to say that pedagogies give rise to a single style, or that pedagogies may not be repudiated in practice: in fact, we will witness all these possibilities below.

It is clear from a perusal of the curriculum that one of the eight branches of Ayurveda called *bhūtavidyā,* which may be variously (and contentiously) translated as the science (or knowledge) of *bhūta* (literally a "being," ghost, demon, spirit, or as a technical term just "past tense" in Sanskrit grammar) has either fallen by the wayside, and/or is translated sometimes as "infection" and at other times as pertaining to "psychiatry" (*bhūtavidyā*).[13] Both these translations are equally instructive. The first retains the causal arrow pointing from the outside to the inside, in so far as infections are caused by a Being, in this case germs, which as Ludwik Fleck pointed out a long time ago[14], is nothing other than the new avatar of the Devil (a Being, an external agent), or the new appellation for an old figure which provides the modern practitioner with a causal format and the ontological certitude of a Being against which one can

---

13   Frederick Smith, in his magnum opus on possession (2006), to which I will return, calls it aptly enough the "knowledge of non-human entities," and shows how this could range from all those descriptions above to what are now seen to be inanimate entities like the "elements" of earth, water, fire, and so forth, which in Indian philosophy are called the *pañca-mahābhūta-s,* or the five constituent elements (literally the "five great entities"), from which, among other things, the three humours in Ayurveda are constituted. One word that recurs in Smith's opus, as he struggles to come to terms with the phenomenon of "possession," is infestation. In opposition to this notion of possession as an infestation or visitation, a large body of literature emerges, peaking in the 1970s, where possession is recast as a form of ethno-psychiatry. Hence, it is none too surprising that *bhūtavidyā* is recast from the register of infection (a cognate term, as is evident, to infestation (consider helminthology and parasitology) and visitation) to the register of psychiatry.

14   Fleck (1979).

do battle[15]. Its opposite, inaugurated virtually at the same historical moment in European medicine, is what Pasteur called the *terrain*, or in current parlance the "immune system," with endless battles being fought on the pre-eminence of the one or the other, with the most famous being the apocryphal story of Pettenkofer drinking a glass of water loaded with the cholera *vibrio* to prove that it is the *terrain* and not the germ that matters. And the "proof" of Pettenkofer's victory supposedly comes from another apocryphal story, that of Pasteur's moment of epiphany on his death bed, where the last words he supposedly uttered before dying were: "It's the *terrain*, the *terrain!*" The Germ and the Terrain may well be seen as what Canguilhem has called the ontological and the dynamic conceptions of disease in their new form: the two polarities between which contemporary European disease causality, starting with the late nineteenth, and especially from the beginning of the twentieth century, seems to endlessly oscillate, with genetics being arrayed on the side of the *terrain*.[16]

Hence, it is none too surprising that at one historical moment *bhūta* is translated as infection, as it retains in this translation externality, agency and ontology; while the translation of *bhūta*, perhaps at a later historical moment, as pertaining to "psychiatry," completely abolishes ontology in so far as *bhūta* in this latter dispensation becomes a purely intra-psychic phenomenon, supposedly misinterpreted in the past as being caused by external agents.[17] The

---

15 The notion of Being is central, as Foucault (1973) points out, to disease aetiology until the advent of Bichat and the founding of Histology, which is nominally dated in conventional histories to the year 1800. This "birth of clinical medicine," to put it in his terms, is best summed up as a movement from the macabre to the morbid (Foucault (1973)); or, as a movement from an ontology of life to an ontology of death (Jonas (1982)). This is evident from the etymology of the word fever. It comes from the Latin word *februare*, meaning to ritually expel from a house the shades of the dead: Foucault (1973). This is best seen as an expiatory act, purificatory in intention, as fever in this "macabre" world was a sign of a struggle, of an attempt on the part of the body to expel the Being that had "settled down in the organism and laid down local signs": Foucault (1973), p. 183. The advent of pathological anatomy, or histology, attempts to abolish this world and ushers in another world: the world of morbid processes where disease is no longer the sign of a struggle with life taken as a norm (an ontology of life), but as a sign of the advent of death grounded in an ontology of death. The Germ may then be seen as a return of this ontological conception that readily fills the conceptual space vacated by the exit of Being about a hundred years earlier, without of course fully reviving an ontology grounded in life. In the light of this European history, the oscillation of *bhūta* between the poles of infestation or infection and as intra-psychic phenomena may be seen as a replay, albeit with twists, of this history.

16 But see Canguilhem's (1978) prescient disquisition on genetics in his second attempt (1963–66) to grapple with the consequences of the arrival of the twin concepts of the "normal and the pathological" on the European firmament in the mid-nineteenth century.

17 This re-translation is true not only of the word or concept *bhūta*. It is true of virtually the entire Ayurvedic corpus, which in translating Ayurveda into English has often, if not invariably, translated various terms and concepts in the then current "language of science." This "updating" has often meant providing more plausible translations of earlier seemingly implausible ones: the shifting of *bhūta* from the register of infection to psychiatry

latter day translation of *bhūta* as "psychiatry" not only abolishes ontology, but also saves the newly emerging canon, struggling to establish itself as a "science" in the early twentieth century, the embarrassment of attributing aetiology to all those "primitive" things like ghosts, demons, deities and planets, all of which needed to be quickly buried if the new canon was to be taken seriously.[18] The end result of this act of excision, translation and transmutation is that *bhūtavidyā* has never been seriously addressed in pedagogic practice until today and has virtually never been practised in private practice by an MDTM. The newly constituted canon, in an attempt to legitimize itself, made sure that it established itself as a purely material science, with the *materia medica* as its centre, the drug as the new sacrament, and all unseemly Beings like Deities and demons swept into the closet.[19] This resulted not only in relegating

---

may be seen as a symptom of this shift. A study of the successive translation of the *Caraka-Saṃhitā*, in the light of this claim, may warrant a detailed study and I am sure it will make for an interesting history of the "evolution" of Ayurveda in the 20th century. But we should not presume that all these acts of translation, even if they labour under a structural asymmetry, might be captured by a single term. I suspect they will result in forms of mangling whose import, especially in clinical practice, will vary depending on context: whether the practitioner has been formally trained in a university or not, who his patients are, what nosological categories are being addressed, and so forth. Here, we are specifically dealing with what I have christened as an MDTM, formally trained in a "modern" institution, which is increasingly, if not already fully, the norm.

18   The earlier translation of *bhūta* as infection serves the same purpose. For a similar event in China, where *xie*, a rough equivalent of *bhūta*, linked as it was to demonic possession (and to the "invading" by "natural substances" like the "damp wind"), has been abolished for roughly the same reasons, see Lo/Schroer (2005). This play and distinction between the naturalistic and the theurgic, which then spawns several other binaries like body and soul or spirit, and mind and body, with which we are saddled, comes from the fact that we live in a post-sacramental world (Naraindas: Korallen (2011)), inaugurated by Zwingli (Uberoi (1978)), after which it is difficult for us, in our "official" dealings as members of the university, to countenance the possibility of theurgies, that is, "the working of a divine or supernatural agency in human affairs." But as I have tried to show elsewhere, this continues to happen in our "non-official" life, albeit minted in the idiom of the present, leading me to describe it as "techno-sacramentalism": Naraindas: Relics (2011); Naraindas: Korallen (2011).

19   This is a truncated summary of another article that deals with the instauration of 20th century Ayurveda around a professed materialism in India, with the *materia medica* and the written word as its centre, leading ironically enough not only to its spiritualization outside India, but to a valorisation of all that is sought to be excluded in India (regimen/dietetics). Hence, if Ayurveda in India appears largely under a de-spiritualized and fully materialized garb, where the drug rather than the regimen is the new sacrament, in the Euro-American world, it has been, *at least initially*, instituted as an esoteric and spiritualized practice, where diet and regimen are central. The exemplum of this is *Pañcakarma*. Deepak Chopra calls Ayurveda in America "*Pancakarma Ayurveda*", or just PK for short; and in Germany this is the central therapeutic format around which in-patient Ayurveda is practised: Naraindas: Relics (2011). But apart from PK, dietetics and regimen, a number of other practices, like bone setting and *Marma*, were also excluded: Cleetus (2012). Some of these, especially those that are seen as being esoteric like Marma, enjoy popularity outside India with Germany being a good example, where a Marma specialist is "imported" every year for a few months into the Ayurveda Academy at Birstein. For a par-

bhūtavidyā to the periphery, but it resulted in seeing it as a purely "vernacular practice"[20], and was jettisoned by the "upper castes" and the small anglicised minority (often but not always the same group), who in their self-presentation relegated it to the realm of "religion" (respectable and pertaining to themselves and their temples with Sanskrit and vegetarian deities)[21], or superstition and witchcraft (disreputable and coeval with lower castes and carried out in "lower caste" shrines and temples, often with deities that purportedly demand blood sacrifices).[22]

While *bhūtavidyā* represents a clearly "understandable" act of excision and relegation, as its causal premises are intangible entities that are anathema to modern science, what the inclusion of biomedicine does as part of the formal curriculum, even with respect to what may be called "somatic pathology," is

ticularly good overview of these strands in the United States, where Ayurveda is positioned between "medicine and metaphysics," see Reddy (2002; 2004). For its global articulation see the edited collection by Wujastyk/Smith (2008). For India, see Leslie (1976), Leslie/Young (1992) and Langford (2002). For a textual exegesis see Zimmermann (1987); and Zimmermann (1992) for the "greening" of Ayurveda in the West. For a recent account that attempts to situate Ayurveda vis-à-vis biomedicine and religious healing in Kerala, see Halliburton (2009).

20 See Frederick Smith's "The Self Possessed" (2006), the first large and sustained attempt to question its presumed vernacular label by showing that it is squarely part of what in the anthropological/Indological literature is called the Textual, Sanskritic, Brahminic corpus, starting with the "Rig Veda" and practised today in Kerala as a therapeutic form by Nambudiri Brahmins, with the *Poonkudil Mana* being an extant example. Sax/Bhaskar's (2014) article on this practice at Poonkudil, currently under review, is due next year. Smith also gives the lie to this popular self-image by drawing our attention to contemporary ethnographies of possession among a range of castes, including *smārta* Brahmins in South India.

21 This notion of Sanskrit and vegetarian deities is rendered problematic if "Hindu" India is seen from a particular kind of "periphery". I have now realized, having been brought up in South India, that being Brahmin and vegetarian is an illusion if one considers Assam, Bengal, Bihar, Kashmir, Orissa and Uttrakhand. In fact, in that entire contiguous region running from Orissa all the way via Assam and Bihar to Kashmir (except Uttar Pradesh) most Brahmins are meat and/or fish eaters. Despite this, the tacit presumption is that India is largely vegetarian (a entrenched European notion) and that all Brahmins are ipso facto vegetarians. Anthropological theories on caste are fundamentally premised on this Brahmin vegetarian myth that may not hold true for the majority of Brahmins.

22 This statement is, in many ways, wholly untrue, as there have been, and continue to be, several mass movements, sometimes connected to political parties, that have led the tirade against these practices. The most prominent among them is the rationalist movement in South India in the 1920s that led to a concerted political mass movement against all religious practices, especially the practices of Brahmins inside temples, and not merely "lower-caste possession practices." This was the case as this movement was explicitly anti-Brahmin, apart from being anti-British and anti-Bania. Its current avatar in Tamil-Nadu is the DK (Dravida Kazhagam or Dravida Party), which continues to lead this tirade against what are now perceived as lower-caste superstitions, one of them being "possession". The DK's doings are occasionally featured on BBC (2010) in their travel section, which showcases this aspect of India with a portly Englishman in a flowery shirt, straw hat and garland around his neck, providing the "ethnographic" voice-over of Tamil rationalists opposing Tamil superstition. For a fuller account of Indian Rationalism and the rationalists and how they are part of rationalism worldwide, see Quack (2012).

to transform the nature of diagnosis, prognosis and therapeutics in interesting ways. If the excision of *bhūta* results in the excising of a whole branch of medicine and its attendant nosology, similarly, the inclusion, and often a wholesale inclusion of biomedicine, leads to re-articulating the pedagogic, clinical and pharmaceutical practice[23], along with what is called "Ayurvedic research." With this as a truncated backdrop to a much larger therapeutic landscape, made up of inclusions and exclusions that I do not have the space to delineate, we will now look at the practice of a contemporary MDTM called Rishi (pseudonym), practising in Bangalore in the mid 1990s, to see what precisely transpires in the clinic when he confronts a patient. While Rishi, whose practice I observed for about 6 months (and followed for several years), will be the central protagonist, I will also briefly allude to two other practitioners (I will call them by the pseudonyms of Ram and Padma), both of whom were his classmates. It was Rishi who sent me to observe both these practitioners to indicate to me where he was situated vis-à-vis both of them, each of whom represented, by his own reckoning, possible ways in which Ayurveda could be practised by physicians in his generation.

I will now enter Rishi's clinic by examining the case of a young female patient who presented herself one morning with the following symptoms.

The logic of the diagnostic and prescriptive practice

A young woman walked in one morning into Rishi's clinic and said that she was itching all over. It had started in her leg a week ago and had spread in a few days to the rest of her body. Three days earlier, this young lady had seen an allopathic doctor who had prescribed a de-worming medicine. It was and continues to be commonplace for most patients to turn up at the door of an Ayurvedic doctor not as their first port of call. I offer below not the questions posed in direct speech, but a conspectus of what may be called a clinical history taking by the Ayurvedic physician. I further present the "reasoning" behind these questions which were revealed to me immediately after the consultation when I asked him to explicitly explain to me why he had asked what he had asked and what reasoning informed the history taking, diagnosis and prescription. I have put this in tabular form for reasons of convenience.

Questions posed by the doctor	Reasons for doing so
Travel history: none	Food or water infection?
Bowel habits: constipated	Constipation/worms?
Joint pain: none	Thyroid problem/Arthritis?
Urinary tract burning: none	Urinary Tract Infection?

23   For the pharmaceutical side of this story that deals with transformations wrought due to manufacturing processes see Banerjee (2009); for transformations due to its marketing, see Bode (2008).

Gynaecological history: normal   Thyroid?
Weight gain or loss: none   Thyroid?
Mental state: normal   Thyroid?
Night sweats / hot flushes: none   Thyroid?
Appetite: very poor
Caterpillar contact? No

Diagnosis: ĀMA (Undigested residue)

Therapeutic Strategy
Drugs for setting right the above, that is, the *Āma*.
"Blood purifier" to stop the itching.
Purgatives for setting right the bowel habits.

Internal oral administration
Kriminishodini tablet: Purgative + deworming
Churnas (powders): *Nimba* (neem): blood purifier + *Harītakī*: mild purgative: *Bhūmyāmalakī*.
Liver stimulant + *Mustafa*: Blood purifier + 1/2 a tablet of *Pandhara Rasayana*: Blood purifier and *rasayana* (roughly translated as rejuvenator).

External application
Bathing powder of *Basin* (green gram) + *Methi*: good for *rakta* (blood) and *kapha*
What are we to make of this encounter? Are we witnessing an allopathic or an Ayurvedic encounter, or perhaps both or neither? It is evident from the questions posed that the practitioner is primarily ruling out the patient being infested with worms, infection, problems associated with a malfunctioning of the thyroid, urinary tract infection, and caterpillar contact. After ruling out these out possibilities, Rishi arrives at an Ayurvedic diagnosis called Āma, which is translated here as "undigested matter" (this should be seen as a technical term)[24], based on the presenting symptoms along with answers given to questions on the patient's bowel habits and her appetite.

---

24   Here is an example of one of several "translations" of what *Āma* may mean: "Each lunar cycle between menarche and menopause, the proliferation of epithelial cells lining the breast's lobular acini (increasing from one to two layers) occurs during the luteal phase. The breast epithelium, unlike the endometrium of the uterus, cannot be shed at the end of the cycle; regression at the end of the cycle is by apoptosis (self-programmed cell death). **The apoptotic residue (ama)** (emphasis added) is plentiful within the lumens toward the late luteal phase of the cycle. Efficient removal of this material is essential for the breast tissue to remain healthy and vital". Scott Gerson, "The Ayurvedic Approach to Breast Health", http://EzineArticles.com/6789166 (last accessed on May 15, 2013). This is an attempt to "explain" how breast cancer (here called *sannipatika gulma* or malignant tumour, a correlation that is moot) supposedly occurs from an Ayurvedic point of view: a point of view that appears to make āma a "natural" part of on ongoing cycle. This one is particularly interesting and exhaustive, offering the contemporary reader, socialized into "universal school science," an Ayurvedic pathogenesis of breast cancer and the ther-

Rishi, interestingly enough, continues with the therapy prescribed by the allopathic doctor, namely a de-worming tablet, but replaces the allopathic medicine with an Ayurvedic one whose scope is "wider" as it comes with a purgative. He then administers a blood purifier and purgative, a liver stimulant and another blood purifier that doubles up as a *rasāyana* (restorative, rejuvenator)[25], and finally gives an external powder of green gram and fenugreek. These external applications are also blood purifiers and very common in India as stock household remedies which are increasingly falling into disuse. When asked about the choice of these drugs, the Ayurvedic physician said that he had read a research paper that had claimed *Nimba* (neem, or

apeutic protocol to <u>prevent</u> breast cancer (not <u>treat it</u>), where *āma* plays a central role and appears to be the lynchpin around which the narrative is mobilized. I am not aware of any websites, books, articles, and so on, that ever explicitly set out to address and explain how *sānnipātika-gulma* comes about from a biomedical point of view. But a careful reading of the translation above seems to do exactly that: in the process of setting out to explain how breast cancer develops from the Ayurvedic point of view, the author is led to explain *sānnipātika-gulma* from a biomedical point of view, although that is not the express intention. Neither do we know if the unintended import of this explanation is the same, nor whether *sānnipātika-gulma* and malignant tumours are identical. In any case, the intention here is to tell an audience that "knows" the disease called cancer, which as a conceptual category remains undisputed, to explain this nosological category differently. Similarly, what one will find are explanations of how Ayurvedic or TCM drugs, or rarely entire therapeutic protocols, "actually work", namely from a biomedical point of view. This is especially so for acupuncture, and is de rigueur if it is to be paid for by health insurance in Europe. In this very article, one of the Ayurvedic medicines is mentioned as something that addresses cancer and as the author states: "the methanolic leaf extract of Aśvagandhā leaf (*Withania somnifera*) was demonstrated to restore normal p53 function in tumor cells bearing mutated copies". In other words, the addressee is always a biomedical nosological category, a biomedical pharmacological action, or a biomedical physiological or neurological description. Another way of translating this, one that patients have alluded to as part of my fieldwork in Germany, is to translate not *āma* per se, but the process of getting rid of the āma as *entschlacken*. This notion of *entschlacken*, meaning to purge or purify, is an old term that harkens back to Galenic medicine and whose contemporary English rendering, which Germans use too, is "detox". In our conversations, some of the patients suggested that ama may be described as *Schlacken*, which is translated as slag in the context of mining, and at the other extreme as waste products. They said that this was how āma was often translated in their Ayurveda cooking course. Thus, while Schlacken is not an easily and readily used term, entschlacken certainly is. The other possible pair, found in the information brochure of my *Kur* clinic, is the term "Ablagerungen" for *āma*, and the term "ausgeleitet" instead of *entschlacken*. It is thus evident that in the European context Ayurveda is often made sense of by templates other than the Anglo-American variant of biomedicine: Naraindas: Relics (2011). This seems to be particularly true in the German context, where the notion of the Kur (poorly translated as spa), with its variety of *entschlacken*, provides a ready template for the embedding of Ayurveda, and where the *Kur* is, unlike in the Anglo-American world, on the margins of, but nevertheless part of, biomedicine: Naraindas: Relics (2011).

25 All these are problematic translations to say the least. All Ayurvedic terms may require, like *āma* above, a sustained attempt at translation which may well "fail," but which happen all the time in pedagogic, clinical and pharmaceutical practice, apart from research, quite as it does in this paper.

Azadirachta indica) in combination with *Bhūmyāmalakī* was good for treating auto-immune disorders affecting the skin. What are we to make of this diagnosis and prescription? What precisely is the practitioner seeking to accomplish through the prescription that he writes for the young lady? As is evident, I am here not concerned with what *she* makes of the prescription, but I am primarily concerned with the practitioner and the reasons for his actions.

Nosopolitics: Mangling and the production of a Creole?

There are two broad ways in which one can proceed with treatment in Ayurveda. The first, which is quotidian, is called *śamana-cikitsā* (pacifying treatment) and the second is called *śamana-cikitsā* (eliminating or eliminative treatment). The first is usually done with drugs and a regimen that centrally considers diet and other habits or bodily dispositions, such as sleep and physical or mental activity, all of which are seen to have a bearing on the disease. This is not to be understood as a pious or moral homily, but as directly causing the disease and hence directly responsible for turning it around. The second, *śamana-cikitsā*, may also be done with drugs, but the protocol is different from the first. But *śamana-cikitsā* is increasingly done via the long drawn-out, time-consuming and often expensive procedure called *pañcakarma* which consists of emetics, enemas, purgatives, bloodletting and nasal errhines. These are preceded by the *pūrvakarma-s* (preparatory actions/procedures) of oleation (popularly known as oil massage) and sudation, which is done by fomenting the oleated body with warm herbal poultices. This is followed by either simply sitting in the sun, sweating in a special sauna (where the patient's head is kept uncovered and cool) and/or with the help of a hot shower.

The *pūrvakrama-s* are themselves preceded, ideally, by *pācana* or the cooking of the undigested residue (*āma*). This *pācana* may take from several days to several weeks and may be something as seemingly simple as consuming a hot infusion of ginger, or even plain hot water, which has the properties of *dīpana* (stoking the *agni* or digestive fire) and *āma-pācana* (or cooking the undigested residue). These *pūrvakarmas* are then followed by the *pañcakarmas* which then are ideally followed by the *paścāt-karma-s* of *saṃsarjana*, *śamana* and *rasāyana*.[26]

What we are supposedly witnessing here is a *śamana-cikitsā*, because in the case of a *śodhana-cikitsā* done only with drugs the *rasāyana* generally may not be given until the peccant humour has been completely eliminated. This is done by "cooking the disease" until it progresses from one stage to the next and then through this "cooking or ripening" to allow the disease to run its course without reaching its last stages where it spreads throughout the body, often leading to dangerous and untreatable complications. Some diseases may warrant such a procedure, for example a running skin ulcer which, if it is to be

---

26 *Saṃsarjana* may be translated as a "graded administration of diet". It consists of a specially prepared diet designed to re-establish full digestive capacity and prevent the formation of new *āma*.

successfully treated, should initially be made to run even more. This depends on the age, strength and constitution of the patient, among other things, which may determine the doctor's choice of protocol.

In a typical *śamana-cikitsā*, for example of a patient who appears at a doctor's chamber with a bad cold, running nose, and so on, the doctor (especially in Kerala and in some parts of South India) may give the patient (depending on his or her constitution) a medicine called *daśamūla-kaṭutraya-kaṣāyam* (a decoction made of 14 ingredients). This is good for addressing the deranged humour that has caused the cold. Since the humour is not confined to the head and chest, the medicine too will act on the deranged humour throughout the body. Hence, to localize the medicine in the "upper clavicle region," part two of the prescription would be a *vadagam* or an *anupānam*, which is like "tying a knot", so that the effect of the first medicine is localized, preserved and at times even amplified. Since all treatment protocols are exhausting and since even the most pacifying of treatments attempt to eliminate the offending humour, they invariably have purgatives as part of the concoction (or formulation which is a carefully chosen union – yoga – of several drugs that act by a kind of therapeutic logic). These purgatives, in the act of eliminating the humour, exhaust or waste the patient, unless of course the patient is already wasted from a disease, in which case one needs to tread more carefully or reverse the protocol depending on several factors. Therefore, the third part of the prescription is a *rasāyana* or restorative that rebuilds the patient which in the case of a *śamana-cikitsā* can also double up as a medicine that addresses the disease. This seems to be the bare bones of a contemporary Ayurvedic practice, especially of a *paramparic* physician[27] in Kerala and parts of South India. This prescription will be hedged in by a regimen consisting of dietary "restrictions" and other behavioural injunctions like going to sleep early and waking up by sunrise; not consuming cold drinks; ruling out citrus fruits or, more precisely, anything that is sour, including yoghurt; avoiding salads or, more accurately, raw food of any kind; making sure the patient exercises if that seems warranted, and so on. These instructions are based on careful reasoning

---

27   This is roughly how a doctor called Theresa (see Naraindas (2006) practises in Madras. The delineation of this logic was carefully and patiently explained to me by a young BAMS physician, who himself came from a family of physicians. Apart from training with Theresa, he had trained for a while at Vaidyamadam. Vaidyamadam is now one of the few extant forms of Ayurvedic practice in Kerala that is based on family learning (*parampara*), whose current senior physician Narayan Namboodri, is seen by many as the among the last of a breed who were not trained in the university. The young physician (now well established) pointed out to me how in a "traditional practice" each of the 14 would be written out by the vaidya and the patients were expected to either fetch, pick or buy these herbs and prepare the decoction at home. This writing out of the prescription, rather than giving the patients a manufactured preparation in a bottle, as is the case now, allowed them to vary the proportion of the individual ingredients depending, for example, on the constitution of the patient. The seemingly simple act of bottling the drug had robbed them of this possibility.

about each humour and their likely effects, in the context of the patient's constitution (*prakṛti*) and his or her present condition (*vikṛti*).

This choice of drugs, diet, and comportment will depend on the disease and the stage of the disease (there are 6 stages). It will also be based on the affected *dhātu*s (tissues) and *doṣa*s (humours, both of which are problematic translations), the constitution of the patient, his or her strength to bear the treatment, the place of treatment, the place from which the patient hails if he or she is not long domiciled, the season and, if possible, the place from which the drugs are procured.

For this protocol to take effect the first act is of course a correct diagnosis. This is largely done through a detailed patient history and may include, at least in theory, reading the pulse, palpation, examining the tongue, eyes, urine, and so on. But the most important of this, or the most common, is the detailed patient history, revealed through the specific questions by the doctor whose aim is to identify what the problem is through a kind of looping and iterative process. It stands to reason that this "clinical history" is best elucidated according to the genius of the treating system if the doctor is to reach a correct diagnosis.

What we witness in the case above is a mode of questioning which, by the doctor's own admission, gives primacy to biomedical reasoning to rule out a number of conditions, namely a malfunctioning thyroid, urinary tract infection, food or water borne infection, worms, constipation and, finally, possible contact with a caterpillar or insects. While this mode of questioning is commendable, it seems to have little to do with arriving at an Ayurvedic diagnosis, except as a residual category.

Styles and Contexts

Rishi's clinical practice may be best understood as a particular stance or style at a particular historical juncture and in a particular social milieu. This is without claiming that the styles on offer here are either exhaustive, or perhaps even indicative, though I would certainly like to believe that it would be the latter, at least of a particular time and place. I indicated earlier that Rishi had sent me to observe two of his classmates, as part of my brief was to study the relationship between pedagogy and practice.

It appeared to me that Rishi was some kind of a half-way house between both his classmates. Like Ram, he always wore a white coat, carried a stethoscope and had a blood pressure machine. But unlike Ram, he invariably ran his patient through an elaborate (allopathic) clinical examination that seemed to be "straight from the book". When asked why he did so, he said it was very important as he had to carefully rule out a host of important possibilities (according to an allopathic nosology) for which Ayurveda was of no help. He said that Ayurveda, both as theory and as a mode of clinical craft, gave him no sense of the "inside of the body;" and since he was primarily interested in the patient's welfare, he had to go through such a protocol as Ayurveda was simply wrong on many counts if not downright ridiculous in several respects.[28] Finally, and most importantly, again unlike Ram, he only prescribed Ayurvedic medicines.

Ram, on the contrary, did not run his patients through an elaborate clinical examination and, most importantly, prescribed allopathic medicines. All three of them, and several others, including the almost 300 students that I spoke to over the three years during which I returned to observe and follow their practice, agreed that Ram's practice was indeed the norm, unless one was affiliated by some kind of contract or choice to an Ayurvedic drug making company. Ram, it turned out, not only prescribed allopathic medicines almost exclusively, but also seemed to operate largely with what may be called a "5A" repertoire: antibiotics, analgesics, antihistamines, anti-inflammatory and anti-pyretic drugs, with the only Ayurvedic medicines being sundry "Ayurvedic tonics".

It appeared to me that Ram did not find it necessary to run his patients through an elaborate clinical examination (neither did most allopathic doctors) as he referred all "complicated cases" to allopathic "specialists" (Facharzt) or to the allopathic hospital. He practised in a lower middle class neighbourhood, did not advertise himself as an Ayurvedic doctor, had a substantial Muslim clientele and a decent practice. He saw himself as the first port of call for his patients in the area and competed with other allopathic doctors in the same neighbourhood whose clinics looked no different from his. He said that these MBBS doctors (the rough equivalent of an Arzt in Germany) saw him and other BAMS doctors as their competitors, while the allopathic MDs (Facharzt) liked him and his ilk as they referred many of their patients to these specialists.

At the other extreme was another classmate whom Rishi grudgingly respected but disagreed with. She was the poorest of the lot and practised in a very modest clinic. She categorically told me that she only practised Ayurveda and nothing else and proceeded to tell me that she often treated chronic and complicated cases like paraplegia with just an external application of medicated oil, a dietary regimen and exercise, and had made her paraplegic sit up and walk. She was again, by common consent of the students who all

---

28 This is similar to what C. Dwakaranath says to Brass (1972) during his interview. He says that all those things in Ayurveda that do not accord with modern anatomy (for example) have to be either minimally revised or jettisoned, with the example that he offers being the untenable conception of the heart in Ayurveda. Leslie finds this same gentleman to be more traditional than Shiv Sharma (who he evidently disliked) in his 1976 essay on "Syncretism". While this may well be true, it hardly helps and, in retrospect, there is probably little to choose between the two of them as what Dwarakanath proposes to Brass had either already come to pass or has come to pass most categorically in the present. It is almost impossible for a "modern subject" not be saddled with an "anatomical cartography of the body", however inaccurate it may be for a layperson. Please see footnote 50 further down on this cartography as a kind of inescapable basis for the very notion of syncretism that Leslie argues for.

knew her well, part of a small minority. She belonged to an esoteric circle of students built around one of her professors who was the superintendent of the teaching hospital (modelled on an allopathic teaching hospital) where they had all studied: a professor and a circle that most students thought was interesting but quite out of step with the times.

The "times" saw most Ayurvedic doctors practise allopathy like Ram, that is, more or less like the allopathic doctor next door, or be employed in small private allopathic hospitals as night duty doctors at half pay.[29] While these jobs brought more or less money, for many of them this was an embarrassment and clearly indicated the asymmetry between allopathy and Ayurveda. In fact, most had wanted to be allopathic doctors, but had scored marks in a common entrance exam that were not good enough for them to be admitted to an allopathic programme. Hence, they were acutely aware of the pecking order as they were living embodiments of it. For these students, Rishi was a possible future as he seemingly attempted to marry the best of both worlds. In fact, Rishi had a large fan following with many of his classmates and juniors crowding his clinic for advice and tips and often hoping to formally intern with him at little or no pay. Rishi was widely read, charismatic, supremely confident and used allopathy extensively as a diagnostic tool, but prescribed only Ayurvedic medicines. When asked why, he gave several reasons: he was not legally allowed to prescribe allopathic drugs (but most of his fraternity did and, in fact, it was then, and continues to be now, a legally ambiguous issue).[30]

29 Another option for them is to join the government medical service and be posted in far-flung Primary Health Centres (PHCs) of rural India, places that allopathic doctors are reluctant to go to. These examples are indicative of the asymmetry. They should not be read as either being exhaustive or as the only possibilities, although both earlier and current studies (Waxler-Morrison (1988); Nisula (2006)) seem to show that the majority of Ayurvedic doctors are like Ram and largely practise allopathy. Many Ayurvedic doctors, often the children of Ayurvedic family physicians, have a roaring practice, but they often have to "unlearn" what they had learnt in these colleges that they see as a necessary evil as they now need a degree to practise. Some migrate to Tokyo, Heidelberg or Amsterdam to pursue anthropology and practise Ayurveda as well. Others enter the increasingly lucrative and booming Ayurvedic spa industry (this was nascent in the 1990s) where regimen and dietetics, once jettisoned in everyday practice, now comes back as the therapeutic mainstay, especially the procedure called *pañcakarma*. A privileged few become consultants and advisors to the proprietary medicine drug industry and get elected to the Indian National Science Academy, and a handful become, or try to become, Ayurvedic drug making barons.

30 Here is the latest controversy and a verdict on this issue: "CHENNAI: The police cannot interfere with doctors qualified to practise Siddha or Ayurveda or homeopathy or Unani, when they prescribe allopathy treatment, the Madurai Bench of the Madras High Court has ruled again. Reiterating the orders passed last year by a division bench on similar issues, Justice K Chandru said that no proceedings could be initiated against any of those registered practitioners, who were eligible to practise, irrespective of the respective system, also with modern scientific medicine, including surgery, gynaecology, obstetrics, ENT, ophthalmology, etc. The judge was disposing of a batch of writ petitions from TN Siddha Medical Graduates Association, Thamizhaga Homeopathy and Siddha (Ayush) Doctors Association and Rural Medical Private Practitioners Associations and others

Furthermore, it was not necessary. Finally, the therapeutic arsenal of Ayurveda was adequate if rightly and carefully handled, without, of course, pre-
suming that either he, or Ayurveda, could treat all diseases. I followed Rishi's
career intermittently for a decade and saw him rise from a small clinic in a
middle class neighbourhood to a large clinic of a major pharmaceutical company at one of the most prominent crossroads in Bangalore where he was the
contracted resident physician. In such a clinic, or more precisely "pharmacy",
many, if not most patients, come to buy Ayurvedic drugs without consulting a
physician. Most of them, like the pharmaceutical company, were from Kerala,
and knew the company's products through a long process of socialization,
spanning over at least two generations. But they always had the choice to consult an Ayurvedic doctor. When they did so, they did not pay for the consultation, but only for the medicines. Rishi, in his earlier avatar as a private physician, seemed tied to this particular pharmaceutical company, although he did
have other products and did prescribe drugs of other companies. But in the
latter instance, when he was the physician or the company's "resident doctor"
– one of the two best-known Ayurvedic pharmaceutical drug making companies from South India – he was, I suspect, precluded by his contract from
prescribing anything other than what the firm manufactured, which was *śāstric*
preparations[31], unless it was absolutely warranted. It is interesting that he
never adduced this as a possible reason for only prescribing Ayurvedic drugs.
He eventually became the proprietor of his own company that made "proprietary medicines". These medicines were newly formulated and their recipes
were not in the public domain in the traditional pharmacopoeias; hence, they
were different from the *śāstric* medicines (medicines in the public domain endorsed by the Indian State) that Rishi had largely prescribed until then. When
I last met Rishi, he occupied a suite of offices in a multi-storeyed corporate
tower that rose majestically over downtown Bangalore, thus fulfilling both his
own dreams and those of his classmates who had seen him as a role model
and had wanted to emulate him. Nevertheless, he still stayed with Ayurvedic
drugs, but now they were of his own making. In fact, these proprietary medicines were the best embodiment of his earlier clinical practice as they too, like
him, combined Ayurveda and allopathy by making Ayurvedic medicines for
a biomedical nosology. It is as if, as a "proprietary medicine maker", he had
reached the logical and financial culmination of his style of practice.

seeking to restrain the government and the police from taking any action against them
under the Anti-Quackery Act." http://ayurbhishak.wordpress.com/2011/02/12/%E2%
99%A3-indian-medicine-doctors-can-practise-allopathy/ (last accessed on May 15, 2013).

31 *Śāstric* medicines are recipes in the public domain and endorsed by the Indian State
through a formulary drawn from 57 canonical texts that were canonised by a committee
of probably highly erudite physicians. An ethnography of the making of this formulary in
post-independent India will make for a fascinating article, if not a whole monograph. I
deal with the movement from *śāstric* to proprietary medicines in a forthcoming paper.

From Conceptual Bilingualism to Creolisation?

In an earlier article I characterised the MDTMs (I did not use this acronym then) as being privy to a form of "conceptual bilingualism" through their "pedagogic training"[32], and I claimed that this bilingualism was equally true of pharmaceutical practices, "thus dovetailing diagnosis and prescription"[33]. This is eminently possible, especially in the case of the practitioner called Theresa who was the subject of that paper and who attempted to interrogate if not repudiate this bilingualism. In the context of this article, while this bilingualism is nominally present and may well work in some or several instances with the practitioner going back and forth, what we witness is a mangling of registers and, as I will presently argue, a process of Creolization through this mangling. I am, in fact, inclined to now argue that this kind of conceptual bilingualism is quite unlike the case of language use between two languages where one can be fully competent in two languages and switch effortlessly between them without having to translate between them. But in the case of the clinical practice above, it leads Ayurvedic practitioners not merely to switch but to translate between them. Apart from the pedagogic training that leads them to do this, there is the fact that most patients arrive at the door of an Ayurvedic doctor pre-diagnosed and often with a "fat biomedical archive" and want the practitioner to take account of this archive.[34] This imposed translation, which nominally may be repudiated, is in most instances readily resorted to and becomes the basis of a diagnostic and therapeutic path resulting in the kind of mangling that we have witnessed above. As Serres has pointed out[35], acts of translation perforce imply comparison, and through this comparison hitherto disparate things are brought together, resulting in displacement and substitution, leading to loss and gain and, more importantly, transformation and transmutation.

This is doubly evident in Rishi's style of practice where the attempt is to elicit a history followed by a clinical examination that either confirms or rules out an allopathic diagnosis. In the case above, it was the latter. Having done so, Rishi seemingly proceeds to treat according to an Ayurvedic protocol, which too, on close examination, seems to be moot. He replaces the allopathic de-worming tablet with an Ayurvedic one. Since skin conditions are often caused by what in Ayurveda is called "*raktavātam*", namely the vitiation of the blood and *vāta*, several of the drugs are "blood purifiers", which again is a particular kind of translation. But again Rishi's choice of the main *cūrṇa* is based on a research paper that claimed that the two main ingredients were

---

32 Naraindas (2006), p. 2659.
33 Naraindas (2006), p. 2659. Abraham (2009, p 74), Sujatha and Abraham (2009, p. 42) and Lang (2013, p. 35), have evidently found the concept "conceptual bilingualism" useful, as a way of characterising the practices of what I have here called MDTMs, in their respective ethnographic settings.
34 Naraindas (2006), p. 2667.
35 Serres (1982).

good for treating auto-immune disorders of the skin. Research of this kind, often state sponsored in both universities and in specialised institutes, is an instance of using the Ayurvedic pharmacopeia to address a biomedical nosology. This is the stock-in-trade of MD theses, a post-graduate degree in Ayurveda where one specialises in a particular branch of Ayurveda and writes a thesis as part of the training. In most instances the Ayurvedic pharmacopeia is used like a cookie jar into which one dips to address an allopathic nosology and through a kind of symptomatic correlation one picks candidate drugs to address a disease category or syndrome that is not native to Ayurveda. This kind of "Ayurvedic research," which, according to a class of physicians like Padma, does nothing to advance Ayurveda as a form of diagnosis and prognosis, is now re-imported by Rishi and becomes part of his protocol that seems to simultaneously address a seemingly Ayurvedic diagnosis and a possible allopathic diagnosis, although on the face of it an allopathic diagnosis has been ruled out. In other instances, Rishi functions directly with an allopathic diagnosis and again, through an act of translation based on symptomatic correlation, chooses a set of drugs. In one instance, when Rishi was confronted by a very seriously ill woman with what he called "primary pulmonary hypertension" (which he described as another auto-immune disorder), he teamed up with a veterinary surgeon and carried out a series of "experiments" on rats to test an Ayurvedic drug that he thought might cure the patient.[36]

It is evident from this brief foray that the two systems, Ayurvedic and biomedical, are being mangled rather than the practitioner simply switching back and forth between two conceptual systems, although at first sight that may seem to be the case. But what, if any, is the logic of this mangling? What exactly is being produced in the bargain? Is this a form of Creolization? If Creole is to be defined as a naturalized pidgin, that is, a "simplified"[37] language in one generation that for the next generation is a language or Creole, the question is which is the language that is being simplified and transformed? While I fully realize that I have opened a Pandora's box by introducing the notion of Creolization as there is an enormous body of literature wrestling with this process, the reason for importing it is that it furnishes us with a model of what is called a superstrate language. This is the dominant language, invariably a European language, from which one borrows a lexical part that is then welded to a substrate grammar, usually of an African language. Is this what is happening here: a biomedical lexicon given by a biomedical nosology welded to an Ayurvedic grammar on the basis of which the therapy proceeds? Or do we see the opposite, namely an allopathic grammar, which is encoded by its nosol-

---

36 I accompanied him on two occasions to see how the guinea pigs were doing.

37 As Mol (2002) demonstrates in another context, a context where she compares two treatment modalities within biomedicine, simplifying may not be seen as a mere loss. It is a complex process where some things are lost and other things gained. We can certainly see that in Rishi's moves: certain complexities are lost, certain things are flattened out, but only to be replaced by other forms of complexity brought about by attempting to suture, through translation, the āma and the skin condition to auto-immune disorders.

ogy, leading to the picking of Ayurvedic drugs to address this nosology, lead-ing to the jettisoning of an Ayurvedic grammar consisting of the elaborate therapeutic protocols that we had outlined earlier? In the second instance the Ayurvedic drugs may then be seen as the vocabulary that addresses an allo-pathic grammar and become specifics against disease entities instead of being embedded in a complex protocol that includes a regimen. Or do we see both processes at work? For example, this could be the case when we say, in the case here, that *nimba* in combination with *bhūmyāmalakī* is good for auto-im-mune disorders where these two drugs, which otherwise would be part of a complex therapeutic format (the grammar) based on several things, are re-duced to "specifics" against a particular syndrome, which in turn has been chosen by some kind of correlation of symptoms. The acme of this latter kind of logic is the proprietary medicine. They are "recipes" (combinations accord-ing to a formulary logic or *yogam*) that clearly address a nosology that is not native to Ayurveda. And when these proprietary medicines are sold over the counter (OTCs) in the pharmacies directly to the customer, we reach the logi-cal culmination of this move: the patient's specificity is now replaced by "uni-versal" disease specificity. Here one is simplifying a complex grammar (Ayur-vedic therapeutics) to address a lexicon (disease category) that is from the su-perstrate language, namely biomedicine. In either case, whether we see the biomedical nosological category as a lexical term, or as a term that is an index of a biomedical grammar, the end result seems to be the "simplification" and transformation of the Ayurvedic therapeutic protocol to address a biomedical nosological category.

In the particular instance above, although Rishi seemed to work with an Ayurvedic diagnosis, his protocol did not suggest either "cooking" this undi-gested matter (āma) or addressing it in both the long and short term with things other than drugs. And the "proof of this pudding" was that he virtually never prescribed or addressed the regimen, including diet, seemingly so cardi-nal to Ayurveda, as he thought it was simply a ruse used by physicians to lay an escape route for themselves: "If their treatment doesn't work they can tell the patient that they violated the *pathya* (regimen) and hence the treatment failed. This is ridiculous. The drugs should work, with or without a *pathya*."[38]

38   While this was what Rishi personally felt and used as justification, the actual clinical prac-tice varied from patient to patient. If patients did not raise questions about diet, neither did he; but for others, especially older patients, or for a breed of well-heeled neophytes, for whom the hallmark of a good Ayurvedic consultation was the regimen, Rishi made a concession. He also said that if he laid down a strict regimen as prescribed in the text, most of his patients would "run away" and he would have to close down his practice. A perceived economic necessity is thus welded to a mode of therapeutic reasoning where the "drug is king" and where what we seem to get is a mangling of registers, prompted by several considerations. The most important fact in this was not alluded to: namely, Rishi was a resident physician, during my second stint with him, at an Ayurvedic pharmaceuti-cal company and was more or less duty bound to prescribe their drugs and, more impor-tantly, prescribe drugs. However, I certainly would not want to reduce Rishi's entire stance to this fact, as drugs were and are the mainstay of most clinical practices irrespec-

But here *āma*, while a "technical term" did in part connote "undigested matter" in some literal sense, and this undigested matter needed to be "cooked" and eliminated. This process of "cooking" and especially eliminating, as we have pointed out earlier, is captured rather well by the term *entschlacken*. Thus āma is often the result of the patient's habits which in turn may be an index of his *habitus*. This might include several things, but cardinally diet, comportment, disposition, and so forth. If these remain unaddressed, it would simply prolong the treatment, and even if the treatment were successful, it would presumably land the patient in the same situation. Hence, leaving diet and regimen unaddressed and relying only on the drugs (the "new sacrament") was also cardinally indicative of particular style of therapeutics that seemed to be partially a mimicry of allopathy.

It is thus evident from the above how different registers or languages are being mangled in ways that are not easy to delineate. The notion of Creole furnishes us with a notion of hierarchy or stratification between superstrate and substrate languages. The proof of this hierarchy, apart from the disciplinary exclusions I started the paper with, is that the opposite never seems to occur: the simplification of an allopathic therapeutic grammar to address an Ayurvedic nosology. This is clear since there is apparently only one "universal nosology", the biomedical nosology.[39] Furthermore, even the attempt to treat

tive of whether practitioners were resident doctors of pharmaceutical companies or not, or whether they trained in the university or not. The exception to this is what may be called spa Ayurveda, both in India and abroad, where what is central here is jettisoned there, partly due to regulatory regimes (especially abroad) that may make it difficult to procure and hence prescribe drugs, and partly for other reasons (cf. Naraindas: Relics (2011) for the German case). Finally, the question of diet may appear to be rather different from the patients' point of view. A particular class of patients might "supply" and practise a regimen even if it has not been prescribed, as it might be part of their "home socialization" as opposed to their "school socialization," quite like playing Indian games in one's neighborhood as opposed to cricket and basketball at school. For such patients a statement like "have a light diet" may encapsulate a whole regimen that they may put into play, while for others a diet, even if made imperative, rather than being therapeutically intrinsic may appear as a homily, cf. Naraindas (2006; 2014).

39 In 2011, a move was made to teach a module on Ayurveda as part of the biomedical curriculum in Maharashtra. We will have to wait and see the result. A few years ago, the secretary of a drug-making co-operative, run by Indian medical practitioners in South India, told me how his fraternity had successfully lobbied against a proposal by the Tamil Nadu government to offer an MD (a postgraduate degree in medicine in India) in Ayurveda for MBBS (biomedical) doctors. They had pointed out to the government that the measure being contemplated was appalling: offering MBBS doctors an MD in Ayurveda "when they had no basic training in Ayurveda and did not know the ABC of it." His fraternity petitioned the government to abandon this move, or if it insisted on doing so (under pressure from the allopathic lobby), they told the government that it should also allow BAMS doctors to do an MD in allopathy, and in specialities like cardiovascular surgery or paediatric neurosurgery. He said that the reverse claim settled the issue and the government abandoned the move. He was certain, however, that this was only a temporary reprieve and saw such moves as attempts to expropriate Ayurveda. The 2011 move in Maharashtra seems to bear out his fears. The exception to this seems to be the

the superstrate lexicon, that is, a biomedical disease category, by a complex substrate grammar, or an Ayurvedic therapeutic protocol, while certainly possible is increasingly rare[40], precisely because of the kind of pedagogic training and the therapeutic landscape that I began the article with. Part symptom, if not proof, of this comes from what Rishi seems to be doing, which is a kind of mangling of diagnostic and therapeutic registers that is difficult to pin down. His attempts give the impression he is addressing symptoms rather than underlying processes; and his therapeutic protocol, by relying only on drugs, seems not to address what in Ayurveda is called *nidāna-parivarjanam*, that is, an attempt to address root causes, which may include a faulty diet and a regimen. The attempt to address these root causes is motivated by the fact that if one did not "turn these habits around" then the disease would simply recur in the long run and, in the short run, it would either prolong the treatment or the treatment may well fail.

The closest comparison that one could possibly draw to what Rishi is doing is perhaps the supposed transformation of homeopathy from its so-called "classical form" and the use of a single drug to the use of several homeopathic drugs prescribed simultaneously to address several symptoms, resulting in their mere suppression. I am here paraphrasing a Swiss homeopathic *Heilpraktikerin* whom I interviewed in Kassel in 2011 and who was there for an Ayurvedic *Kur*. Listening to her, one had the impression that homeopathic nosology may be read as a medico-social commentary of allopathy whose epistemic premises and clinical practice, which seemed to be to wage war and suppress symptoms according to her, had resulted in both cancer and a host of chronic conditions that contemporary Europeans suffer from. In other words, current European (and by now global) disorders were the result of allopathic iatrogenesis; and contemporary homeopathy in addressing symptoms rather than "constitutions" had fallen prey to the same logic and had not only joined the allopathic bandwagon, but also now caused its own form of iatrogenesis. While this picture of homeopathy is contentious to say the least – the argument being that the posited "classical" form was a therapeutic strategy meant only for chronic conditions and that Hahnemann himself regularly treated patients symptomatically[41] – what this invoking and supposed simplification

Banaras Hindu University where, for a substantial period of time only MBBS doctors were admitted to an MD Ayurveda, with supposedly some exceptions made for students from the Sanskrit college. This is what Dr. Ananda Samir Chopra (personal communication on September 10, 2012) discovered while there in the 1990s, and tells me that this was a diktat laid down by K. N. Udupa, after whom the famous Udupa commission was set up to enquire into the state of Ayurveda.

40 However, this is possible, and this was what Padma above would do. I have dealt with this possibility in another article based on another physician like Padma in Madras: Naraindas (2006).

41 One of the arguments is that Hahnemann would not have survived financially as a practitioner if he had only resorted to what is now called "classical homeopathy". Martin Dinges informs me that this conception of "classical homeopathy" was invented in the 1960s: "the term 'classical homeopathy' is an invention of the 1960s, referring to the re-

does is signal another therapeutic possibility that distinguishes homeopathy from allopathy and allows, as is the case with the interlocutor above, to practise it, and the rest to jettison it. But the difference is that homeopathy does not operate with an entirely different nosology and, at least in non-chronic conditions, recognises a nosology that it shares with allopathy. While with Ayurveda there is the possibility of another nosology, and even if the diseases are addressed symptomatically, as they sometimes are, they need not have to contend with a nosology that is alien to it and devise a therapeutic protocol to address this alien lexicon.

However, it is evident that this is no longer really possible for what I have called MDTMs. This largely appears to be because of their pedagogic training, unless they make strenuous efforts to swim against the tide, as Padma did. But as it turned out, she belonged to an esoteric circle whose purpose was to partially, if not fully, repudiate the curriculum.[42] For the rest, the easiest way was to altogether jettison Ayurveda, as Ram did, or, like Rishi, to create a Creole under the shadow of another language that seemed to rule the roost, exemplified in various ways, ranging from prestige, salary, profits, government budgets, truth value, cognitive supremacy and the ability to save lives in an "emergency" (this is what Latour would call a network).[43] The proof of this was a one and-a-half year course in what was called "emergency medicine," a perfectly apposite term for allopathy, portrayed as it was in cinema in this particular mode. This course was taught for several years in this college in Bangalore to the students after finishing their BAMS. They eagerly looked

discovery of the high dilutions at the end of the 1940s" (personal communication, June 2012). Cf. Dinges (2007). But he also says that the use of more than a single drug, which my Swiss *Heilpraktiker* sees as the hallmark of "classical" homeopathy, was discussed during Hahnemann's time. Let me quote Dinges here: "The debate around double medication in homeopathy is documented in the correspondence of Hahnemann with Aegidi in: Vigoureux, Ralf: Karl Julius Aegidi. Leben und Werk des homöopathischen Arztes. Heidelberg 2001, p. 83. It was a debate between three physicians, considering themselves as the elite of homeopathy – and then with the colleagues meeting at Hahnemann's birthday. Hahnemann refrained from double medications after protestations of the colleagues that the identity of homeopathy would be endangered and that the adversaries would jubilate [celebrate] if he allows such a modification" (personal communication, June 2012). From this it is evident that certain contemporary renderings of homeopathy's "purity" as being tied to a single drug (or in Dinges's rendering non-"double medication") has historical roots and that Hahnemann's ardent acolytes (quite like the Swiss homeopath I allude to) established it as its distinguishing mark. We may presume from this that this has continued to be a strand of homeopathic thought and practice according to some, while others may have "evidence" to dismiss it.

42 I have elsewhere dealt with another physician called Theresa who, like Padma, although trained as an MDTM, set out to repudiate what her curriculum had imposed on her. This is more easily said than done, as patients, especially middle class patients, are often an enormous impediment and challenge, as they have been socialized through 12 years of schooling and subsequently through the university into a "universal science" and a biomedical nosology and often demand evidence of cure in biomedical terms, cf. Naraindas (2006).

43 Latour (2007).

forward to it, as this was their "finishing school". It "licensed" them and allowed them, by their own admission, to practise allopathy with confidence. During my fieldwork this course had been suspended, supposedly under pressure from the allopathic lobby, and the students were furious about it.[44] In fact, in the state of Karnataka, this course legally allowed them to practise allopathy, as it allowed them to be registered as practitioners of integrated medicine, which was maintained as a separate register.

It is therefore evident that a concatenation of circumstances, all products of a particular kind of history, has a bearing on diagnostic and therapeutic styles. And Rishi's style (and it is possible that Padma and her "circle", despite their best efforts and intentions, may not have succeeded in fully repudiating the curriculum) is clearly a kind of Creolization: a word that I have chosen consciously in opposition to words like domestication, hybridisation, incorporation, and appropriation, or that well-worn term "syncretism"[45] for which South Asia is justly famous. While all these processes may be at work, and in fact from an emic point of view may be a more apt description in certain particular and limited instances, they are unable to capture what appears to be a structural asymmetry. In fact, from an emic point of view, what Rishi is trained to do and is attempting to do is best captured by the seemingly neutral and official term "integration" that I alluded to earlier on when I pointed out what BAMS may be interpreted as. For a period of time prior to the BAMS, the degree awarded to the doctors of Indian systems of medicine was called BIMS (in Karnataka GIMS, Graduate Course in Integrated Medicine and Surgery), or "Bachelor in Integrated Medicine and Surgery".[46] This notion of "integra-

44   This student fury, in the form of repeated and widespread strikes, is what Brass (1972) painstakingly investigates and records in post-independent India up till the 70s, where there is a continuous demand for what he calls a "condensed version" of the MBBS course after graduating from their Ayurveda programme. It is evident that the students, who had not succeeded in this demand for a condensed course when Brass published his essay, eventually managed to have their demand fulfilled, even if temporarily. The fact that the last word on this has not been written is evident from this latest "breaking news": "BANGALORE: If everything goes well, Ayurveda graduates and practitioners will get to study a short term course in allopathy to handle patients in emergency cases. Speaking at a programme organized to release the Rajiv Gandhi University of Health Sciences (RGUHS) Journal of Ayush Sciences on Monday, RGUHS Vice Chancellor Dr S Ramananda Shetty said many Ayurvedic doctors were migrating to allopathy nowadays [...] In this regard, the RGUHS is examining a proposal to introduce a short-term course to handle emergency situations." http://ayurbhishak.wordpress.com/2011/06/28/allopathy-course-for-ayurveda-graduates/ (last accessed on May 15, 2013).

45   Leslie (1976).

46   This statement is also a simplification. There are more than 100 universities offering degrees in the AYUSH disciplines. If one were to examine only the titles of the degrees awarded in each of these universities over the last 100 years, or even post-independence, one will be saddled with a confusing maze of degrees. If one were to examine the curriculum too, it is likely to be even more challenging; and as to how these curriculums were and are translated into living pedagogic practice is anybody's guess. But for a useful look at its origins in the context of early twentieth-century Kerala, where one of the seeds of this "integrated" form is sown, see Cleetus (2012). For a good history of the evolution

tion" was one of the two dominant strands in the debate on how the Indian systems of medicine should be organised and taught in the future.[47] Hence, if Rishi is representative of this trend, Padma may be seen as being representative of the trend that attempts to practise what in the literature has been called *shuddha* (literally clean or pure, or, without being "mixed up" or "mangled" in the context of this paper) Ayurveda. These two trends are clearly visible in the division of the faculty, with one of the professors and his acolytes, one of whom was Padma, representing this point of view. These two strands are part of an ongoing dialogue, whose roots go back to the early twentieth century, and societies of BIMS doctors still exist currently in India as the term continues to enjoy currency worldwide as one "official way" of "integrating" biomedicine and alternative medicine.[48] But this official and consciously articulated term by the Ayurvedic doctors, while it is certainly indicative of a claiming of rights by a subordinated profession[49], a right which argues for allowing them to practise and integrate both Ayurveda and allopathy, as this is what the very acronym BAMS seems to indicate if not promise, it does not preclude us from subjecting the term and its implications to scrutiny. That it has been scrutinised is borne out by all the other terms invoked above: syncretism, domestication, hybridisation, incorporation, and so on, or descriptive ones such as

until about 1970, see the essay by Brass (1972) which quite clearly demonstrates how, for all practical purposes, the integrationists won the day and partly so as the *shuddha* camp, called upon to prepare a pure Ayurveda syllabus, develop cold feet and did a *volte face* by including allopathic content in their "pure" Ayurveda curriculum. Later studies (Waxler-Morrison (1988), Naraindas (2006), Nisula (2006) and Wujastyk/Smith (2008)) bear witness to the preponderance of both allopathy in the curriculum and the fact that the majority largely practise allopathy, thus testifying to the fact that the *shudda* position, though persistent, is a minor trend.

47 Brass (1972); Leslie (1976).

48 Here is one of several such worldwide variants and one that is particularly apt: "Given the present contiguity of Chinese and western medicine, there is a growing need for the two forms of medicine to be integrated as regards both theory and practice. The Graduate Institute of Integrated Medicine was established in 1999 [...] Our goal is to train professionals in the practice, the teaching, and the research of integrated medicine [...] Our institute is the first one of Chinese and western medical integration in Taiwan, therefore, it becomes our responsibility to promote Chinese medicine and integrate *it with western medicine* (emphasis added). It is hoped that in the future *a new form of medicine* (emphasis added) will be created", http://cmucacwa.cmu.edu.tw/introduction.html (last accessed on May 15, 2013). For a cognate analysis of integration in the case of Tibetan medicine, where Vincenne Adams asks whether "integration" mean erasure, see Adams (2002); Adams/Fei-Fei (2008). For other accounts that wrestle with this problem, especially with Chinese medicine, see Jingfeng (1988); Fan/Holliday (2007); Kim (2007); and for Ayurveda, see Sujatha (2011). In other contexts, for example in Australia, integration may mean teaching biomedical doctors a bit of CAM. While what is likely to transpire in the Taiwanese and Australian case is moot, it is evident from the studies alluded to above, that integration will invariably lead to a creolized TCM in Taiwan, while in Australia the premises of biomedicine are unlikely to be creolized by the presence of CAM.

49 There is a whole journal devoted to this endeavour called the *Journal of Ayurveda and Integrative Medicine*.

pluralism and diversity. While these are all useful terms and have analytic power, especially the first set of terms that attempt to describe and analyse what I have here called mangling, they nevertheless seem to rob the process that they attempt to describe of the extenuating circumstances, both historically and in the present, under which the transformation of Ayurveda (or Unani, Siddha, and so on), happened and continues to happen. Equally importantly, they sometimes seem innocent of the fact that this mangling involves excisions and inclusions on the epistemic and ontological registers. In other words, these terms appear to defang what is clearly a form of nosopolitics based on a structural asymmetry.[50] The word creolization, on the contrary, while it can easily subsume these processes within itself, points to the emergence, at least at this historical juncture, of a new lexicon and a therapeutic protocol under conditions of unequal contest marked initially by colonialism, rather than a mere continuation of Ayurveda with twists. A new lexicon that may well grow into a vast lexicon with a complex grammar of its own and one which, being allied with state craft, science and industry, may increasingly police[51], evaluate and regulate all the other subordinated lexicons such as *bhūta*, possession, folk and vernacular practices which have been either ex-

50   One example of this de-fanging is provided by Leslie (1976) in his essay on "Syncretisn" where he provides three case studies: a kind of textual and theoretical act of synthesis by Dwarakanath, who as we have pointed out earlier (see footnote 28 above), irrespective of his erudition and sophistication, was quite clear that all those tenets of Ayurveda that did not accord with some fundamentals of modern anatomy (for example) had to go, quite like the principal protagonist Rishi in our narrative. The third example that Leslie adduces does not count for the argument here as he uses the case of a non-university educated village physician from Nichter's work, where he examines the relationship between Ayurveda and astrology and how they are cognate, similar and part of a network. While this is well taken, it is of no interest to us here, as it does not address the presumed syncretism between allopathy and Ayurveda. The second case study, where he draws on Tabor's work, is based on clinical practice in a hospital setting. It is evident from this example that once again the anatomical atlas, as given by allopathy, and its physiological functions have to be taken account of. There is no way around this. Leslie is able to see this as being syncretic, as he too tacitly, if not explicitly, presumes that there is indeed no way around this. In fact, in his rendering this is the way forward and has presumably always been the case. When one is presented with such a *fait accompli*, this certainly appears to be the case. I suspect that this is the way most people see it. But in the bargain it robs it of its politics, de-fangs it and, most importantly, disallows the possibility of imagining either a situation in reverse ("integrating" allopathy into Ayurveda on terms dictated by Ayurveda, whatever that may mean) or, at the least, imagining other possibilities where allopathic anatomy, physiology and nosology are not the *sine qua non* of a possible dialogue. It is thus evident why the word creolization works better than syncretism (or other terms like hybridisation), as it carries the burden of the asymmetry clearly and unambiguously and it points to the emergence of a new language that is neither the one nor the other, but on terms dictated by the politics of the encounter. Hence nosopolitics.

51   This what Burton Cleetus has to say about one of the professors of Ayurveda in Kerala: "He despised local healers and indigenous medical practitioners as quacks, who were not trained in the academic curriculum imparted through the Ayurveda colleges, and held them responsible for bringing disrespect to Ayurveda. Potty explained at length his role in leading court cases against medical practitioners who held no university certificates

cised from this creolized form and/or now appear as residual categories. The proof, to repeat again, of this act of creolization is that the opposite process, namely, the emergence of a new biomedical language or therapeutic protocol to address an Ayurvedic nosology, never seems to happen. To put this plainly and unambiguously, there are no moves, for example, to devise an antibiotic protocol to treat *āma* or *raktavātam*; no neurosurgery is being concocted to excise *bhūta*: and no MD theses are being written in allopathic institutions, such as the All India Institute of Medical Sciences, to see what candidate drugs from the biomedical pharmacopeia can be used to address, through a correlation of symptoms, *śvāsa-kāsam*. I suspect that no such thesis will be allowed in such an institution.

Is this nosopolitics only true of Ayurveda? This is evidently not the case, as the BSc in herbal medicine at Middlesex University also needs to contend with it. From what we have said above this seems to be the very basis of homeopathy too, at least in certain renderings. Is it possible for the substrate language to completely occlude the superstrate language? Perhaps it is, as this seems to be case with Indian naturopathy shutting out its German roots. Is that because it is a battle between two substrate languages? Perhaps not, if English is treated as a Creole. It may be claimed that it was a language that was abandoned after the Norman Conquest to be spoken only by the hoi polloi who supposedly simplified it and sheared it or, as the English may now argue, transformed it and enriched it. Its subsequent renaissance, probably after the Reformation, meant an enormous borrowing from several other languages, principally "superior" French and German, especially as spoken by the elite, and thereafter from several other languages through its global spread as the language of Empire, making it perhaps a versatile and comprehensive language. Its continuing growth worldwide may well be an instance of world dominance of what became, for an extended period of time, the language of "uneducated people." If this rendering is indeed true, it is also possible that other languages, like the language of Ayurveda, which at a historical juncture are reduced to "inferior languages," are similarly sheared, transformed and creolized in conversation with a superstrate language, which in this case is the language of "science" spoken in an European tongue which in India was and still is principally English. And it is eminently possible that this Creole may rise to be an independent language (as some indeed have and with a flourishing literature) and may well be the language that puts the world into place.[52]

and expressed his delight as a crusader in preserving the scientific character of Ayurveda." Cleetus (2012).

52   For another instance of "putting a world into place", see Withers (1995) who argues for the importance of language, in this case English and Latin, through which the Scottish Highlands are "catalogued" and "put into place" through the tours of the natural historians, whose taxonomies of English/Latin incorporate these remote Scottish regions into the British economic system and thus make them "productive." As Withers points out, the Scottish Highlands in the 18th century were as strange as the Outer Hebrides (or India?). The Great Indian Surveys are part of the same move to produce an atlas of the

Again, as Latour (1993, 2007) would say[53], we need to put the networks that make this possible and sustainable into place for this to happen. And they may well happen. But for the moment, as far as Ayurveda is concerned, we are at a particular historical juncture where this possibility seems unlikely. I have attempted to address this juncture, though the gigantic growth of the Ayurvedic pharmaceutical industry and its creolized Ayurveda[54] may well put a new world into place.

Bibliography

Internet Links

http://www.drsnpandey.com/Origin%20of%20naturopathy.html (last accessed on May 15, 2013)

http://www.mdx.ac.uk/courses/undergraduate/complementary_health/herbal_medicine_bsc.aspx (last accessed on May 15, 2013)

http://EzineArticles.com/6789166 (last accessed on May 15, 2013)

http://cmucacwa.cmu.edu.tw/introduction.html (last accessed on May 15, 2013)

http://ayurbhishak.wordpress.com/2011/02/12/%E2%99%A3-indian-medicine-doctors-can-practise-allopathy/ (last accessed on May 15, 2013)

http://ayurbhishak.wordpress.com/2011/06/28/allopathy-course-for-ayurveda-graduates/ (last accessed on May 15, 2013)

http://ayurbhishak.wordpress.com/2012/05/14/kerala-dc-raids-3-big-ayurveda-cos-for-violating-magic-remedies-act-may-lose-licences/ (last accessed on May 15, 2013)

world and are homologous to the anatomical atlas. These cartographies are now a given. Hence, it is next to impossible to imagine a "normal" body without a heart.

53 Latour (1993; 2007).

54 The fact that this creolized Ayurveda is increasingly the norm is partly borne out by the fact that close to 90 percent of industrially manufactured Ayurvedic products are pharmaceuticals, cf. Bode (2008). An increasing share of these is Ayurvedic neutraceuticals and Ayurvedic cosmoceuticals. This means that *sastric* medicines are by now a small part of the market share. I address their formulary logic in another article and argue that these creolized Ayurvedic "ceuticals" (pharma, cosmo and neutra) are best described as "polyherbals", as they are often of a piece with the global herbal industry *also* in terms of their formulary logic. The easy proofs of this creolized pudding are of course the cosmo and neutraceutical, which, according to the drug controller, are sometimes based on "spurious claims." These have led the drug controllers in Kerala to carry out raids on a number of factories producing these ceuticals and threatening them with closure. The latest of these was in 13 districts of Kerala on 10 April 2012, resulting in the seizing of products worth 5, 211,700 rupees: http://ayurbhishak.wordpress.com/2012/05/14/kerala-dc-raids-3-big-ayurveda-cos-for-violating-magic-remedies-act-may-lose-licences/ (last accessed on May 15, 2013).

Literature

Abraham, Leena: Medicine as Culture: Indigenous Medicine in Cosmopolitan Mumbai. In: Economic and Political Weekly 16, (2009), pp. 68–75.

Adams, Vincanne: Randomised Controlled Crime: Postcolonial Sciences in Alternative Medicine Research. In: Social Studies of Science 32 (2002), pp. 659–690.

Adams, Vincanne; Fei-Fei, Li: Integration or erasure? Modernising medicine at Lhasa's Mentsikhang. In: Pordié, Laurent (ed.): Tibetan medicine in the Contemporary world. Global politics of medical knowledge and practice. London 2008, pp. 105–131.

Alter, Joseph: Gandhi's body: sex, diet, and the politics of nationalism. Philadelphia 2000.

Banerjee, Madhulika: Power, Knowledge, Medicine: Ayurvedic Pharmaceuticals at Home and in the World. Hyderabad et al. 2009.

Bode, Maarten: Taking Traditional Knowledge to the Market: The Modern Image of the Ayurvedic and Unani Industry, 1980–2000. Hyderabad 2008.

Brass, Paul: The politics of Ayurvedic education: A case study of revivalism and modernization in India. In: Rudolph, Susanne Hoeber; Rudolph, Lloyd I. (eds.): Education and politics in India: Studies in organization, society and policy. Cambridge 1972, pp. 342–371.

Burke, Kenneth: A Rhetoric of Motives. Cambridge 1969.

Canguilhem, Georges: On the normal and the pathological. Boston 1978.

Cleetus, Burton: Negotiating western science and the state: The case of indigenous medical revivalism in Kerala. Paper presented at the Pharmasud workshop, Rio de Janeiro, March 2012.

Dinges, Martin: Klassische Homöopathie in Deutschland – Rückblick auf die ersten Jahrzehnte eines langen Weges. In: Zeitschrift für Klassische Homöopathie 51 (2007), Sonderheft, pp. 5–19.

Fan, Ruiping; Holliday, Ian: Which medicine? Whose standard? Critical reflections on medical integration in China. In: Journal of Medical Ethics 33 (2007), pp. 454–461.

Fleck, Ludwik: Genesis and Development of a Scientific Fact. Chicago 1979.

Foucault, Michel: The birth of the clinic. An archaeology of medical perception. London 1973.

Halliburton, Murphy: Mudpacks and Prozac: Experiencing Ayurvedic, Biomedical and Religious Healing. Walnut Creek, California 2009.

Jingfeng, Cai: Integration of traditional Chinese medicine with western medicine – Right or wrong? In: Social Science & Medicine 27 (1988), pp. 521–529.

Jonas, Hans: The phenomenon of life: toward a philosophical biology. Chicago et al. 1982.

Kim, Jongyoung: Alternative medicine's encounter with laboratory science: The scientific construction of Korean medicine in a Global age. In: Social Studies of Science 37 (2007), pp. 855–880.

Kumar, Anil: Medicine and the Raj: British medical policy in India, 1835–1911. Walnut Creek, California 1998.

Lang, Claudia and Eva Jansen: Appropriating Depression: Biomedicalizing Ayurvedic Psychiatry in Kerala, India. In: Medical Anthropology 32 (2013) no. 1, pp. 25–45.

Langford, Jean: Fluent Bodies: Ayurvedic Remedies for Postcolonial Imbalance. Durham, NC 2002.

Latour, Bruno: We have never been modern. Trans. by Catherine Porter. New York 1993.

Latour, Bruno: Reassembling the Social: An Introduction to Actor-Network-Theory. Oxford 2007.

Leslie, Charles: Asian Medical Systems: a Comparative Study. Berkeley 1976.

Leslie, Charles: Interpretations of illness: Syncretism in modern Ayurveda. In: Leslie, Charles; Young, Allan (eds.): Paths to Asian Medical Knowledge. Berkeley 1992, pp. 177–208.

Leslie, Charles; Young, Allan (eds.): Paths to Asian Medical Knowledge. Berkeley 1992.

Lo, Vivienne; Schroer, Sylvia: Deviant Airs in "Traditional" Chinese Medicine. In: Alter, Joseph (ed.): Asian Medicine and Globalization. Philadelphia 2005, pp. 45–67.

Malamoud, Charles: Cooking the World. Ritual and Thought in Ancient India. Translated from the French by David White. Delhi 1996.

Mol, Annmarie: Cutting surgeons and walking patients: Some complexities involved in comparing. In: Mol, Annmarie; Law, John (eds.): Complexities. Social studies of knowledge practices. Durham; London 2002, pp. 191–217.

Naraindas, Harish: Poisons, Putrescence and the Weather: A Genealogy of the Advent of Tropical Medicine. In: Contributions to Indian Sociology 30 (1996), no. 1, pp. 1–35.

Naraindas, Harish: Of Spineless Babies and Folic Acid: Evidence and Efficacy in Biomedicine and Ayurvedic Medicine. In: Social Science & Medicine 62 (2006), no. 11, pp. 2658–2669.

Naraindas, Harish: Korallen, Chipkarten, medizinische Informationen und die Jungfrau Maria: Heilpraktiker in Deutschland und die Aneignung der Ayurveda-Therapie. In: Zeitschrift für Ethnologie 136 (2011), pp. 93–114.

Naraindas, Harish: Of Relics, Body Parts and Laser Beams: The German Heilpraktiker and his Ayurvedic Spa. In: Anthropology and Medicine 18 (2011), no. 1, pp. 67–86.

Naraindas, Harish: My Vaidya and my Gynaecologist: Narrative of a Post-modern Birth. In: Naraindas, Harish; Quack, Johannes; Sax, William (eds.): Asymmetrical Conversations: Contestations, Circumventions and the Blurring of Therapeutic Boundaries (forthcoming, 2013).

Nisula, Tapio: In the presence of biomedicine: Ayurveda, medical integration and health seeking in Mysore, South India. In: Anthropology & Medicine 13 (2006), pp. 207–224.

Quack, Johannes: Disenchanting India: Organized Rationalism and Criticism of Religion in India. Oxford 2012.

Reddy, Sita: Asian Medicine in America: The Ayurvedic Case. In: Annals of the American Academy of Political and Social Science: Global Perspectives on Complementary and Alternative Medicine 583 (September 2002), pp. 97–121.

Reddy, Sita: The Politics and Poetics of "Magazine Medicine": New Age Ayurveda in the Print Media. In: Johnston, Robert (ed.): The Politics of Healing: Histories of Alternative Medicine in Twentieth-Century North America. London 2004, pp. 207–231.

Sax, William; Bhaskar, Hari: A Non-modern Healing Practice in Kerala. In: Naraindas, Harish; Quack, Johannes; Sax, William (eds.): Asymmetrical Conversations: Contestations, Circumventions and the Blurring of Therapeutic Boundaries. New York 2014.

Scheid, Volker: Shaping Chinese medicine: Two case studies from contemporary China. In: Hsu, Elisabeth (ed.): Innovation in Chinese medicine. Cambridge 2001, pp. 370–404.

Serres, Michel: Hermes: Literature, Philosophy and Science. Ed. by Josué V. Harari and David F. Bell. Baltimore 1982.

Smith, Frederick: The Self Possessed: Deity and Spirit Possession in South Asian Literature and Civilization. Columbia 2006.

Spiegel, Andrew; Sponheuer, Silke: Transforming Musical Soul into Bodily Practice. Tone Eurythmy, Anthroposophy and Underlying Structures. In: Fedele, Anna; Blanes, Ruy Llera (eds.): Encounters of Body and Soul in Contemporary Religious Practices. Anthropological Reflections. New York 2011, pp. 179–202.

Sujatha, V.: What could 'integrative' medicine mean? Social science perspectives on contemporary Ayurveda. In: Journal of Ayurveda and Integrative Medicine 2 (2012), pp. 115–123.

Sujatha, V. and Leena Abraham: Medicine state and society. In: Economic and Political Weekly 16), (2009), pp. 35–43

Tabor, Daniel: Ripe and unripe. Concepts of health and sickness. In: Social Science & Medicine 15 (1981), pp. 439–455.

Uberoi, Jitendra Pal Singh: Science and Culture. Delhi 1978.

Waxler-Morrison, Nancy: Plural medicine in Srilanka: Do ayurvedic and western medical practices differ? In: Social Science & Medicine 27 (1988), pp. 531–544.

West, Albert: In The Early Days With Gandhi, URL: http://www.mkgandhi-sarvodaya.org/articles/earlydays.htm (last accessed on May 15, 2013)

Withers, Charles W.J.: Geography, Natural History and the eighteenth century Enlightenment: putting the world in place. In: History Workshop Journal 39 (1995), no. 1, pp. 137–164.

Wujastyk, Dagmar; Smith, Frederick: Modern and Global Ayurveda: Pluralism and Paradigms. Albany 2008.

Zimmermann, Francis: The Jungle and the Aroma of Meats: An Ecological Theme in Hindu Medicine. Berkeley 1987.

Zimmermann, Francis: Gentle Purge: The Flower Power of Ayurveda. In: Leslie, Charles; Young, Allan (eds.): Paths to Asian Medical Knowledge. Berkeley 1992, pp. 209–223.

The Quest for Another Recognition.
Ethnography of an homeopath in Tamil Nadu

Hugues Dusausoit

This paper is based on an ethnographic study which took place in 2005 in the south of India and which was part of a larger research project entitled "Diffusion and adjustment of homeopathic medicine in India: comparative anthropology based on the example of Belgium".[1] In that project, my role was more specifically to focus on the question of why India, more than any other country, is today so receptive to homeopathy.[2] While some answers have already been put forward to this question, it appears that most of them are based on theoretical considerations rather than on actual observations. In contrast to such an approach, I was able to attend for three months the daily consultations of an Indian homeopath who practises in a government hospital and in his own "private clinic". In this paper, I will give an account of my field observations and I will suggest that the reasons for the success of homeopathy in India might not always be found where expected.

India and homeopathy, a spiritual connection?

Carrying out the "ethnography of an homeopath in Tamil Nadu" requires many skills, of which I see at least three: being an ethnologist, knowing homeopathy and speaking Tamil. I have none of these skills, and the few months I worked on this research were undoubtedly not enough for me to acquire them. When the opportunity arose for me to do this ethnographic work, I was finishing my degree in philosophy and, although I had already lived in India, it had not been in Tamil Nadu. Moreover, I knew almost nothing about homeopathy. And yet, in this paper, I claim to have done such ethnographic research. All I can do is warn the reader about its substantial limitations.

---

1   "Diffusion et ajustement de la médecine homéopathique en Inde : anthropologie comparée sur l'exemple de la Belgique". This research was directed by Olivier Schmitz and financed by the "Agence Universitaire de la Francophonie (AUF)". It involved the Catholic University of Louvain-la-Neuve (Centre d'Etudes de l'Inde), the University Jawaharlal Nehru and the French Institute of Pondicherry. Cf. Hoyez/Schmitz (2007). I wish here to warmly thank Robert Deliège and Olivier Schmitz for having introduced me to ethnology, for having put their trust in me and for having always supported me.

2   While Belgium considers homeopathy as a "non-conventional medicine", India has fully recognised it among its "national systems of medicine" and does not seem to be concerned by the debate around its efficacy. That is at least what appears on the AYUSH department's website which proposes a real plea for this medicine: "It [homeopathy] has been serving suffering humanity for over two centuries and has withstood the upheavals of time and emerged as a time-tested therapy, for the scientific principles propounded by Hahnemann are natural and well proven and continue to be followed with success even today". Cf. http://www.indianmedicine.nic.in (last accessed on May 15, 2013).

I started my research with some reading in order to best prepare my field-work and I realised that there was at least one thing on which people seemed to agree unanimously with regard to homeopathy. Those in favour of it as well as those against both recognised that this medicine offers an alternative concept of health. More precisely, it appears that, in opposition to biomedicine, which reduces the patient to a simple body-object, homeopathy considers every patient in his or her singularity and globality. Thus, homeopaths are "known for listening attentively to their patients" and for their "thorough clinical examination" that gives rise to "a special relationship between the doctor and the patient".[3] This "humanism" is put forward by the promoters of homeopathy as well as by its detractors. Indeed, those with doubts about the intrinsic effectiveness of homeopathic remedies see the reason for its success in precisely the attention that patients get from their doctor. The "thorough clinical examination" would then work as a kind of psychotherapy and the relief of the patient could be explained with the fact that the patient is encouraged to speak about his or her sufferings and, in doing so, achieve a certain distance from them.

There was another reason why my attention became focused on this alternative health concept. In my readings, it appeared that this concept was likely to explain why homeopathy became so successful in India, why it "has blended so well into the roots and traditions of the country".[4] India has often been considered a privileged place for the development of mystical thoughts, and the same can be said about the health concept defended by homeopathy.[5] It is therefore not astonishing that some authors thought it possible to establish between India and homeopathy what could be called a "spiritual connection". For example, some suggested that "the homeopathic concept of the vital force [was] familiar to Indians".[6]

3   Sarembaud (1999). I refer to the following extracts and translate from French: "les mé-decins homéopathes sont connus et reconnus pour l'écoute attentive qu'ils accordent à leurs patients" (p. 56); "le thérapeute, dans le cadre d'une écoute attentive et au moyen d'un examen clinique approfondi, cherche le médicament actif sur la globalité du patient. Ainsi, dans le cours de son enquête, l'homéopathe inclut les troubles rejetés par le dis-cours médical habituel. Par ailleurs, une relation particulière médecin-malade s'installe: le patient est écouté jusque dans ses signes les plus singuliers et le thérapeute recherche toutes les causalités, y compris les facteurs émotionnels." (p. 85).

4   "It's more than a century and a half now that homeopathy is being practised in India. It has blended so well into the roots and traditions of the country that it has been recognised as one of the National Systems of Medicine and plays an important role in providing health care to a large number of people".
     Cf. http://www.indianmedicine.nic.in (last accessed on May 15, 2013).

5   Cf. Sarembaud (1999), pp. 107–108.

6   In "Towards an ethnography of Indian homeopathy", Frank and Ecks enumerate briefly the different works which have tried to explain the "remarkable success" of homeopathy in India with the closeness between "homeopathy's conceptual features" and "Indian (medical) culture". Among these works: "Pfleiderer perceived the homeopathic concept of the vital force to be familiar to Indians". Cf. Frank/Ecks (2004).

As a result of my preparatory reading on homeopathy, I was convinced that I was going to India to explore this humanism coloured by mysticism.

Biomedicine and homeopathy: "what is the difference?"

On arriving at the French Institute of Pondicherry, I soon met a colleague who came from a city in Tamil Nadu. He knew a homeopath there and, given that he was about to go back to his hometown for a few days, he suggested that I join him and meet this doctor. He mentioned that the latter was working in a government hospital and I thought that this was an opportunity not to be missed. With the help of my colleague, I immediately obtained all the authorisation required to work there and I decided to settle in that city for three months.

The first thing I noticed was the separation between the AYUSH department and the rest of the hospital. The government hospital was composed of several buildings concentrated around the city centre, in a busy area. However, as my colleague told me, they were all exclusively dedicated to "English medicine". What was still called the "Indian Systems of Medicine and homeopathy"[7] was established in a small building located in a quiet peripheral area. If one compares these two parts of the hospital, the building dedicated to Indian medicines and homeopathy looked like a very small annexe of the hospital. Nevertheless, the area was much more pleasant than that of the city centre, and the building was less cramped and less crowded than the other hospital buildings.

Inside the AYUSH department's building, every unit had a room of exactly the same size: around 20 square metres. In the homeopathy unit, that space was divided into two unequal parts. The main one was the office where the doctor gave his consultations. The other part, much smaller, was a little pharmacy where an assistant prepared and dispensed the remedies.

When entering the office, my attention was immediately drawn to the portrait of Hahnemann on the wall, who seemed to be watching over the room. A little later, I noticed the more discreet presence of a bas-relief in plastic representing three Hindu deities. Also, doors, windows and many objects bore signs of the recent Saraswathi pooja. The room was furnished with the doctor's desk, many chairs and a stool for the patient. On the desk, I noticed a

This kind of argumentation can also be found on the AYUSH department's website: "Homeopathy is one of the scientific systems of medicine based on the Principle 'Similia Similibus Curentur' which means, 'let likes be treated by likes'. [...] This concept is similar to the 'Samam Samenah Shanti' concept of Indian thought".
Cf. http://www.indianmedicine.nic.in (last accessed on May 15, 2013).

7   Before becoming the "Department of AYUSH (Ayurveda, Yoga and naturopathy, Unani, Siddha, and Homeopathy)" in November 2003, this department was known as "Department of Indian Systems of Medicine and Homeopathy (ISM&H)".

stethoscope, a sphygmomanometer, a torch, an old repertory, and a frame with the picture of a guru.

Despite the fact that my colleague from the Institute knew the doctor, we had a cold reception. My colleague introduced me as someone working on "the philosophy of homeopathy". The doctor seemed very sceptical and kept asking what a student in philosophy who has no knowledge about medical sciences would be able to observe from his practice. Referring to my first readings, I answered that I wanted to study the new concept of health involved in homeopathy and look at the differences that it implied, mainly in comparison with biomedical practice. The doctor did not seem to understand. His reaction surprised me: "what is the difference?"

The unexpected exemplarity of the biomedical approach

Although I had obtained the authorisation required to attend the doctor's daily consultations, it was clear at this point that I was not really a welcome presence. My ignorance of medical sciences brought out the doctor's scepticism. At best, this scepticism manifested itself in his indifference towards me; at worst, in his jokes about my presence. The doctor remained suspicious and, after a few days, he requested a meeting with my director. Finally it was decided that we would do a round trip to Pondicherry.

Upon arriving at the French Institute of Pondicherry, the doctor looked very surprised by the prestigious building and his contemplation of the colonial architecture made it necessary for me to slow down my pace. Then, apparently refreshed by the air-conditioning of my director's office, the doctor immediately abandoned the high position adopted in the hospital. He looked shy and deferential. My director generously praised my research, then he organised a visit of the institute's library and computer labs for us. The doctor now seemed absolutely convinced: "intellectuals like you have to study and show us the way to practise". This reaction revealed that the doctor did not seem to have really understood my director's speech about the value of an anthropological approach. Nevertheless, I gained the legitimacy required to pursue my research and was even invited by the doctor to attend the consultations he gave on the side in his own "private clinic".

Back in Tamil Nadu, I suddenly became the doctor's ally in what I understood to be his major concern: the development of homeopathy. Of course, the doctor believed in the effectiveness of homeopathy. Otherwise, as he always argued, how would it be possible to explain that it still existed after so many years and that so many people were using it? According to him, that was not the issue. The issue that mattered to the doctor was how to spread the practice of homeopathy.[8]

8   The development of homeopathy was a permanent concern for the doctor who always described it as a long and difficult struggle. I was often asked to think of new ways to develop it and to promote it with local authorities in order to obtain new funds. Patients

In this perspective, pragmatic argumentation[9] will not suffice. According to the doctor, biomedicine is not so successful because it works better than homeopathy, but because it can explain how it works. The same thing should be done in homeopathy and that was precisely what the doctor believed I should work on.

Waiting for my explanatory theory, the doctor explained his own notions about how other kinds of research should be done in the field of homeopathy. The starting point should be what is certain, namely the effectiveness of this medicine. Admittedly, the doctor recognised some of its limits and the need to turn to biomedicine at times. Nevertheless, according to him, this could be avoided if, like in biomedicine, homeopaths could measure and forecast exactly the therapeutic effectiveness of their treatments. Based on this assessment, the doctor suggested the following research project: of the patients entering the emergency department, a part should be treated with homeopathy and closely monitored with very precise analyses (blood, urine, …). These analyses would be carried out at regular intervals, before, during, and after treatment. Such research, done on a large scale, would then provide statistics that would be compiled in a big book. The generations to come would then know the precise effects of every remedy as well as its rate of therapeutic efficacy.

The research project proposed by the doctor led me to start asking myself a question. I was not particularly convinced that the emergency department was the best place for "thorough clinical examination", nor were statistics the best way to consider the singularity of the patients. Therefore, remembering the doctor's question "what is the difference?", I started to wonder myself whether his medical approach differed from the biomedical approach.

Another question could be raised here. Apart from the issue of how to develop homeopathy, why did the doctor want to develop it? It appeared that, according to the doctor, there was only one reason to do so: the quality of its remedies. The doctor never mentioned that homeopathy should be developed in order to add an alternative approach to the biomedical one, an alternative that would be more humanist, or an approach coloured with Indian mysticism. The only reason mentioned was that homeopathic remedies are effective, cheap and without side effects.[10]

---

satisfied with their treatment were asked to promote the doctor in their circle. They were also invited to ask the authorities for the opening of a homeopathic dispensary in their neighbourhood.

9   For example, the doctor had medical pictures taken before and after treatment. According to him, they could prove the effectiveness of the homeopathic remedies to all the "rascals" who would dare to have doubts about it.

10 This argumentation was not only used to justify homeopathy towards the biomedical approach. It was also often used against the other medicines of the AYUSH department, especially Siddha medicine which was said to be very costly and ineffective. Originally from Tamil Nadu and very popular in that part of the country, Siddha medicine was often criticised by the doctor and tensions between the two units were frequent. For example,

One might recall here that obvious religious signs had been noticed in the doctor's office, like the portrait of a guru and a Hindu bas-relief. I could add that a pooja in honour of Hahnemann is organised on every 10th April, the date of his birth. Nevertheless, it would be a mistake to deduce from these signs, which are very common in India, that religion was omnipresent. Actually, the doctor never mentioned religion in his practice. It is true that he was a religious person (he never hid the fact), but this aspect seemed to simply overlap the medical one without mixing with it. For example, the doctor never tried to suggest a synthesis, or even a single link, between the two. It is significant to mention here the doctor's interpretation of the concept of "vital force". This concept had inspired mystical interpretations of homeopathy, but the doctor rejected such interpretations. He preferred to credit Hahnemann with this "beautiful discovery" and to link it with the concept of "acid-base balance" in biomedicine.[11]

Thus, it is surprising to notice that the doctor did not refer to what is usually mentioned in explaining the success of homeopathy in India. His research project, and more generally his speech, never suggested the need to adopt an alternative approach to biomedicine. On the contrary, he seemed to hold the view that homeopathy should copy the biomedical approach. With hindsight, this might be observed in the doctor's sudden collaboration with my research. At first, while doing my preparatory readings, I believed that my degree in philosophy would help me to enter into contact with homeopaths, especially in India where philosophy is still often considered from a religious perspective, but it appeared that I was wrong. It was only after visiting the impressive French Institute of Pondicherry that the doctor thought it appropriate to work with me. Also, it was not with philosophy or religion that the doctor hoped to develop homeopathy. According to him, any development would only be possible with a scientific explanation and, in such a quest, "English medicine" might be the very model.

---

each unit tried to be more visible than the other by using bigger signs and in putting them in the places designated for the other.

11   The doctor never spontaneously mentioned this concept of "vital force" and, if I had not asked him about it at the end of my research stay, he would probably never have talked to me about it.

The consultations, in theory and in practice

With regard to the consultations, the doctor always talked about the importance of symptoms: "Symptoms, symptoms, symptoms, that's all [...] If you miss the symptoms, you miss the remedy". Not doubting the effectiveness of the homeopathic remedies, the doctor explained every lack of results with a mistake in the "similia" choice. It is to avoid such mistakes, the doctor insisted many times, that very meticulous recording of symptoms is required. Several times, he explained to me how to proceed with the "case taking": "First of all, the chief complaints". Then, the precise determination of the problem with questions about the sensations (what are the sensations, the pains, …?), their places (where are they located, …?) and their evolution (how do they evolve – getting worse or better – during the day – before, during, and after meals, …?). The doctor often added that the "rural people" were unable to express their symptoms and that it was therefore necessary to "come down to their level". Also, according to the doctor, the "mind symptoms" were the most important and their repertorisation required that the patient had confidence in his doctor. Once all this information was collected, the treatment had to be found from the totality of the symptoms and, if ever the patient remained anxious, it was important to explain to him the nature of his disorders. Of course, concluded the doctor, the practice of homeopathy required many years of practice and a high degree of modesty to agree to question the treatment in case there was no improvement.

But I was not only able to hear the doctor talk about his consultations, I was also attending them. The consultations at the government hospital took place every morning. Then, in the evening, the doctor also had consultations in his "private clinic", an office located in the city centre and reserved for those he called the "VIPs". There, in contrast to what happened in the hospital, the consultations (which were not very different from the ones in the hospital) and the remedies (which were directly imported from the hospital) were not free.[12] Maybe this is why the "VIPs" almost never came. I attended the two kinds of consultation, but I will here focus on the hospital consultations.[13]

12 His consultations and his remedies being free at the hospital, the doctor told me that he was hated by all the homeopaths and the pharmacists of the city. Concerning his private consultations, the doctor never told me directly that they were not for free. He preferred to tell me that patients thanked him with "some sweets". It emerged later that the doctor charged between fifty to one hundred rupees per consultation. The remedies were included in the price, but not directly available. It was necessary to come back the next day, the time it took for the remedies to be prepared at the hospital.

13 Not speaking Tamil and not having a translator, I can only refer to what I could see during the consultations. With most of the patients not speaking English, I also had to abandon the idea of meeting them. Nevertheless, I tried to find out more about the content of the consultations and submitted to the doctor a table to fill in with every patient's age, sex, symptoms and treatment. I thought it would demonstrate to him the scientific clout that he was looking for, but he was not cooperative at all. Although sometimes I could convince him to fill in the table, I quickly gave up because he was paying more attention

Concerning the private consultations, the desperate waiting for patients gave me the chance to speak to the doctor for longer and to obtain the information that will be mentioned in the last part of this paper.

What surprised me on the very first day at the hospital was that I was not the only observer of the consultations. I do not refer here to the people, relatives or friends who often came with the patient. I refer to the doctor's acquaintances who attended the consultations and talked with him between them, if not during them. Most of these people, who entered and left the office freely, had the doctor's respect. Sitting in chairs reserved for them, these people were politicians that might help to develop homeopathy, religious people bringing documentation about the guru displayed on the doctor's desk, doctors from the hospital who had been converted to homeopathy[14], and some other "good friends".[15]

Another observation, also very surprising to me, was the length of the consultations, at least when they were given.[16] I learned later that, even in homeopathy, brief consultations were very common in India and that I should not have been surprised by the minimum of fifteen minutes mentioned by the doctor. Nevertheless, the fact is that those fifteen minutes were far more than the time actually given to the patients. When it came to his hospital consultations, the doctor would say: "it has to go"; and very often, even during an initial consultation, the prescription was given by the doctor in the very first minutes, or even sometimes in less than a minute.[17] The progress of the con-

---

to it than to the consultation itself. I also found it too risky to try to guess the patients' social class or religion based only on their appearance. I could not check if, like the doctor told me, patients were from all castes, classes, and religions. I also did not have any reliable data concerning the kind of complaints treated. I can nevertheless mention that many patients came because of chronic diseases, particularly arthritis and asthma. Many others came with skin diseases like ulcers, eczema, vitiligo and, above all, warts. In the latter case, patients were sent most of the time to the doctor from the "skin department" of the hospital.

14   The doctor was particularly proud to introduce me to these allopaths who consulted him. Also, he was always very happy to inform me when a patient was sent by another department (which only happened with the "skin department") or when a patient came to him after the failure of other medical treatments.

15   It quickly emerged that, when all these people were coming for a consultation, they did not have to queue to see the doctor nor to get their remedies. The quantity of drugs received was also much bigger than for any other patient.

16   It was not rare for the doctor to leave his office for an hour or two despite being on duty. He always mentioned "personal reasons" like, for example, going to the bank. When this happened, it was the assistant from the unit's pharmacy who, although he had no degree in homeopathy, prescribed the treatments. The doctor was not much more diligent during the evening consultations at his "private clinic".

17   The "it has to go" explanation, suggesting that a crowd is waiting for a consultation and that the doctor is running out of time, might not be sufficient here. Indeed, the doctor saw around 15 patients (this number can be multiplied by two on Saturday, or divided by two on days of heavy rain, the eve of festivals, …) every weekday morning (theoretically the unit is open from 8am to 2pm, in practice the consultations started at 9am and finished before noon). Instead of spreading the consultations over the whole morning, the doctor

sultation seemed in fact to depend mostly on the personality of the patient rather than on his symptoms. If a patient came and showed his foot with his hand without saying anything, the doctor did not consider it useful to talk either. The patient would leave thirty seconds later with a prescription in his hand but without a single word having been exchanged. On the contrary, a loquacious and confident patient might be able to impose himself for a few minutes, even if it was a follow-up consultation. Sometimes, it also happened that the doctor himself decided to be less expeditious, especially with women, children and "good friends". Nevertheless, a longer consultation rarely meant that the doctor was more involved from a medical point of view. Although some privileged patients had longer consultations, sometimes much longer, their prescriptions were written as quickly as those for any other patient.[18] The doctor almost never looked in his repertory, and used his instruments arbitrarily and carelessly. Actually, the doctor only really seemed concerned with the most serious cases (e.g. cases that "English medicine" has given up hope of curing). In these very rare situations, the doctor always showed real enthusiasm, seeing in them opportunities to "test" his remedies.

Subsequently, I have to say that I did not really see the "thorough clinical examination" or the "special relationship between the doctor and the patients"

always concentrated them in the first half (mostly from 9am to 10.30am), and then saw almost nobody. That second half was usually the time for him to complain about the remote location of the unit that would prevent him from having more patients. Therefore, the doctor was not running out of time, he was running out of patients. Also, a patient breaking the boredom of the late morning would not get a different kind of consultation than if he had come in the early morning rush.

Another explanation suggested by some other studies about the brevity of the consultation is that patients do not expect nor want the consultation to be longer. Since I was not able to interact with the patients, I find it difficult to comment on this.

18   This is why, despite mostly having no knowledge of the content of the consultations, I still claim here that the length of these does not seem to depend on the patients' symptoms. The same can be said about the evening consultations in the "private clinic" of the doctor. There too, the doctor rapidly wrote a prescription, and then the consultation seemed to turn into a conversation led by the patient. Since there was more or less only one patient coming to the evening consultations, this again illustrates that the time taken to determine treatment does not depend on the time available.

As for the prescriptions, it can be added here that, apart from very rare exceptions, the doctor's consultations almost always ended with a prescription. The latter never contained more than a single remedy, which shows his sympathy for the "Hahnemannian" or "unicist" tendency. Besides, remedies mixing several drugs were criticized by the doctor because, according to him, they did not respect the genuine spirit of homeopathy. Nevertheless, he explained to me that this unicist tendency was a problem for him because his patients were used to getting a much larger quantity and number of drugs from the other medicines (and, here again, Siddha medicine is the main target). As a result, even if taking a single remedy was sufficient, the doctor believed that the patients would not be satisfied. He then prescribed "empty pills". The doctor also told me that he prescribed "empty pills" when, after a first consultation, he could not decide on the proper treatment, notably because the patient was under the effect of allopathic drugs. Two-three weeks with "empty pills" would then "clean" the patient and make it possible for the doctor to find the appropriate treatment.

that I was expecting from my preparatory readings. The doctor's practice not only contradicted my picture of homeopathy, it also contradicted his own discourse about it. How can it be explained that, although he insisted on the need to develop homeopathy and offer its benefits to more and more patients, the doctor seemed to care so little about those coming to his consultations? How can it be explained that, while praising the effectiveness of scientific rigour, the doctor showed so much nonchalance in his practice? The literature on homeopathy often insists on the singularity of every patient and on the need to have a global approach. This might also be true for the doctor. I would therefore like to suggest here that these questions might find some answers in the doctor's personal story.

The trader who dreamt of being a doctor

The doctor told me that he belonged to a caste of traders. His father was doing good business in their village and the family belonged to the middle class. However, he did not want to take over his father's business, he wanted to be a doctor. Unfortunately, he failed the entrance exam in medicine. He was then advised to take a degree (MBS) in homeopathy. According to him, it was a risky choice because no one really knew what it was, himself included. He told me that the risk was worth taking because it could make his dream of becoming a doctor come true. Also, he said, it would give him a "high social status".

It is interesting to note that the doctor did not know what homeopathy was when he started to study it at medical college. Also, his faith in this medicine did not come while studying it but with personal experience. Indeed, the doctor told me that, while in the last year of his degree, he suffered from stomach pains that nothing seemed to relieve. After several biomedical treatments, he finally decided to try homeopathy. It cured him and from this recovery his faith in homeopathy grew.

The doctor then started to give consultations as a "general practitioner" in a little town. These were hard times for him. Homeopathy was not known and his office did not attract many people. He was struggling to earn enough to live on while his colleagues in biomedicine were already all driving "big cars".

According to him, he passed the UPSC (Union Public Service Commission) exam with flying colours a few years later and this gave him the opportunity to obtain a position at the government hospital. When I asked about the reason for this choice, he mentioned: a "better salary", a "better pension" and, faithful to his initial aspirations, "more prestige". He also told me that he should have been able to teach at university, but that posts there had to be bought and he did not have enough money. Anyway, the doctor said he had no regrets and was fully satisfied with his practice at the hospital. He added that he saw more "cases" than if he had given the same lecture every year at university and that, moreover, he was better paid than a professor.

How could this biographical sketch help to shed light on the questions previously raised in this paper? During my stay, I met another homeopath who told me something that might be very significant here. According to her, the students in medical sciences did not think very highly of their colleagues studying homeopathy. The homeopath who told me this did not seem to care much about such disdain. Homeopathy had worked wonders in her family and, since her youth, she had always wanted to study and practise it. She even went to study it in Calcutta[19], at the National Institute of Homeopathy, to be sure to get the best education[20]. But how did the doctor from the government hospital cope with this disrespect from his colleagues in biomedicine? What if his degree in homeopathy was not recognised as a real degree in medicine?

In the "world-capital of homeopathy"[21], where homeopathy is taught in colleges, a homeopathy graduate might still not be considered a proper doctor. Therefore, achieving scientific recognition for homeopathy might well be the only way for the homeopath presented here to finally become a proper doctor, and the only way for him to silence the roar of the "big cars" which has taunted him for so many years and which seems to have made him deaf to the moaning of the unwell.

Limits and prospects

Besides the substantial limitations mentioned at the beginning of this paper, it has been said that I have not been studying a "real" homeopath and that, as a result, focusing on him was a mistake. Instead, I should have seen many other homeopaths in order to get a more accurate picture of the contemporary practice of homeopathy in India. Of course, this study has never claimed to offer such a picture since it is not an ethnography of Indian homeopathy but an ethnography of one Indian homeopath. Maybe the homeopath described in this paper is just an isolated case. If that were true, this paper would still remind us that there might be differences between what a doctor says about his practice and what his practice actually is, and that we might need to have a closer look at the latter. But perhaps this homeopath is not just an isolated case. Perhaps it is not so improbable that part of the success of homeopathy in

19   While the doctor was interested in the "case taking" approach, this one was more interested in that of the "materia medica". It appeared that, according to the latter, this difference refers to the two schools of homeopathy in India, the Bengali school and the Bombay school. The first, her own, was the best, the one which is truly faithful to the original philosophy of homeopathy. The other one, which was also the European one, was disdainfully considered as being of a "teaching or college level". It was not practical, took too much time (minimum an hour per case) and should only be used for complicated cases. To illustrate this point, the Bengali homeopath mentioned the image of a lock and a bunch of keys. While the school of Bombay would try every key, the school of Calcutta would first select the keys of a plausible size and shape (Cf. the diathesis).
20   According to her, there were no good colleges for homeopathy in Tamil Nadu.
21   I take this expression used by R. Jütte and quoted in Frank/Ecks (2004), p. 308.

India can be explained by the fact that to study homeopathy there is an easier and a faster way to become a doctor than to study medicine. Such motivation would then be likely to have consequences for the understanding and practice of homeopathy. If this last hypothesis were to be confirmed, it might be necessary to start considering these non "real" homeopaths.

Bibliography

Internet Link

http://www.indianmedicine.nic.in (last accessed on May 15, 2013)

Literature

Frank, Robert; Ecks, Stefan: Towards an ethnography of Indian Homeopathy. In: Anthropology & Medicine 11 (2004), pp. 307–326.
Hoyez, Anne-Cécile; Schmitz, Olivier: Les voies indiennes de l'homéopathie. Diffusion et ajustement d'une médecine alternative européenne en Asie. In: Revue transcontinentales. Sociétés, idéologies, système mondial 5 (2007), pp. 97–112.
Sarembaud, Alain: L'homéopathie. Paris 1999.

The Patients' Choice – How and Why Sick People Used Homeopathy in 19ᵗʰ Century Münster

Marion Baschin

200 years ago, Samuel Hahnemann published the "Organon der rationellen Heilkunde" in which he formulated the principles of the healing method he called homeopathy. His treatments differed completely from "academic medicine" and were meant as an "alternative" to the methods taught at the beginning of the 19ᵗʰ century. When one asks patients today why they use homeopathy, a wide range of motives are found, mainly the avoidance of critical side-effects of today's medicine and the impersonality of the machine-based treatments. People appreciate homeopathy as a "gentle" method, especially in those cases in which "conventional" medicine has so far shown no positive result, for example in the case of chronic diseases.[1]

Unfortunately, finding out why people used homeopathy in the past is not as easy. One cannot turn back time and ask them to respond to a questionnaire. But a special historical source still offers the possibility of detailing how and why sick people turned to the method of Samuel Hahnemann. This refers to patient journals which document the practice of doctors. These journals are even available for the 19ᵗʰ century.

This essay will introduce the homeopaths Clemens and Friedrich von Bönninghausen. Father and son practised from 1829 to 1910 in the city of Münster in Westphalia. They left behind more than 149 patient journals, which offer a rich source for historical research into their practices in general and especially into their patients.[2] After having described these journals, the "medical market" of Münster will be sketched out. Only by knowing which different medical treatments were available for the sick people, can we evaluate their behaviour in case of an illness. The homeopaths asked their patients which therapies they had tried before. Therefore, it is possible to describe what the sick people had already tried to get well before they went to see one of the homeopaths. By taking into account how long the patients used the service of the homeopaths and how often they came to their practices, we will be able to learn more about the use of this method. In the conclusion, some considerations will be made about the motives for consulting one of the homeopaths, and in which way this "alternative" method was used.

---

1   Günther/Römermann (2002), Sharma (1995), pp. 24–26, and concerning the consultation of "Heilpraktiker": Leonhard (1984), pp. 183–185.
2   These journals are kept in the Homeopathy Archives of the Institute for the History of Medicine of the Robert Bosch Foundation in Stuttgart. IGM, P 1–149. Clemens von Bönninghausens also used three additional journals. See Baschin (2010), p. 46.

Clemens and Friedrich von Bönninghausen

Clemens Maria Franz von Bönninghausen (1785–1864)

Clemens Maria Franz von Bönninghausen was born in March 1785. He studied law and later worked for Louis Napoleon, King of Holland. After Louis Napoleon abdicated in 1810, he returned to his home region of Westphalia. He worked there for the Prussian administration and earned his living as a member of the land registry service ("Katasterkontrolleur"). He was very interested in botany and agriculture as well. In 1827, he became so gravely ill that all of his friends, and even all the doctors, thought he would not survive. So he wrote a goodbye to a friend who was, unbeknown to Bönninghausen, also a homeopathic doctor – the very first in Westphalia. This physician advised Bönninghausen of some remedies and he got better. Due to this miraculous healing, Bönninghausen became interested in the therapy, which had saved his life, and studied it himself. In 1829, he started his first official casebook named: Trials in Homeopathic Healing ("Homöopathische HeilungsVersuche").[3] His first patient was the famous German poet Annette von Droste-Hülshoff.[4] More patients followed. But, as Bönninghausen had never studied medicine and was not approved as a legal medical physician, his treatments soon provoked criticism. In 1836, the Prussian Government prohibited him from practising homeopathy. But he never stopped his service and kept on treating those who sought his help. In 1843 he was officially allowed to practise as a lay homeopath by an extraordinary permission of the Prussian king. He did so in his home town of Münster in Westphalia until he died on January 26, 1864.[5]

Friedrich Paul Joseph von Bönninghausen (1828–1910)

Friedrich Paul Joseph was born in April 1828 as the fourth son of Clemens von Bönninghausen. Like his father, he studied law. But, having finished, he added a proper medical degree in Bonn and Berlin. Friedrich concluded with an MD about "Diabetes mellitus" in 1859. Therefore Friedrich was a fully trained physician and he was legally approved as a "doctor, surgeon and obstetrician" [Arzt, Wundarzt und Geburtshelfer] in the city of Münster in 1862. Until 1864 he trained and helped in the practice of his father and, on the death of Clemens, he took over the practice and also some of the clientele. Friedrich was also allowed to dispense the homeopathic remedies himself. He married in 1888, but a son born in the same year lived only for a day. In 1907, Friedrich von Bönninghausen was given the title of a "Sanitätsrat" to honour him for his long medical activity. But Bönninghausen obviously was never part of a medi-

---

3   This journal has been published: Bönninghausen (2011).
4   Dinges/Holzapfel (2004).
5   For more details about the life of Clemens von Bönninghausen, see Kottwitz (1985).

cal society, neither homeopathic nor allopathic, and he also never published any essays or books. He seems to have concentrated on his medical services in his private practice. And he did so until his death in August 1910.[6]

In most cases, both healers used high potencies (C200) in their treatments and they therefore belong to the classical branch of homeopathy. In the case of Friedrich, this is quite interesting because most of the homeopaths in Germany in the late 19th century were adherents of the scientific-critical approach of the method, which meant that they preferred low potencies.

The Journals

Since homeopathy requires a lot of details concerning all the symptoms of an illness, it is very difficult to remember everything the sick people mention during an anamnesis. Homeopaths therefore very soon started keeping records. In the "Organon", Samuel Hahnemann gave instructions as to how a doctor should behave whilst questioning the patients and about how the information was to be written down. Hahnemann also followed his own suggestions and, every single day, he noted the symptoms the patients described to him.[7]

Clemens von Bönninghausen also followed the suggestions, but he developed a different system of record-keeping. His son Friedrich took over the journals and the way of taking notes. These more than 149 journals are kept in the Homeopathy Archives of the Institute for the History of Medicine of the Robert Bosch Foundation in Stuttgart. For the research about 77 of the 149 journals had to be chosen because going through all of them would have been a colossal task.[8]

The books the Bönninghausens used were imprinted and therefore standardised. They used a whole page for each patient, starting with general information about the sick person, such as name, age, place of residence, profession and marital status. In the upper half of the page there is also a line listing the remedies and cures already received. And the first anamnesis would be written down there as well. A comment was even made on whether or not the homeopath had actually seen the patient.

In the second half of the page, there are three columns. First, one for the prescribed homeopathic remedies and the appointments. Second, a column,

---

6 There is no biography of Friedrich von Bönninghausen available. For brief information, see Schroers (2006), p. 16. A biography with these and more details will be published in a monograph at the end of the current project "Ärztliche Praxis (17.-19. Jahrhundert)". For more details, see the webpage of the project: http://www.medizingeschichte.uni-wuerzburg.de/aerztliche_praxis/beteiligte_projekte.html (last accessed on May 22, 2013).

7 Details on case taking in homeopathy Jütte (1998) and in general Gillis (2006).

8 Baschin (2010) and the current project dealing with the practice of Friedrich von Bönninghausen, see http://www.igm-bosch.de/content/language2/html/12298.asp (last accessed on May 22, 2013). All following results concerning the practice and the patients of Clemens von Bönninghausen are part of and published in the named book. The other results will be published in a monograph at the end of the research project.

for the dose and the amount of "globules" to be taken and then a third one containing further remarks concerning changes in the state of the sick person, whether the symptoms improved, vanished or new complaints arose.

With the help of this source, a database was developed, adhering very closely to the original. There are several fields containing the original information and others dealing with and structuring these original words. The database was the main instrument for obtaining quantitative and qualitative access to the mass of information. In the case of the practice of Clemens von Bönninghausen, the database contains the stories of more than 14,200 patients, their diseases and their behaviour. In the case of Friedrich's practice about 6,830 files were transcribed.[9]

Regarding the purpose of the investigation – how and why people used homeopathy – it has to be kept in mind that only those pieces of information were written down by the Bönninghausens which they were told by the patients and which the homeopaths thought necessary to prescribe the right remedy. With regard to the therapies the sick people had tried before seeing the homeopaths, this means, that, in several cases, these efforts might not have been fully revealed. And of course we know nothing about the behaviour of all the other sick people who never decided to use the "alternative" treatment.[10]

The "medical market" in Münster

The city of Münster is located in Central Western Germany. It was a former Hanseatic City and seat of a Prince-Bishopric ("Fürstbistum Münster"). In 1815 it became Prussian and was made the capital of the newly-formed Province of Westphalia. The main university of the region was, and still is, located there and offers students courses in medicine. Although most of the inhabitants were members of the lower social classes, many nobles and clerics chose to live in Münster. As the town was also the administrative centre, civil servants also made up an important part of the population.[11]

Therefore, the city was very attractive for doctors and barber-surgeons offering good opportunities for income. During the 19th century, the average number of inhabitants per doctor was much higher than for the whole province or the Prussian kingdom in general. When Clemens von Bönninghausen started his healing activities in 1829, 28 doctors were offering their medical services to the 18,502 inhabitants of Münster. This means a ratio of about 660

---

9   For more details on the methodological proceedings see Baschin (2010), pp. 45–57, and Baschin (2011).
10   In this context the word "alternative" is anachronistic, but had to be used due to the lack of appropriate terms. It is meant to describe all those methods which were not approved by the educated and trained doctors in the 19th century. For an explanation of the word "alternative methods" see Jütte (1996), pp. 11–65.
11   Krabbe (1983); Teuteberg (1993).

inhabitants to each doctor. In Prussia at that time, a doctor had to take care of about 3,000 people on average. When Friedrich was approved as a lawful doctor in 1862, he was one of 34 doctors who were in charge of approximately 700 inhabitants each. As the city grew in the following years, the number of people per doctor increased. And, during the 1880s, a practitioner had to look after about 1,200 inhabitants.[12]

As Münster was a regional capital city, medical "innovations" were also available at an early stage. From 1875 onwards, several specialised physicians offered their services. There was, for example, an ophthalmologist, a dermatologist or even someone who offered treatments with the then newly-developed X-rays. Midwives were also employed and helped the women to deliver their babies. But the birth rate was low in Münster compared to the Province in general, and the profession of the midwife was not well regarded.

Beside these approved medical people, lay healers and "quacks" offered various treatments. But it is difficult to give information about their number. In addition, nothing is known about their therapies. Clemens von Bönninghausen was also able to "convert" some of the doctors in Münster to homeopathy. But they all died before his son took over the practice. Until 1878, Friedrich was the only homeopath in Münster itself. But, in the following years, four other homeopaths subsequently joined the medical market. In addition, other "alternative methods" such as electricity, water cures or magnetism were available.

Münster had six hospitals and institutions in which sick people were taken care of. By 1900, some smaller, but specialised, hospitals opened and the others grew. Five pharmacies also existed and, by 1900, seven offered the possibility of buying a range of drugs. Some spas were also located in the vicinity of Münster.

This is why inhabitants were able to choose from a variety of medical services. The city of Münster offered a lot of medical services and possibilities, even for poor people, to receive medical care.[13] In particular, in the second half of the 19th century, characteristics of a "progressive" medical market, typical for a bigger city, emerge. It is quite remarkable that Clemens von Bönninghausen was able to have a flourishing homeopathic practice without being a trained physician. Friedrich was also successful, although he faced competition from several other homeopaths in Münster. But what kind of cures had the sick people already tried?

12   In 1862, 23,124 inhabitants lived in Münster. In 1881, 33 physicians were available for 41,135 inhabitants of the city.
13   For more details about the medical situation in Münster in the 19th century Schwanitz (1990), Teuteberg (1993) and Baschin (2010), pp. 73–82.

Before using homeopathy – patients in the "medical market"

The homeopaths were interested in those remedies and treatments the sick people had tried to get well before turning to them, because these could have changed the original symptoms. But, to prescribe the right homeopathic remedy, it is necessary to know the symptoms in the form in which they first occurred. The information given in response to the question as to what the patients had already tried in order to get well again enables us to discover how people moved self-confidently through the different medical fields which were available.[14]

When feeling sick, people normally start treating themselves with "home remedies".[15] In most cases, they also ask family members or acquaintances for advice. But, when given the name of some remedy in the patient records, one can only guess whether certain plasters, pills, ointments or drops were bought by the patients themselves or were taken on the instruction of an approved medical practitioner. Drugs such as quinine, mercury or sulphur belonged to the Materia Medica of the approved doctors or could be easily bought in a pharmacy.[16] One could also produce one's own plasters and ointments. Several volumes of "lay advisory literature" offer thousands of recipes on the subject.[17] The same applies to baths, showers and even teas. Table 1 provides some figures regarding the number of patients who said that they used a particular drug or remedy before. It is quite interesting that there was a decline in the use of sulphur and mercury between Clemens and Friedrich. Maybe the patients had realized that these remedies often did more harm than good.

Table 1: Patients in the "medical market" (Absolute numbers and percentage per total number of patients in each practice, own data)

"Therapies" used by patients before consulting a homeopath	Clemens von Bönninghausen (14,266 patients)	Friedrich von Bönninghausen (6,832 patients)
Information given concerning previous therapies	9,851 (69%)	3,623 (53%)
Drugs/Remedies in general	5,568 (39%)	2,953 (43.2%)

14 The files of Friedrich give in 53.0% of cases (3,623 patients) clues about the cures already received. Clemens von Bönninghausen noted such information in 69% (9,851) of his patients.
15 The drugs or remedies people had taken to improve their status were given in 5,568 cases in the files of Clemens (39.0%) and 2,953 patient stories of Friedrich (43.2%).
16 In Clemens' practice 998 patients had taken sulphur (7.0%), 906 mercury (6.4%) and 547 quinine (3.8%). In Friedrich's practice 110 patients had used sulphur (1.6%), 15 mercury (0.2%) and 105 quinine (1.5%).
17 Plasters were used by 36 of Friedrich's patients and by 118 of Clemens'. Ointments were used by 286 patients in Friedrich's practice and by 461 in the practice of Clemens.

Plasters	118 (0.8%)	36 (0.5%)
Ointments	461 (3.2%)	286 (4.2%)
"Home remedies"	281 (2.0%)	89 (1.3%)
Sulphur	998 (7.0%)	110 (1.6%)
Mercury	906 (6.4%)	15 (0.2%)
Quinine	547 (3.8%)	105 (1.5%)

The mention of food, such as potatoes, bacon or porridge, and mostly alcoholic drinks, like beer, wine and spirits, strongly suggests the use of "home remedies".[18] Several other patients only say they had taken "home remedies" or "quackeries" without indicating what they had used in particular.[19]

According to claims by "allopathic" doctors, lay healers were practically everywhere, treating sick people and preventing them from seeing a "proper" physician. But in only a few cases did people admit on their first encounter with the homeopaths that they had consulted a lay healer before. Even fewer people had done so before visiting the practice of Friedrich, which leaves the question whether "popular" or "lay medicine" were really not used any more or whether the people did not want to admit to having used them. Table 2 gives an overview of the different therapists and institutions the patients had tried before they turned to either of the homeopaths.

Table 2: Patients in the "medical market" (Absolute numbers and percentage per total number of patients in each practice, own data)

"Therapies" used by patients before consulting a homeopath	Clemens von Bönninghausen (14,266 patients)	Friedrich von Bönninghausen (6,832 patients)
Lay healers, "alternative methods"	46 (0.3%)	21 (0.5%)
Homeopathy	261 (1.8%)	83 (1.2%)
Midwife	8 (0.1%)	2 (0%)
Surgeon or operation	95 (0.7%)	143 (2.1%)
Doctor	1,210 (8.5%)	537 (7.9%)

---

18   Alcoholic beverages were used by 93 patients who later consulted Clemens and by 31 consulting Friedrich. For the use of food as medicine by the patients of Clemens, see Baschin (2010), pp. 96–97. In the case of Friedrich's practice, an overview cannot be given because of the variety of foods used. But the range is approximately the same as in the practice of Clemens.

19   The phrase "Hausmittel" ("home remedies") is used in 281 cases in Clemens' journals and in 89 in Friedrich's journals.

Legally-approved medical people in general	1,313 (9.2 %)	682 (10.0 %)
Venesection	149 (1.0 %)	21 (0.3 %)
Pharmacy	89 (0.6 %)	6 (0.1 %)
Hospital	79 (0.6 %)	32 (0.5 %)
Spa	93 (0.7 %)	72 (1.1 %)

Not only homeopathy is to be counted under the "alternative" methods of the 19th century. The use of electricity or magnetism is to be mentioned here as well. But only very few sick people experienced those forms of therapy. Those patients, in fact, suffered from severe and long-term ailments, which points to the conclusion that, in these cases, everything had been tried to achieve a cure. About 261 people had already used the method of Samuel Hahnemann before consulting Clemens, and the same applies to 83 of Friedrich's patients. These stories reveal that the beginning of a homeopathic treatment was by no means a "one-way" process. Many of them had returned to "allopathic" treatment or even to lay healers before giving homeopathy another chance.

Legally approved medical staff was of course also asked for advice. Only a few patients said that they had consulted a midwife. In these cases, in particular, people might stay silent about having used the service of a midwife, because her assistance during birth was not seen as "allopathic" treatment.[20]

Several sick people had seen surgeons or even undergone surgery before turning to one of the homeopaths.[21] But, in most cases, the operations were not difficult ones. Most had experienced the extraction of teeth or inflammations that had been opened. Some of the sick people hoped to avoid surgery with the help of the homeopathic remedies. In other cases, the Bönninghausens had to treat the negative side effects of operations, such as wounds which were still bleeding or stiff parts of the body. Interestingly enough, the method of "blood letting" was still used in the 19th century.[22] The number of patients who said that they had "venesection" before seeing either of the Bönninghausens decreased over the years, while other methods, such as cupping, were still used.[23]

About 1,210 sick people told Clemens von Bönninghausen that they had seen one or even two or three doctors before, often giving the exact name. Friedrich von Bönninghausen was consulted by 537 patients who had tried

20 Eight sick people had called in a midwife in the case of Clemens' journals and only two in the stories of Friedrich. See Baschin (2010), pp. 115–117, with regard to this problem.
21 Surgical activities in the broadest sense were mentioned 95 of Clemens' (0.7 %) and by 143 (2.1 %) of Friedrich's patients.
22 Maibaum (1983).
23 149 of Clemens' patients (1.0 %) had had venesection as opposed to 21 of Friedrich's (0.3 %). Cupping was mentioned by 35 of Clemens' patients (0.2 %) and by 32 (0.5 %) of Friedrich's. Leeches were used by 39 of Friedrich's patients (0.6 %) and by 62 in the practice of Clemens (0.4 %).

treatment by an "allopathic" physician. If the sick people did not live in the city of Münster they had usually consulted the doctors in or near their home town. In particular, when people were suffering from longer-term ailments, several doctors had been consulted. Only after that did they consider the long journey to Münster. Many doctors offering their services in Münster had also been consulted but had obviously not satisfied the patients.

Only a few patients mentioned pharmacies as the place where they received their drugs. Some patients had already been to spas or to hospitals. Interestingly enough, more people mention a visit to a spa than to a hospital. But even today most illnesses are treated without the need for staying in hospital. Visits to spas were also very popular in the 19th century. Unsurprisingly, it was mostly wealthy people who had been to spas. However, some of the places had special areas for "poor" people. 93 patients had been to a spa before seeing Clemens and 72 before consulting Friedrich. The visit to a spa need not contradict a homeopathic cure, since, for example, in the spa of Lippspringe, a homeopathic doctor took care of the patients.[24] In the case of Clemens, 79 sick people had been to hospital before, and the same applies to 32 of Friedrich's patients. Some of them had stayed for several weeks. Some men had been to a military hospital. The majority had been to the Clemenshospital, the biggest and oldest hospital in Münster.

In fact, the majority of the sick people visiting one of the Bönninghausens had had experience of "allopathic" medicine, either by self-medication or under the guidance of an approved medical person. Therefore they cannot be counted as convinced users of homeopathy at the time when they started their treatment.

Using homeopathy – Treatments by the Bönninghausens

In total, Clemens and Friedrich von Bönninghausen treated about 39,000 people between 1829 and 1889.[25] In specific years, more than 1,000 patients asked for homeopathic therapy, in other years there were less. On average, Clemens received 711 new patients per year and Friedrich could offer his services to about 427 sick people per year. These averages changed during the years under consideration. While Clemens was able to augment his practice, Friedrich obviously received fewer patients during his time of practice, as is illustrated in Chart 1.[26]

24 See Baschin (2010), p. 134, for further literature.
25 This is an estimated number according to all the patient stories recorded in the journals. In total Clemens von Bönninghausen treated about 27,500 patients between 1829 and 1864 and Friedrich saw about 11,500 patients up to 1889.
26 In the years under consideration, Clemens and Friedrich had the following average number of new patients (P) and consultations (C): Clemens 1829/33 237 (P), 1,091.4 (C); 1839/43 904.8 (P), 3,011.2 (C); 1849/53 898.2 (P), 3,741.6 (C); 1859/64 802.8 (P), 2,675 (C); Friedrich 1864/67 903 (P), 2,811 (C); 1872/75 475.3 (P), 1,756 (C); 1879/82 147.5 (P), 551.8 (C); 1886/88 155.3 (P), 515.8 (C).

Chart 1: Patients and consultations in the practices of the homeopaths von Bönninghausen (until 1864 Clemens, from 1864 Friedrich) (Average numbers, own data)

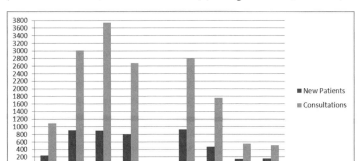

But the sick people did not stop having their own opinion when they entered the rooms of the homeopaths. Moreover, they were still self-confident, deciding for themselves how long and how often they would have homeopathic treatment. In fact, the majority of patients only stayed for a short time.

Considering the length of the therapies, most people only continued them for up to a year, as can be seen in Table 3. In the case of Clemens, about 72 % of the sick people came within this period of time and in the practice of Friedrich this applied to 78 %. About 12 % of Clemens von Bönninghausen's patients, and about 11 % of Friedrich's received treatment over two years. Even fewer continued to see one of the homeopaths for a period of three years. This is the case in about 3 % of the treatments in either of the practices. Slightly more patients went to see Friedrich for about four years, 2.6 %, while this applied to only 2.1 % in the practice of Clemens. Five-year-treatment was given to 1.6 % of Clemens' patients and to 1.9 % of Friedrich's.

Table 3: Length of treatments in years in the practices of the homeopaths von Bönninghausen (percentages per total number of patients in the practices, own data)

Years/Percentage of all patients	Practice Clemens (14,266 patients)	Practice Friedrich (6,832 patients)
One year	72.1	78.0
Two years	12.2	10.6
Three years	3.2	3.0
Four years	2.1	2.6
Five years	1.6	1.9
Total	91.2	96.1

Most of the patients, indeed, came only once or twice and then abandoned homeopathic therapy. In the practice of Friedrich, even more sick people came only once, about 38.4 %, compared to the practice of Clemens with about 34.0%. 20.3% of patients asked Friedrich twice for advice and the same applied to 22.3% of Clemens' clientele. This phenomenon is however not seen only in homeopathic practices. With other, for example "allopathic" doctors, most patients only stayed for a short-term treatment as well.[27] About 8% of the sick people seeing Clemens had more than ten consultations and 6.6% of those seeing Friedrich. On average, a therapy included 4.4 consultations with Clemens and 3.9 with Friedrich. Some patients even came to see their homeopath more than 100 times. In those cases, it is very likely that the patients were convinced of the homeopathic treatments. These patterns of consultation behaviour are shown in Chart 2.

Chart 2: Consultations per patient in the practices of the homeopaths von Bönninghausen (Percentage per total number of patients in the practices, own data)

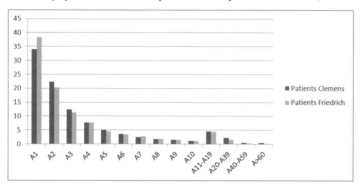

A therapy that lasted for years or that consisted of several consultations does not necessarily mean that all the patients were converted to homeopathy. As the patient journals reveal, the sick people did not stop having their own opinion when they saw a homeopath. Normally, a homeopathic treatment was accompanied by dietary suggestions, such as not drinking alcohol or coffee or avoiding spicy meals. But a lot of people disregarded such advice or they did not feel the necessity to follow the homeopathic treatment only.[28] Several people still used allopathic remedies whilst in the care of the Bönninghausens. Some visited spas, whilst others used plasters or ointments.[29] Such behaviour

---

27   Schuricht (2004), p. 11. 37% of the sick people came only once, 25.6% had between two and four consultations. In the first journal of Samuel Hahnemann, more than 50% of the patients came only once. Hörsten (2004), pp. 51–52. For a Belgian homeopath see Baal (2004), p. 179. The same applies to the practices of "allopaths" such as Haller (22.6% came only once), Boschung (1996), p. 8, or a doctor called Kortum (59.9% had only one consultation), Balster (1990), p. 123, or a doctor from the Harz region (73.6% came once), Thümmler (2004), p. 40.

28   Such behaviour of neglecting dietary suggestions could be found in at least 44 patient histories of Clemens and 35 of those of Friedrich.

29   At least 35 patients first ended their homoeopathic treatment and consulted other "allopathic" doctors before returning to Clemens von Bönninghausen. The same applies to 84 of the patients of Friedrich.

could mean the end of the therapy, but did not in all cases. This kind of "diso-bedient" behaviour was, however, not reported for many patients.[30] In gen-eral, sick people did not only behave that way in the practices of the homeo-paths von Bönninghausen. They did the same in "allopathic" practices.[31]

Just "shoppers"? – Concluding remarks on how and why sick people used homeopathy

Clemens and Friedrich von Bönninghausen were by no means the only peo-ple who offered health care services to the population in and around Münster. On the contrary, they both faced a very busy "medical market". Therefore, the question of why sick people decided to see either of the homeopaths needs to be asked. Without doubt, it was known that both of the Bönninghausens treated according to homeopathic principles.[32] One can therefore expect that the decision to use the "alternative" concept was a more or less conscious one. Conclusions cannot be drawn in every case as to the particular motives that led to the consultation of a homeopath, but some conclusions are possible from the various files.[33]

---

30 In general, some sort of "disobedient" behaviour is reported in the stories of 251 patients of Clemens and in the stories of 115 patients of Friedrich. It is likely that this figure may actually have been higher than reported.

31 The parallel use of homoeopathic and "allopathic" treatment is proven in the journals of Samuel Hahnemann: Schuricht (2004), p. 27, Sauerbeck (1989), and a Belgian homeo-path as well Baal (2004), p. 110. In the casebooks of the following "allopathic" doctors also other cures are mentioned: Balster (1990), pp. 202–208; Jütte (1991), pp. 97–99; Lachmund/Stollberg (1995), pp. 106–112; Lindemann (1996), p. 365; Loetz (1993), p. 244; McCray Beier (1987), p. 57; Oberhofer (2008), p. 171.

32 This was not always the case as Baal (2002), pp. 252–253, and Gijswijt-Hofstra (2002), pp. 214–215, prove.

33 With regard to the pattern of use of homeopathy, different types of "users" have been described. These "types" have to be seen as "idealistic types" to structure the pattern of use of a certain method by the patients, they do not necessarily occur in reality and of course the "lables" are not used in the sources. Dinges (2002), pp. 18–20, separates be-tween "random patients", "shoppers", "habitual patients", "converts" and "activists". The following remarks are orientated to this distinction. But, due to the source of the patient journals, "activists" are not to be found, because a public commitment to homeopathy is not documented there. The same applies to the "habitual patients", as it is not reported how the adult patients were treated in their childhood and, only in few cases, sick chil-dren who were brought to a homoeopath stayed in their care after growing up. With re-gard to the "random patient", the pattern seems not to fit the situation in Münster. As Dinges states: "The random patient is often the product of a local supply situation: where there is only one doctor or non-medical practitioner and that person practises homeopa-thy, it is simply a matter of convenience for the patient to visit that homeopath." But, as was shown here for Münster, sick people could choose from a variety of medical services and, if they were afraid or total opponents of homeopathy, they were not forced to use that method by local circumstances. Moreover, as it is not quite clear whether people were "converted" to homeopathy by their treatments or other circumstances, the term

In summary it can be said that the majority of the patients arriving in the practices of the Bönninghausens had experienced some sort of "allopathic" treatment before. Therefore, they were not convinced users of homeopathy at the beginning of the therapy. This might apply only to those few who had already undergone another homeopathic treatment. But, even in their histories, it becomes clear that they were not completely loyal adherents of this method.

It is plausible to suggest that most patients were not satisfied by the "cures" they had received so far. This is explicitly shown in those files which state that all previous attempts had been unsuccessful or had even worsened the symptoms.[34] If homeopathy then was chosen as a last attempt to find a cure or whether there were other reasons for turning to this method cannot be decided. But, in most cases, homeopathy might have been the last resort.[35]

Surgery with disastrous results or the death of relatives as a consequence of an obviously failed "allopathic" treatment were, indeed, strong motives for searching for another therapy. If, for example, an ophthalmic operation led to the loss of an eye, it was quite logical for the patient to look for another method of treatment. Or, if parents had already lost a child to whooping cough under the care of an "allopathic" practitioner, one can well understand why they now used homeopathic remedies for the other children who displayed the same symptoms.[36]

If doctors, who had been consulted, told their patients that their illness was incurable or that they had no hope for them, they clearly turned to the homeopaths as a last resort. The same applies to patients who hoped to escape surgery or even amputation of a part of the body. These patients might have hoped that the homeopathic remedies would improve their situation.[37] In all these cases, the turning to homeopathic treatment was probably the "last resort" for the sufferers who can therefore be seen as "shoppers" on the "medical market". For a better orientation, the number of cases in which the motives mentioned played a part are given in Table 4.

"convinced" is used instead. For other suggestions for describing users of "complementary" medicine, see Sharma (1995), pp. 47–53.

34 In the files of Clemens the phrase "o. E.", which means "without success" appears 1,177 times. But it can only be found in about ten cases in the journal entries of Friedrich.

35 But homeopaths in the 19th century often knew that they were the "last resort" and had no illusion about this fact. Baschin (2010), p. 143.

36 Unsuccessful surgery was mentioned by eleven patients who asked Friedrich for advice. The death of relatives suffering from a similar ailment as the one with which they consulted the homeopath was mentioned in 18 cases. The files of Clemens von Bönninghausen have not been searched with direct focus on such motives. But the death of relatives in connection with the current illness was mentioned by 58 patients and unsuccessful surgery was mentioned in about 14 cases, although there might have been more. See Baschin (2010), p. 121 and p. 265.

37 Six patients of Friedrich had been told that their ailment was incurable and seven tried to avoid amputation or surgery. In the practice of Clemens, about 26 sick people had been told that their ailment was incurable and at least five tried to avoid surgery. See Baschin (2010), pp. 121–122.

Table 4: Motives for the use of homeopathy mentioned in the files (Total numbers, own data)

Motives for the use of home-opathy mentioned in the files	In the practice of Clemens	In the practice of Friedrich
Previous therapies without success ("o. E.")	1,177	10 (at least, could not be counted)
Death of relatives during "allopathic" treatment	58	18
Unsuccessful surgery	14	11
Declared "incurable" by the doctors	26	6
Attempt to avoid an operation or amputation	5	7

There was another motive that is not proved by the journals: the financial one. Clemens von Bönninghausen treated all his patients for free until 1835. But up to that time the majority of his patients had been wealthy nobles who could have easily afforded treatment. Moreover, the percentage of patients from the lower social classes increased during his years of practice up to 1864. Obviously, the cost of homeopathic treatment was no hindrance for those poorer patients.[38] Clemens, and later Friedrich as well, adapted the fee they asked for their therapies to the financial means of their patients. In some cases, they also accepted payment in kind. In general, their cures were not necessarily cheaper than those of the other practitioners in Münster. There is therefore no evidence that there was an economic motive for choosing homeopathy. According to the patient journals, which give only little indication concerning the costs and payments of the homeopathic therapies, the financial argument cannot be entirely excluded.

When dealing with the question of whether the sick people were "shoppers" or convinced users, the question of "how" sick people made use of homeopathy has to be taken into account as well. As could be seen, most of them only saw the homeopath once or twice. In these cases, the use was highly sporadic. Although some of the patients continued their therapies over several years, it cannot be said for sure that they were loyal adherents of the method although that is possible. In general, it is very difficult to find out from the notes in the journals whether the sick people became converted users of homeopathy during a treatment. In most cases, we only learn that someone came, had some consultations and vanished again. He or she might return, but the homeopaths rarely provide information as to what these people did in between. Even if the first treatment was successful, some patients returned to the "allopathic" remedies instead of consulting a homeopath straight away. In

---

38   Baschin (2010), pp. 368–382, for the question of fees and payments for homeopathic treatment.

most cases, the historian is left guessing what the sick people did when they were not seeing a homeopath. They might have stayed healthy or they might have called on an "allopathic" doctor again. It is also impossible to find out whether some people used the homeopathic remedies only for certain symptoms. The duration of a treatment and the amount of consultations during a therapy, therefore, do not seem to be appropriate measurements of the sure conviction of a certain method. However, there is the possibility that, with increasing length and increasing amounts of consultations, people became convinced of and converted to the homeopathic method.

Therefore, in most cases, the consultations of the homeopaths von Bönninghausen can be traced back to the fact, that, besides a lot of other possibilities, homeopathy was tried as well. Most sick people "shopped around" searching for a cure, whatever it might have been. In view of this result, homeopathy cannot be regarded as an "alternative" in the medical market of Münster, but more as a "complementary" offer.[39]

Bibliography

Internet Links

http://www.medizingeschichte.uni-wuerzburg.de/aerztliche_praxis/beteiligte_projekte.html
(last accessed on May 22, 2013)
http://www.igm-bosch.de/content/language2/html/12298.asp (last accessed on May 22, 2013)

Literature

Baal, Anne van: Homoeopathy in Nineteenth-Century Flanders. The Patients of Ghent Gustave A. van den Berghe (1869–1902). In: Dinges, Martin (ed.): Patients in the History of Homoeopathy. (=European Association for the History of Medicine and Health Network Series 5) Sheffield 2002, pp. 237–258.

Baal, Anne van: In Search of a Cure. The Patients of the Ghent Homoeopathic Physician Gustave A. van den Berghe (1837–1902). Diss. phil. Amsterdam 2004.

Balster, Wolfgang: Medizinische Wissenschaft und ärztliche Praxis im Leben des Bochumer Arztes Karl Arnold Kortum (1745–1824). Diss. med. Bochum 1990.

Baschin, Marion: Wer lässt sich von einem Homöopathen behandeln? Die Patienten des Clemens Maria Franz von Bönninghausen (1785–1864). (=Medizin, Gesellschaft und Geschichte, Beiheft 37) Stuttgart 2010.

Baschin, Marion: How patients built the practice of the lay homoeopath Clemens von Bönninghausen. Quantitative and qualitative aspects of patient history. In: Dynamis 31 (2011), no. 2, pp. 475–495.

39 Even today homeopathic patients do not fully rely on the method of Hahnemann alone. See Günther/Römermann (2002); Sharma (1995), pp. 24–26 and pp. 53–59. This also applies for the patients of Samuel Hahnemann himself, Schreiber (2002), p. 135. The difficulty of finding out precisely why people actually use "complementary" medicine is also shown in Bishop/Yardley/Lewith (2007); Günther/Römermann (2002), pp. 295–296. There seem to be many more motives and especially a mixture of different ones that lead to the use of "complementary" or "alternative" medicines.

Bishop, Felicity; Yardley, Lucy; Lewith, George: A Systematic Review of Beliefs Involved in the Use of Complementary and Alternative Medicine. In: Journal of Health Psychology 12 (2007), pp. 851–867.

Bönninghausen, Clemens von: Das erste Krankenjournal (1829–1830). Edited by Luise Kunkle. (=Quellen und Studien zur Homöopathiegeschichte 14) Essen 2011.

Boschung, Urs: Albrecht Haller's Patient Records (Berne 1731–1736). In: Gesnerus 53 (1996), pp. 5–14.

Dinges, Martin: Introduction. Patients in the History of Homoeopathy. In: Dinges, Martin (ed.): Patients in the History of Homoeopathy. (=European Association for the History of Medicine and Health Network Series 5) Sheffield 2002, pp. 1–32.

Dinges, Martin; Holzapfel, Klaus: Von Fall zu Fall. Falldokumentation und Fallredaktion Clemens von Bönninghausen und Annette von Droste-Hülshoff. In: Zeitschrift für Klassische Homöopathie 48 (2004), pp. 149–167.

Gijswijt-Hofstra, Marijke: The Haverhoeks and their Patients. The Popularity of Unqualified Homoeopaths in the Netherlands in the Early Twentieth Century. In: Dinges, Martin (ed.): Patients in the History of Homoeopathy. (=European Association for the History of Medicine and Health Network Series 5) Sheffield 2002, pp. 213–235.

Gillis, Jonathan: The History of the Patient History since 1850. In: Bulletin of the History of Medicine 80 (2006), pp. 490–511.

Günther, Martina; Römermann, Hans: The Homoeopathic Patient in General Practice. Findings of a Comparative Poll of Patients in Conventional Medical Practices and Homoeopathic Private and Health Insurance Scheme Practices. In: Dinges, Martin (ed.): Patients in the History of Homoeopathy. (=European Association for the History of Medicine and Health Network Series 5) Sheffield 2002, pp. 281–299.

Hörsten, Iris von: Samuel Hahnemann. Krankenjournal D2-D4 (1801–1803). Kommentarband zur Transkription. Heidelberg 2004.

Jütte, Robert: Ärzte, Heiler und Patienten. Medizinischer Alltag in der frühen Neuzeit. Munich; Zürich 1991.

Jütte, Robert: Geschichte der Alternativen Medizin. Von der Volksmedizin zu den unkonventionellen Therapien von heute. Munich 1996.

Jütte, Robert: Case Taking in Homeopathy in the 19th and 20th Centuries. In: British Homoeopathic Journal 87 (1998), pp. 39–47.

Kottwitz, Friedrich: Bönninghausens Leben. Hahnemanns Lieblingsschüler. Berg 1985.

Krabbe, Wolfgang: Wirtschafts- und Sozialstruktur einer Verwaltungsstadt des 19. Jahrhunderts. Das Beispiel der Provinzialhauptstadt Münster. In: Düwell, Kurt; Köllmann, Wolfgang (eds.): Rheinland-Westfalen im Industriezeitalter. Vol. 1: Von der Entstehung der Provinzen bis zur Reichsgründung. Wuppertal 1983, pp. 197–206.

Lachmund, Jens; Stollberg, Gunnar: Patientenwelten. Krankheit und Medizin vom späten 18. bis zum frühen 20. Jahrhundert im Spiegel von Autobiographien. Opladen 1995.

Leonhard, Joachim: Motive zum Heilpraktikerbesuch. Eine empirische Untersuchung über die sozialen Aspekte und die Krankengeschichte als Hintergrund eines Entscheidungsprozesses. Teningen 1984.

Lindemann, Mary: Health and Healing in Eighteenth-Century Germany. Baltimore 1996.

Loetz, Francisca: Vom Kranken zum Patienten. "Medikalisierung" und medizinische Vergesellschaftung am Beispiel Badens 1750–1850. (=Medizin, Gesellschaft und Geschichte, Beiheft 2) Stuttgart 1993.

Maibaum, Elke: Der therapeutische Aderlaß von der Entdeckung des Kreislaufs bis zum Beginn des 20. Jahrhunderts. (=Studien zur Medizin-, Kunst- und Literaturgeschichte 2) Herzogenrath 1983.

McCray Beier, Lucinda: Sufferers and Healers. The Experience of Illness in Seventeenth-Century England. London; New York 1987.

Oberhofer, Andreas: Eine Landarztpraxis im 19. Jahrhundert am Beispiel der Ordination des Dr. Franz von Ottenthal (1818–1899). In: Dietrich-Daum, Elisabeth; Dinges, Martin; Jütte,

Robert; Roilo, Christine (eds.): Arztpraxen im Vergleich. 18.-20. Jahrhundert. (=Veröffentlichungen des Südtiroler Landesarchivs 26) Innsbruck; Vienna; Bozen 2008, pp. 167–192.

Sauerbeck, Karl-Otto: Der späte Hahnemann und sein ärztliches Umfeld. Maschinenschriftliches Vortragsmanuskript, gehalten 1989 (IGM, Sign.: H/k/Saue/1989,2).

Schreiber, Kathrin: Samuel Hahnemann in Leipzig. Die Entwicklung der Homöopathie zwischen 1811 und 1821, Förderer, Gegner und Patienten. (=Quellen und Studien zur Homöopathiegeschichte 8) Stuttgart 2002.

Schroers, Fritz: Lexikon deutschsprachiger Homöopathen. Stuttgart 2006.

Schuricht, Ulrich: Samuel Hahnemann. Krankenjournal D16 (1817–1818). Kommentarband zur Transkription. Heidelberg 2004.

Schwanitz, Hedwig: Krankheit, Armut, Alter. Gesundheitsfürsorge und Medizinalwesen in Münster während des 19. Jahrhunderts. (=Quellen und Forschungen zur Geschichte der Stadt Münster, Neue Folge 14) Münster 1990.

Sharma, Ursula: Complementary Medicine Today. Practitioners and Patients. 2nd ed. London; New York 1995.

Teuteberg, Hans-Jürgen: Bevölkerungsentwicklung und Eingemeindungen (1816–1945). In: Jakobi, Franz-Josef (ed.): Geschichte der Stadt Münster. Vol. 2. Münster 1993, pp. 331–386.

Thümmler, Andrea: Rekonstruktion des Alltags eines thüringischen Arztes im 18. Jahrhundert anhand seines Praxistagebuches 1750–1763. Diss. med. Berlin 2004.

Patients' Trend in Choosing the Homeopathic Medical System in India

Rahul Tewari, Ramachandran Valavan

Introduction

India knowingly or unknowingly follows pluralism in healthcare. It has an eclectic health system that incorporates biomedical as well as traditional, complementary and alternative medicine (TCAM)[1] which in India is called as Indian Systems of Medicine and Homeopathy (ISM&H). Currently, India is the country with the second largest population in the world (surpassed only by China) and is estimated to have about 1.21 billion people: more than one-sixth of the world population.[2] Medical systems in India are broadly divided into allopathy (modern system of medicine) and complementary and alternative medicine (CAM) systems. The Ministry of Health and Family Welfare regulates education and practice of all the systems. Within the Ministry, the Department of AYUSH regulates CAM systems including Ayurveda, Yoga and Naturopathy, Unani, Siddha and Homeopathy.

Historical background and present status of homeopathy in India

Some historians say that the history of homeopathy in India is somewhat unclear. According to the historiographer Dr Eshwara Das[3] homeopathy was brought to India in 1810, by German missionaries. However Poldas has definitely demonstrated that there are no documents for homeopathy in Calcutta for 1810. The first document is from 1851. There are only unproven assumptions that a German geologist and some German missionaries brought homeopathy to Calcutta as early as 1810.[4] The credit of receiving official patronage goes to Dr. John Martin Honigberger who was called as a physician to the Court of Maharaja Ranjeet Singh in 1839. After independence an homeopathy enquiry committee was formed by the Government of India in the year 1948, followed by the homeopathy advisory committee in the year 1952. The system was recognized in 1962 and integrated into the Drugs Act in 1969. The Homeopathy Central Council (HCC) Act came into force and the Central Council of Homeopathy (CCH) was formed in 1984 in India. Other important landmarks in homeopathy include the formation of the Homeopathic Phar-

---

1   Broom/Doron/Tovey (2009).
2   http://censusindia.gov.in/2011census/censusinfodashboard/index.html (last accessed on May 22, 2013).
3   Das (2005), pp. 101–113.
4   Poldas (2010), p. 41.

macopoeia Laboratory (HPL) in 1975 and the formation of the Central Council for Research in Homeopathy (CCRH) in 1978.[5]

At present the homeopathic industry is growing faster than the mainstream medical industry. Homeopathy in India is growing at around 25%[6] whereas the conventional system of medicine is reported to be growing at a rate of 8–9%[7]. The Indian homeopathic market is estimated at around Rs. 27.58 billion. It is reported that about 50 million people opted for homeopathy in 2006–07 and their number grew to 100–120 million in 2010.[8] According to the administration of the Delhi Government's homeopathy division, 1.36 million patients visited their 82 homeopathic dispensaries in 2006. Their number rose to 1.5–1.6 million patients in the subsequent years 2007 and 2008.[9] The country's leading educational institute, the National Institute of Homeopathy registered over 235,000 patients in the year 2010.[10]

With 230,000 homeopaths India is presently estimated to have the largest number compared to any other country. The homeopathic infrastructure under the Government of India is well established. There are 3,071 hospitals with 9,366 beds, 6,030 dispensaries, 184 colleges with a capacity of 13,385 on undergraduate courses, 1,260 places on postgraduate courses and 398 manufacturers in the country.[11]

Popularity of homeopathy in India

According to J.T.H.J. Dekkers, the popularity of homeopathy in India is high. As a reason he cites: "The principles and philosophy of homeopathy have found fundamental parallels with Indian culture of medicine and existing indigenous therapies, such as Ayurveda". He further states that

Since the 1960s the government has always been a strong supporter of homeopathy. For almost 50 years now, homeopathy is fully recognized, financed, politically embraced, and to a large extent equated with the other medical systems, which makes the position of homeopathy in India unique in the medical world.[12]

However, there could be other reasons such as the cost-effectiveness linked to a huge proportion of the population falling below the poverty line,

---

5   Central Council of Homoeopathy's website: http://cchindia.com/history.htm (last accessed on May 22, 2013).
6   ASSOCHAM (2007; 2011).
7   Confederation of Indian Industry (2012).
8   ASSOCHAM (2007; 2011).
9   Government of NCT of Delhi (2006; 2007; 2008).
10 Eswara Das, Consultant – Homoeopathy, Department of AYUSH, Government of India, his personal communication to the authors about the total number of registered patients in the National Institute of Homoeopathy, Kolkatta in 2010.
11 Department of AYUSH (2010).
12 Dekkers (2009), p. 40.

the choice of homeopathy as an option in their charitable activities by trusts, etc.

Use of Indian Systems of Medicine & Homeopathy (ISM & H)

The use of these systems of medicine has been surveyed in the past. In 1986–87, a survey was conducted by the National Sample Survey Organization (NSSO) on 'Morbidity and Utilization of Medical Services' which indicated that 96% of the sick persons who sought treatment were treated within the allopathic system. The survey also revealed that about 14% of sick persons (18.5% in rural and 11% in urban areas) did not seek any treatment.[13] There was another survey done by the National Council of Applied Economic Research (NCAER) in the early 1990s, covering a comparatively higher proportion of samples from big cities, towns and villages. It revealed that about 8% of illness episodes were treated by the Indigenous Systems of Medicine & Homeopathy (ISM&H).[14]

Later, a detailed survey was conducted by the Institute for Research in Medical Statistics, functioning under the Indian Council of Medical Research, Government of India, which was published in 2005. About 45,000 sick persons from 33,666 households from 35 districts were covered. The preference of ISM&H was about 33% with common ailments, while only 18% preferred to use these systems in case of serious ailments in the country. The proportion of sick persons actually seeking ISM&H treatment was about 14%.[15]

Objective

The popularity of a medical system may vary from time to time. Sometimes it depends on the economic background of the people, place, religion, education, promotion and support by the Government, availability of practitioners, medicine, cost, disease/condition for which the treatment is sought, stage of the disease/condition, scope of the system in a particular disease/condition, popularity of the physician, patients' belief, etc. The trend may vary from urban to rural areas. Furthermore, the decision of the patient to stick to a certain medication depends on his or her trust in the doctor, the overall relief the patient feels from his ailments, the doctor's past experience, his influence in society, etc. In rural areas, the choice of treatment further depends to a large extent on other unique factors like availability, distance, cost-effectiveness, belief (either one's own belief or that of others), etc. Even though the trend may depend on these factors, it is not clear which factor is more important. All the above cited studies have been conducted on both ISM & H. But the trend of

13   National Sample Survey Organization (1986–87).
14   National Council of Applied Economic Research (1993).
15   Singh/Yadav/Pandey (2005).

homeopathy alone and the large potential for ISM&H in India, including the socio-economical status, referrals, educational status, rural and urban, etc have not been surveyed extensively so far. Hence, the authors have decided to carry out a survey to explore patient trends in choosing the homeopathy system in India.

Methodology

Questionnaire

A structured questionnaire was formulated with the objective mentioned above. The questionnaire has 11 closed questions (Appendix 1). It was translated into two native languages to make it easier for the respondents to understand (Appendix 2).

Choosing the survey field and conducting the survey

The randomized survey method was adopted and questionnaires were distributed in 14 homeopathic centers (Appendix 3). To maintain geographical diversity the centers were chosen from different areas and states of the country. The eight places chosen were (i) Asansol (West Bengal), (ii) East Delhi – Mayur Vihar Phase 3, (National Capital Territory of Delhi), (iii) Ghaziabad (Uttar Pradesh), (iv) Noida (Uttar Pradesh), (v) Panchkula (Haryana), (vi) Raipur (Chattisgarh), (vii) Chinna Seeragapadi, District Salem (Tamil Nadu) and (viii) Shegaon (Maharashtra), covering 7 states as can be seen from the information in brackets. It was not only circulated in the top clinics and hospitals, but also in the charitable clinics and Government hospitals where people from low socio-economic background go. Although we tried to maintain a balance between villages and towns, 6 out of 8 centers were located in towns of more than 500,000 inhabitants. Asansol (West Bengal) and Panchkula (Haryana) have almost equal numbers of inhabitants viz. 564,491[16] and 558,890[17] respectively. Whereas East Delhi (1,707,725)[18], Noida (1,674,714)[19] and Raipur (1,010,087)[20] each have a population of over 1 million and Ghaziabad

16   http://en.wikipedia.org/wiki/Asansol (last accessed on May 22, 2013).
17   Census of India 2011, http://www.censusindia.gov.in/2011-prov-results/paper2/data_files/Haryana/8-pop-decadal-15-19.pdf (last accessed on May 22, 2013).
18   Census of India 2011, http://www.censusindia.gov.in/2011-prov-results/paper2/data_files/delhi/Data%20Sheet_%20PPT%20Paper-2_%20NCT%20of%20Delhi.pdf (last accessed on May 22, 2013).
19   Census of India 2011, http://www.censusindia.gov.in/2011-prov-results/paper2/data_files/UP/7-pop-12-22.pdf (last accessed on May 22, 2013).
20   Census of India 2011, http://www.censusindia.gov.in/2011-prov-results/paper2/data_files/India2/Table_2_PR_Cities_1Lakh_and_Above.pdf (last accessed on May 22, 2013).

$(4,661,452)$[21] has over 4 million people. We could not get the population data for the two villages Chinna Seeragapadi in the Salem District and Shegaon in the Buldhana District, since they are smaller villages or towns. The questions were asked while the respondents were waiting either to see the doctor or when they came to collect their medicines. The responses were collected only after obtaining verbal consent from the participants and after it had been explained to them that the survey was confidential.

Results and discussion

The results of the survey are depicted below.

Table 1: Circulated questionnaire and obtained responses

Number of questionnaires circulated	2,500
Number of completed questionnaires	1,822

Chart 1: Male female ratio | n = 1822

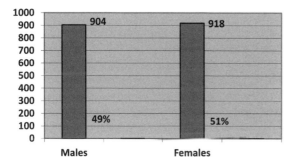

A total of 2,500 individuals participated. 678 incomplete questionnaires were excluded from analysis. From the remaining 1822 participants the male-female ratio is close to equal, i. e. 904 (49%) males and 918 (51%) females (Chart 1). It slightly differs from the country's gender ratio of 48.45% females.[22] But this male-female ratio differs greatly from earlier studies[23], a fact that is discussed in detail under 'Possible biases and limitations' further down in this paper. From the 1,822 participants, 733 (40%) were first time attendants of a homeopathic clinic and 1,089 (60%) were follow-up patients (Chart 2).

21   Census of India 2011, http://www.censusindia.gov.in/2011-prov-results/paper2/data_
     files/ UP/7-pop-12-22.pdf (last accessed on May 22, 2013).
22   Census of India 2011, http://www.censusindia.gov.in/2011-prov-results/paper2/data_
     files/Haryana/8-pop-decadal-15-19.pdf (last accessed on May 22, 2013).
23   Frank (2002); Singh/Singh (2010).

Chart 2: First time vs. follow-up users | n = 1822

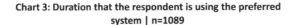

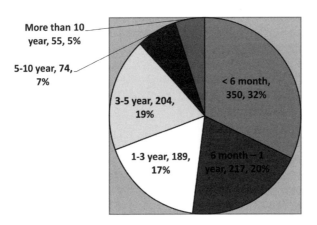

Chart 3: Duration that the respondent is using the preferred system | n=1089

With regard to the time period of using homeopathy, more respondents (350 or 32%) have been using homeopathic treatment for less than 6 months (Chart 3). If we look at all respondents who have been using homeopathy for the last 5 years (less than 6 months + 6 months to 1 year + 1 to 3 years + 3 to 5 years), the cumulative figure comes to 960 (88%). Whereas only 129 or 12% of respondents have been using homeopathy for more than 5 years. This indicates that more new users have come to homeopathy in the last 5 years. The finding roughly corresponds to the data of two reports published by ASSOCHAM[24] in 2006–07 and 2009–10 as reported above. According to these reports 40 to 50 million people opted for homeopathy in 2006–07 and 100–120 million in 2009–10, which corresponds to a 100% growth in the usage over 3 years.

---

24 ASSOCHAM (2007; 2011).

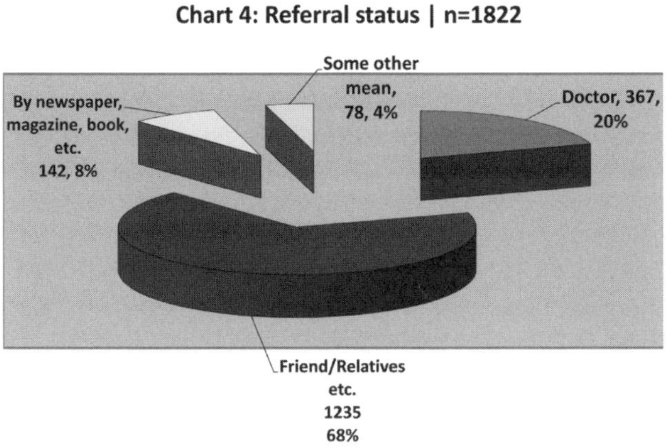

Chart 4: Referral status | n=1822

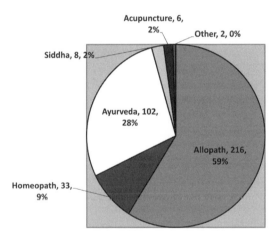

Some other
mean,
78, 4%

By newspaper,
magazine, book,
etc.
142, 8%

Doctor, 367,
20%

Friend/Relatives
etc.
1235
68%

Chart 5: Referred by type of doctor | n=367

Acupuncture, 6,
2%

Other, 2, 0%

Siddha, 8, 2%

Ayurveda, 102,
28%

Allopath, 216,
59%

Homeopath, 33,
9%

Among the first-time users, the majority (1235, 68 %) were referred by friends and relatives (Chart 4). It is a well-known fact in medical sociology that reference by the people who have experienced a treatment has more influence than others. This survey supports this fact. A significant number (367, 21 %) of respondents were referred by doctors. This is in contrast to the belief of most homeopaths, who think their patients have not been referred by their professional colleagues. Only a very few (142 8 %) respondents found out about homeopathy through newspapers, magazines, books and other printed media.

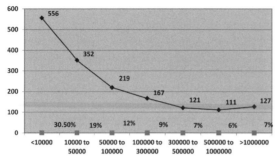

Chart 6: Economic background | Income in Rupees per annum | n=1653*

*169 children and housewives who do not know their family income were not included.

In this survey, the majority of doctor referrals (216, 59%) are from allopaths, followed by a significant number (102 or 28%) from Ayurvedic practitioners (Chart 5). It is interesting to note that there are cross referrals also between homeopaths (33 or 9%).

While the questionnaires were sorted and the incomplete ones excluded, a small number of responses (from children and housewives who did not know the family income and did not respond to the question regarding their economic background) were not treated as incomplete and hence included. They were however excluded from analysis of economic background. The total number of respondents who have given their economic status is 1,653. The graph shows clearly that, as the income rises the number of users goes down (Chart 6). Around 30% of users are from the very low income bracket. The pattern shown in this graph differs from the report by Padam Singh et al.[25], where a higher preference was seen in both lower and higher income groups for common ailments, and a step-ladder pattern for serious ailments. The majority of the centers selected for this randomized survey are towns, but not the metropolitan cities. The average income of the individuals in these cities is usually lower. The fact that the high income group is generally low in these populations is reflected in this survey too.

25   Singh/Yadav/Pandey (2005).

Chart 7: Educational qualification | n=1822

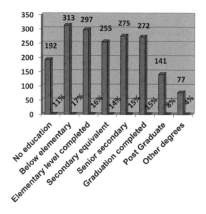

All in all there are fewer users of homeopathy among educated people (Chart 7). This is not astonishing as their number in the total population is low. The number of users of homeopathy is also significantly lower in the 'no education' category. According to Padam Singh et al.[26], the pattern initially goes down and then rises, clearly showing the higher usage of homeopathy among the educated.

Chart 8: Rural vs. urban area | n=822

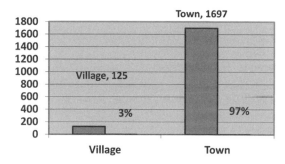

125 (3%) respondents participating in this survey are from villages and 1697 (97%) are from towns (Chart 8). This reflects the fact that the survey has been conducted mostly in the larger towns, as mentioned earlier.

Possible biases and limitations

As stated earlier, the gender ratio hugely differs from the previous studies. It is possible that in this randomized trial, the questionnaires were distributed alternately to male and female, perhaps unconsciously. Since it was conducted

26 Singh/Yadav/Pandey (2005).

on a limited sample and within a limited time period, it is not possible to come to a gender-based conclusion regarding preference of the system.

It is possible that the first time users are slightly over-represented (40%). While conducting the survey, the follow-up patients who had already participated in the survey were not allowed to participate a second time. As a result of this the number of new users might have gone up.

There is a remarkable gap between village and town respondents. As mentioned above, 6 out of 8 places were towns or cities with populations of more than 500,000. There might be another element that further pushed up the town figures. A person who migrated from a village for a brief period (usually this happens after the crops have been harvested) might have claimed to come from a town.

Although we collected more data viz. (i) specific condition for which the respondent has been treated, (ii) religion and (iii) opinion about the system, we chose not to include them in our results, the reason being that the vast number of diseases and opinions given by people made it difficult to quantify and tabulate the responses in a simple manner within the time allocated for analysing the survey.

Conclusion

This survey has shown that almost equal numbers of male and female (49% and 51%) persons seek homeopathy in the centers surveyed. From the 60% of follow-up cases, 88% of the population have sought homeopathic treatment in the last 5 years and 12% of people have used it for more than 5 years. The majority (68%) of patients using the homeopathic system of medicine has been referred by friends and relatives, followed by 21% of patients who have been referred by physicians. A majority of doctor referrals (59%) are from allopaths, followed by ayurvedic physicians (28%). Around 30% of people seeking homeopathy have a poor economic background and only 13% are from the middle or upper class. In this randomized trial there is a slight decrease in the usage of homeopathy among educated people, especially degree-holders over the time period under consideration.

Acknowledgement

The authors thank Dr Eshwara Das, consulting Homeopath for his information and guidance. The authors also thank Mrs. Priti Gupta for her assistance in sorting and analyzing the data. The authors are grateful to Dr. Saurav Arora for his support in making the manuscript and thank Miss. Pooja Rajagopal, Ms. Rituparna Mukherjee and Miss. Vineeta Verma for their help with data entry. The authors are indebted to all the homeopathic centers (Appendix 3) who consented to take part in this survey.

Conflict of interest

The authors declare that there is no conflict of interest in this study. The survey was funded by the authors.

Bibliography

Internet Links

http://en.wikipedia.org/wiki/Asansol (last accessed on May 22, 2013)
http://cchindia.com/history.htm (last accessed in May 22, 2013)
http://censusindia.gov.in/2011census/censusinfodashboard/index.html (last accessed on May 22, 2013)
http://www.censusindia.gov.in/2011-prov-results/paper2/data_files/Haryana/8-pop-decadal-15-19.pdf (last accessed on May 22, 2013)
http://www.censusindia.gov.in/2011-prov-results/paper2/data_files/delhi/Data%20Sheet_%20PPT%20Paper-2_%20NCT%20of%20Delhi.pdf (last accessed on May 22, 2013)
http://www.censusindia.gov.in/2011-prov-results/paper2/data_files/UP/7-pop-12-22.pdf (last accessed on May 22, 2013)
http://www.censusindia.gov.in/2011-prov-results/paper2/data_files/India2/Table_2_PR_Cities_1Lakh_and_Above.pdf (last accessed on May 22, 2013)
http://www.censusindia.gov.in/2011-prov-results/paper2/data_files/UP/7-pop-12-22.pdf (last accessed on May 22, 2013)
http://www.censusindia.gov.in/2011-prov-results/paper2/data_files/Haryana/8-pop-decadal-15-19.pdf (last accessed on May 22, 2013)

Literature

ASSOCHAM: Homeopathy Emerging With Big Bang, Likely To Be Rs. 26 Billion Industry: A Press Release by The Associated Chambers of Commerce and Industry in India, Sunday, December 09, 2007.
ASSOCHAM: Homeopathy Industry Likely to be Rs. 4,600 cr. by 2012: Press Release by Associated Chambers of Commerce and Industry in India, Friday, March 18, 2011.
Broom, Alex; Doron, Assa; Tovey, Philip: The inequalities of medical pluralism: Hierarchies of health, the politics of tradition and the economies of care in Indian oncology. In: Social Science & Medicine 69 (2009), no. 5, pp. 698–706.
Confederation of Indian Industry: A Brief Report on Pharmaceutical Industry in India, March 2012, URL: http://www.cci.in/pdf/surveys_reports/Pharmaceutical-Industry-in-India.pdf (last accessed on May 22, 2013).
Das, Eswara: History and Status of Homeopathy around the World. New Delhi 2005.
Dekkers, Joris Theodorus Hubertus Johannes: What about homeopathy? A comparative investigation into the causes of current popularity of homeopathy in The USA, The UK, India and The Netherlands, URL: http://igitur-archive.library.uu.nl/student-theses/2009–0917–200223/ScriptieJorisDekkers.pdf (last accessed on May 22, 2013).
Department of AYUSH: AYUSH in India – 2010, Section 1, Summary Of All-India Ayush Infrastructure Facilities, Planning & Evaluation Cell, Department of Ayurveda, Yoga & Naturopathy, Unani, Siddha and Homeopathy (AYUSH), Ministry of Health and Family Welfare, Government of India.
Dinges, Martin (ed.): Weltgeschichte der Homöopathie. Länder – Schulen – Heilkundige. Munich 1996.

Frank, R.: Homoeopath and patient – a dyad of harmony. In: Social Science & Medicine 55 (2002), no. 8, pp. 1285–1296.

Government of NCT of Delhi: Delhi Homeopathic Anusandhan Parishad. Yearly Report – Year 2006, URL: http://delhihomeo.com/y2006.htm (last accessed on May 22, 2013).

Government of NCT of Delhi: Delhi Homeopathic Anusandhan Parishad. Yearly Report – Year 2007, URL: http://delhihomeo.com/y2007.htm (last accessed on May 22, 2013).

Government of NCT of Delhi: Delhi Homeopathic Anusandhan Parishad. Yearly Report – Year 2008, URL: http://delhihomeo.com/y2008.htm (last accessed on May 22, 2013).

National Council of Applied Economic Research: Household Survey of Health Care Utilization and Expenditure. New Delhi 1993.

National Sample Survey Organization: Morbidity and Utilization of Medical Services (42nd round). New Delhi 1986–87.

Poldas, Samuel Vijaya Bhaskar: Geschichte der Homöopathie in Indien: von ihrer Einführung bis zur ersten offiziellen Anerkennung 1937. Stuttgart 2010.

Singh, Chandra Mandal; Singh, Subhas: Recent criticism on homoeopathy: retrospection. In: Bulletin of the National Institute of Homeopathy 13 (2010), pp. 157–160.

Singh, Padam; Yadav, R.J.; Pandey, Arvind: Utilization of indigenous systems of medicine & homeopathy in India. In: Indian Journal of Medical Research 122 (August 2005), pp 137–142.

Appendix 1: Questionnaire in English

A Survey for Institute for the History of Medicine of the Robert Bosch Foundation, Germany

Centre/clinic/doctor's name _ _ _ _ _ _ _ _ _

Patient's Gender:

Age:

1. Are you a first time user of this system of medicine?
   - ☐ a. Yes
   - ☐ b. No

2. If not, how long are you using this system?
   - ☐ a. < 6 months
   - ☐ b. 6 months to 1 year
   - ☐ c. 1 year to 3 years
   - ☐ d. 3 years to 5 years
   - ☐ e. 5 years to 10 years
   - ☐ f. > 10 years

3. If you are a first time user, who had referred or how did you come to know about this system?
   - ☐ a. A doctor
   - ☐ b. A friend or relative of mine
   - ☐ c. Came to know through a magazine, newspaper, book, internet, etc.
   - ☐ d. Any other; please specify _ _ _ _ _
   _ _ _ _ _ _ _ _ _ _

4. If a doctor has referred then, is he from the same system or other system of medicine?
   - ☐ a. Same system. Mention the name of the system _ _ _ _ _ _ _ _ _ _ _ _ _ _ _ _
   - ☐ b. Other system

5. If other system means the doctor is from which system of medicine?
   - ☐ a. Allopathy
   - ☐ b. Ayurveda
   - ☐ c. Siddha
   - ☐ d. Acupuncture
   - ☐ e. Etc. Please specify _ _ _ _ _ _ _ _
   _ _ _ _ _ _ _

6. Kindly specify your annual income (it will not be disclosed)
   - ☐ a. < ₹ 10,000
   - ☐ b. ₹ 10,000 to 50,000
   - ☐ c. ₹ 50,000 to 100,000
   - ☐ d. ₹ 100,000 to 300,000
   - ☐ e. ₹ 300,000 to 500,000
   - ☐ f. ₹ 500,000 to 1,000,000
   - ☐ g. > ₹ 1,000,000

7. Please specify your educational background
   - ☐ a. No school education
   - ☐ b. Below elementary level school (4th class)
   - ☐ c. Elementary school completed (5th class)
   - ☐ d. SSLC (10th class or equivalent) completed
   - ☐ e. 12th class completed
   - ☐ f. Graduate
   - ☐ g. Post graduate
   - ☐ h. Other degrees or qualification (M. Phil, IAS, etc.), please specify _ _ _ _ _ _ _ _
   _ _ _ _ _ _ _ _ _ _ _ _ _ _

8. Please specify your disease or condition for which you are seeking treatment

9. Place
   a. Village/town/city: mention appropriately
      i. Village _ _ _ _ _ _ _ _ _ _ _
      _ _ _ _
      ii. Town _ _ _ _ _ _ _ _ _ _ _
      _ _ _
      iii. City _ _ _ _ _ _ _ _ _ _ _ _
      _ _
   b. Taluk _ _ _ _ _ _ _ _ _ _ _ _ _ _ _
   c. District _ _ _ _ _ _ _ _ _ _ _ _ _ _ _
   d. State _ _ _ _ _ _ _ _ _ _ _ _ _ _ _

10. Religion _ _ _ _ _ _ _ _ _ _ _ _ _ _ _

11. What is your opinion towards this system of medicine?

Appendix 2: Questionnaire in Tamil (same has been distributed in Hindi)

மருத்துவ முறை உபயோகம் தொடர்பான சர்வே

நோயாளியின் பாலினம்:_____ வயது:_____

தயவு செய்து கீழே டிக் (✔) செய்யவும்

1. நீங்கள் இந்த மருத்துவ முறையை முதல் முறை உபயோகிப்பவரா?
□ ஆம் □ இல்லை

2. நீண்ட நாளாக உபயோகிப்பவரென்றால் எவ்வளவு காலமாக உபயோகிக்கிறீர்கள்
□ 6 மாதத்திற்கும் குறைவு □ 6 மாதம் முதல் ஒரு வருடம் □ ஒரு வருடம் முதல் மூன்று வருடம்
□ மூன்று வருடம் முதல் 5 வருடம் □ 5 வருடம் முதல் பத்து வருடம் □ பத்து வருடத்திற்கு மேல்

3. நீங்கள் முதல் முறை உபயோகிப்பவரென்றல் உங்களை இந்த மருத்துவ முறையை
உபயோகிக்க பரிந்துரை செய்தவர் யார்? அல்லது உங்களுக்கு எவ்வாறு இந்த மருத்துவ
முறையைப் பற்றி தெரிய வந்தது?
□ வேறொரு மருத்துவ முறை மருத்துவர் □ நண்பர் (அ) உறவினர் □ செய்தித்தாள், புத்தகம், வார
மாத இதழ்கள், இணையம் வாயிலாக □ வேறு வகையில் தெரிய வந்தது (தயவு செய்து
குறிப்பிடவும்) _____

4. வேறொரு மருத்துவர் பரிந்துரைத்தது இருந்தால் அவர் எந்த மருத்துவ முறையைச் சார்ந்தவர்?
□ ஹோமியோபதி □ அலோபதி □ யுனானி □ சித்தா □ அக்குபஞ்சர் □ வேறு மருத்துவம் (தயவு செய்து
குறிப்பிடவும்) _____

5. உங்களின் ஆண்டு வருமானத்தை தயவு செய்து குறிப்பிடவும் (இவ்விவரம் இரகசியமாக
வைக்கப்படும்)
□ பத்தாயிரத்திற்கும் குறைவு □ பத்தாயிரம் முதல் ஐம்பதாயிரம் □ ஐம்பதாயிரம் முதல் ஒரு
லட்சம்
□ ஒரு லட்சம் முதல் மூன்று லட்சம் □ மூன்று லட்சம் முதல் ஐந்து லட்சம் □ ஐந்து லட்சம் முதல்
பத்து லட்சம்
□ பத்து லட்சத்திற்கு மேல்

6. உங்கள் கல்வித்தகுதி:
□ பளளிக்கல்வி அறவே கிடையாது □ துவக்கப்பள்ளிக்கும் குறைவு □ துவக்கப்பள்ளி □ எஸ் எஸ்
எல் சி
□ பன்னிரண்டாவது □ இளநிலை பட்டம் □ முதுநிலை பட்டம் □ மற்றவை (எம் பில், பி ஹெச் டி, இ
அ எஸ். இன்னபிற. தயவு செய்து குறிப்பிடவும்) _____

7. உங்கள் நோயை பற்றிய விவரம் (symptom/diagnosis)

8. உங்கள் ஊர்
கிராமம்/நகரம்/பெருநகரம் _____
வட்டம்/தாலுக்கா _____
மாவட்டம் _____
மாநிலம் _____

9. மதம் _____

10. இந்த மருத்துவ துறையைப் பற்றி உங்கள் கருத்து (தேவையெனில் பின் பக்கம்

உபயோகிக்கவும்)

Appendix 3: List of homeopathic centers/doctors chosen for the survey

1. Banerjee Homeopathic Clinic, Asansol, West Bengal.
2. Central Research Institute, Central Council for Research in Homoeopathy, Noida, Uttar Pradesh
3. Dr Ajay Gajender's clinic, Raipur, Chhattisgarh
4. Dr Arvind Pandey's clinic, Mayur Vihar 3, East Delhi
5. Dr Morkhade's clinic, Shegaon, District Buldana, Maharashtra
6. Dr Pankaj Chandna's clinic, Punchkula, Haryana
7. Dr Prem Lal Sau's clinic, Raipur, Chhattisgarh
8. Dr Sunil Sau's clinic, Raipur, Chhattisgarh
9. Dr Vivekananda's Vision, Ghaziabad and Noida
10. Gurdwara charity clinic, Noida, Uttar Pradesh
11. Mn Homoeo Clinic, Ghaziabad, Uttar Pradesh
12. Noida Homoeopathic Medical Association's free camp, Noida, Uttar Pradesh
13. Sai Dharmarth Chikitsalaya, Noida, Uttar Pradesh
14. Vinayaka Mission's Homeopathic Medical College Hospital, Chinna Seeragapadi, and its 10 rural peripheral centers around Salem, Tamil Nadu

Medical Pluralism and the Patients' Perspective in Germany – Letters to "Natur und Medizin" (1992–2000)

Philipp Eisele

Introduction

In post-war Germany the efficiency and competency of Biomedicine seemed to be unlimited. Incredible technical and scientific progress raised the expectation that it – sooner or later – could cope with any disease and the finding of adequate cures was just a question of time. Today, this former optimism has at least partly disappeared and has been substituted by harsh criticism and decreasing acceptance triggered by the publicly debated negative side-effects, the impersonality of its machine-based treatments, its lack of a more holistic approach towards the human body, and its high costs.[1] Today it seems that orthodox medicine has – at least to some extent – failed to fulfil the changing and sometimes ambitious needs of the modern patient who suffers from a shifting spectrum of illness dominated by chronic diseases.[2]

Simultaneously, the use of CAM (Complementary and Alternative Medicine) among German patients has grown rapidly during the past decades.[3] Although BM (Biomedicine) still dominates the medical market, its hegemonic position is challenged and questioned by various therapeutic systems which have their own concepts of health, illness and healing.[4] An increasing number of dissatisfied patients turn to them in search of better or more adequate treatment. This "silent revolution"[5] in the patients' behaviour has led to a pluralisation and fragmentation of the medical market, where today both, academically and not-academically trained care-givers eagerly offer a large scope of different forms of CAM.[6]

---

1   In historical terms this criticism is not a novel phenomenon. But with regard to its intensity that has increased enormously since the 1970s one might argue that on the one hand today's healthcare system suffers from more serious problems of acceptance than in the 1950s and 1960s. On the other hand this criticism might indicate that the healthcare system is undergoing a period of transition. Cf. Dinges (1996), p. 8.
2   For an overview of the ongoing discussions about the recent changes in the wide field of medicine see the contributions in Schäfer et al. (2008); Michl/Potthast/Wiesing (2008).
3   Although there is a lack of exact numbers concerning the use of CAM among German patients, an increasing demand can be attested. Cf. Willich et al. (2004), p. 1314; Stange/Amhof/Moebus (2006), pp. 209–210. For the increasing use of CAM in Germany and other Western countries cf. Maddalena (2005), pp. 18–23. Taking into account Homeopathy for example, Martin Dinges has also shown a growing demand among patients in Germany and other countries since the 1970s. Cf. Dinges (forthcoming).
4   Cf. Wiesing (2008), p. 459.
5   Dinges (1996), p. 7.
6   In comparison to earlier forms of the phenomenon of 'medical pluralism' the sociologists Sarah Cant and Ursula Sharma define the specific form, which has been emerging since the late twentieth century, as a 'new medical Pluralism'. Some of its key features are:

While the discussion[7] whether to refuse or integrate these therapies into the public healthcare system continues, most patients have recognized that the choice of how to preserve and restore health is their own responsibility.[8] As a consequence, demand for the respective information and advice has grown enormously.[9] Therefore, a multitudinous number of literature dealing with health and illness on the one hand and an increasing quantity of support groups and patients' organisations often sponsored by medical insurance companies, pharmaceutical industries, local authorities and charitable institutions on the other hand are available to patients.[10]

In this context the independent patient organisation "Natur und Medizin e. V." (VNM)[11] provides professional assistance to their more than 30,000 members by academically trained care-givers. Considering, integrating and combining both BM and CAM, it is the announced aim of the organisation to create more transparency concerning the patient's possibilities of choice – especially with reference to homeopathy and naturopathy. Besides offering public lectures, organizing special events and publishing its own members' magazine[12] and other health-related literature, VNM explicitly invites its members to turn to its academically trained health experts with their personal health-related questions. Hence numerous requests by people seeking advice for the optimal treatment of their individual illness are answered every year. Those requests have been partly handed over to the Institute for the History of Medicine of the Robert Bosch Foundation.[13]

Expressing the patients' demands, experiences, judgements, believes and expectations – in the context of the German health system in general and of CAM in particular – these letters allow access to a critical understanding of today's medical care. Analysing them can not only enrich the ongoing discus-

---

"[T]he diversity to which it refers is highly structured. The ways in which this structuring is achieved varies locally, but is not determined entirely by pure market conditions [...]. It is a pluralism in which biomedicine still has a dominant position and still plays a mayor part in the process by which different therapies are accorded different degrees of legitimacy and prestige. [...] Outside the biomedical clinic alternative therapists compete with each other and with the service of biomedical doctors for the patronage of an increasingly sophisticated and consumerist clientele". Cant/Sharma (1999), p. 195.

7   For the current discussion cf. the contributions in Becker et al. (2010); Schweiger (2003); Maddalena (2005).

8   Cf. Coulter/Magee (2004), p. 248.

9   Cf. Coulter/Magee (2004), pp. 245–246.

10 The number of support groups has grown enormously since the 1980s. Cf. Kofahl/ Nickel/Trojan (2011), p. 70.

11 For the following information about this organization cf. "Natur und Medizin e. V.", Pressemappe, http://www.naturundmedizin.de/wuu/presse/NaturundMedizin_Presskit.pdf (last accessed on May 22, 2013).

12 The members' magazine is published six times a year and deals with health-related issues, mainly with homeopathy and naturopathy.

13 The letters written to "Natur und Medizin" between 1992 and 2000 are stored at the Institute for the History of Medicine of the Robert Bosch Foundation in Stuttgart under the signature VNM.

sions about integrating or refusing complementary medicine into the public healthcare system, but can also help to draw attention again to the most important – but often neglected – factor of the debate: the patient himself.

Approaching the patient's perspective this essay will take three steps. First of all it will provide a short overview of the current state of research on patient's demand in Germany. Secondly, it will focus on the letters, outlining the socio-structural features of its authors, the reasons for writing and the spectrum of illnesses the patients suffer from. Thirdly and finally with regard to the claim of the 'informed patient'[14], this essay will examine the way patients gather information about health-related matters. Furthermore, it will not only try to present an attempt of classifying the different types of CAM-users, which can be distinguished in the letters to VNM, but also summarise the attitudes towards and experiences with both BM and CAM.

It is important to note that this essay is an extract of an ongoing PhD project. Therefore, its results have only provisional character.

Current State of Research on Patient Demand

There are only a few studies about the usage of CAM among German patients. However, concerning the recent research work, a growing interest can be attested, but most of those studies are restricted to the question of acceptance, degree of popularity and the market of CAM. For instance, the Allensbach Institute for Public Opinion Research conducted a survey in 2009 about the popularity, use and reputation of Homeopathy.[15] It showed that more than half of the German adults have already tried this therapy and that the total number of users has increased enormously during the last decades. Such studies surely have their credits, but often neglect the individual expectations, experiences, motivations and behaviours of patients using CAM.

In this chapter I will present and discuss three studies that have dealt with these psychosocial components, done by Leonhard in the 1980s, Günther in the 1990s and Köntopp in 2004.[16] Approaching the complex and comprehensive subject of the patient's perspective all three scholars use methods taken from Social Sciences, namely conducting interviews and distributing questionnaires. Leonard and Köntopp solely concentrate on patients who use or have used CAM, whereas Günther also takes patients into account who were treated exclusively in a conventional way. Although their methods concerning the structure and evaluation of their conducted interviews and questionnaires as well as their epistemological interests differed, their final results show a strik-

14 For a discussion about the claim of the 'informed patient' cf. the contributions in Klusen/Fließgarten/Nebling (2009).
15 Cf. Allensbacher Berichte 2009, Nr. 14, "Homöopathische Arzneimittel in Deutschland: Verbreitet genutzt und geschätzt", URL: http://www.ifd-allensbach.de/uploads/tx_reportsndocs/prd_0914.pdf (last accessed on May 22, 2013).
16 Leonhard (1984); Günther (1999); Köntopp (2004).

ing congruence: More women than men use CAM. Its users feature a higher level of education and financial status in comparison to the average German citizen and the individually chosen CAM therapy corresponds to their personal life-style. They appreciate CAM, because of its little side-effects, gentle mode of action and holistic approach. Furthermore, they are convinced that those therapies are effective. Putting emphasis on a positive and patient-oriented relationship between therapist and patient and showing a higher level of compliance are also common features. Finally, CAM users can be characterised by leading a healthier lifestyle in comparison to BM users and by drawing on their social environment in case of health-related questions.[17]

The three studies highlight different aspects among CAM users that the authors considered to be significant. Leonard points out that greater confidence towards non-academically trained care-givers can only be attested when the confidence towards academic health care professionals is slight.[18] He suggests that a possible motive for patients to turn to a non-medical practitioner is triggered by exactly this lack of confidence in physicians. In her summary Günther underlines that dissatisfaction and negative experiences with BM can be seen as the main reasons that make patients start a homeopathic therapy.[19] But holding on to it mainly results in good supervision by the homeopathic physician, a strong belief in its effectiveness, the therapy's equivalence with the patient's own attitudes towards life and finally in greater self-responsibility during the cure.[20] Lastly, Köntopp emphasises the possibility of self-medication. She suggests that the aspects of saving money and time as well as a reticence towards professional medical treatment motivate patients to help themselves rather than visit a physician.[21]

Considering the results of these three publications, one may ask what contribution or new results to this field of research can be provided by an analysis of letters written by patients seeking medical advice from an organisation that supports CAM. The contribution of such analysis is based only to a small extent on the application of new methods and approaches, but rather on the novel and broader perspective on the research subject. This chance is provided by letters as a historical source.[22] In comparison to more or less standardized interviews and questionnaires – often including multiple-choice elements – letters from patients offer abundant information to the historian about their health behaviour in everyday life, their illness perceptions, the way they

17   It should be mentioned that the fact of drawing back on one's social environment in case of health related questions is a common feature of all patients, no matter whether they prefer CAM or BM. Cf. Faltermeier (1994), pp. 151–152.
      The question whether or to what extent the behaviours of CAM users and BM users differ has not been answered yet.
18   Cf. Leonhard (1984), p. 185.
19   Cf. Günther (1999), p. 134.
20   Cf. Günther (1999), p. 134.
21   Cf. Köntopp (2004), p. 283.
22   For the value of letters to the history of medicine cf. for example Dinges/Barras (2007); Schnalke (1997), pp. 13–22; Eckart/Jütte (2007), p. 184; Schweig (2009), pp. 35–36.

choose or neglect different therapies and therapists, their relationship to people who treated them and so on.[23] Since the letters are creative products of individuals, their value is not restricted to answering standardized questions of the researcher, but allows insights into the patient's mind on a much deeper level that goes beyond any standardization. Every letter is the product of a lived experience and an attempted interpretation that contains a large number of aspects that require different approaches from the researcher. Therefore, each letter may present new aspects to the researcher that force him or her to return to the perspective of the individual – the patient.[24]

The Letters of 1992, 1996 and 2000

Content

Although the organisation VNM was already founded in 1983, only letters written between 1992 and 2000 are stored at the IGM. Their exact number can only be estimated, but with regard to my own research more that 25,000 letters are archived. For this essay around 20% of the correspondence written during the years 1992, 1996 and 2000 was selected.[25] Thus, 1,655 letters were used for this analysis, but a majority of them only covered non-medical aspects.

Letters	Number
without medical aspects	$1,143 = 69\%$
with medical aspects	$512 = 31\%$
total	**$1,655 = 100\%$**

Letters that were summarized under the category "without medical aspects" mostly deal with administrative issues or orders of literature published by the organisation. Consequently, with regard to the epistemological interest of this essay, those letters have no significance and have been excluded from the following investigations.

The character of those letters containing medical aspects shows striking diversity with regard to length, manner of writing and the type of request.

---

23 Cf. Dinges/Barras (2007), p. 12.
24 As an extract of an ongoing Ph. D. thesis this essay will primarily present and discuss statistical evaluations.
25 The letters are stored chronologically according to year as well as alphabetically according to the initials of the authors' family names. To create a 20% sample, letters written by people whose names start with *B, O, R* or *T* were selected, because around 20% of German names start with one of those initials. Cf. Statistisches Bundesamt (1977), p. 451. More recently, this relative frequency of family names' initials has also been verified for North Rhine-Westphalia – the most populous federal state of Germany. Cf. Reinders (1996), pp. 652–653. A more recent survey for Germany as a whole does not exist.

Some writers describe their concerns within only a few lines, whereas others need several pages. Moreover, the correspondence is often not factually but emotionally formulated. This fact reveals that many writers did not regard VNM solely as an information centre, but as a trustworthy organisation that could also provide comfort, relief and understanding for their individual problems. In this context the chairwoman of VNM at that time – Dr. Veronica Carstens (1923–2012)[26] – played a special role. She was not only an academically trained physician, but also the wife of Karl Carstens (1914–1992)[27], the former President of the Federal Republic of Germany. Due to her reputation and profession the writers trusted her, relied on her power of judgement and therefore articulated themselves with remarkable forthrightness. She was not only regarded as an adviser but also as a substitute for a real physician. Thus, many letters were written directly to her – sometimes even with the remark 'confidential' – and often contained statements of admiration or even adoration.

Furthermore, the letters do not exclusively deal with medical requests. Many writers used this communication medium to disclose their individual experiences – positive as well as negative – in the context of health and illness.

To demonstrate the various aspects of the letters of the sample used here, the reasons for writing were counted and analysed. Many letters contain more than one reason for writing and all of them have been counted equally. Therefore, the total number of reasons (n) exceeds the number of letters.

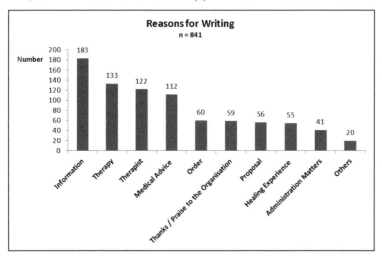

Number of letters including statements: 512

26 For a short biography cf. http://www.bundespraesident.de/DE/Die-Bundespraesidenten/ Karl-Carstens/Veronica-Carstens/veronica-carstens-node.html (last accessed on May 22, 2013).
27 For a short biography cf. http://www.bundespraesident.de/DE/Die-Bundespraesidenten/ Karl-Carstens/karl-carstens-node.html (last accessed on May 22, 2013).

Some categories need further explanation: The chart above also includes reasons for writing that cover non-medical aspects, because people turning to VNM with health related questions often also used their letters to order literature or to clarify administration matters. Furthermore, some letters that were written for non-medical reasons – e.g. cancelation of or application for membership – also contain valuable information about people's health and illness behaviour. Therefore, this letters have also been included in the sample.

As can be seen from the chart, most writers requested general information. For instance, they asked for the mode of action of special medical devices, for suppliers of pharmaceuticals or for information about topics like electromagnetic pollution or heavy-metal-pollution. Under the category of "Therapy" those requests were subsumed that asked what methods of treatments were available or adequate for the patients' specific disease patterns. Requests categorised under 'Therapist' searched for a suitable care-giver that either could offer a distinct treatment or could handle or cure distinct illnesses. Patients who asked for 'medical advice' had precise questions concerning their health and illness, like for instance about the use of a distinct therapy for a distinct illness or the exact dosage of a drug.

The patients' interest covered a wide spectrum of different therapies and therapists who offer them. The spectrum ranges from Ayurveda to Zilgrei[28], whereas Homoeopathy and Naturopathy were the most requested treatments.

Supposing that patients asking for a distinct therapy or a distinct therapist possessed previous knowledge of the method of treatment, it is interesting to note that many patients had no or only a sketchy idea of the treatment or therapist they wanted. Some common requests generally asked for 'possible therapies', for 'alternative therapies', for 'holistic therapies', for 'natural therapies', for 'therapies without surgery and chemistry' or for 'physicians who treat their patients in the sense of VNM'. The mayor part of those patients asking for a suitable therapist demanded an academically trained care-giver. Furthermore, the patients' questions were not restricted to CAM. Some even wished for the recommendation or explanation of therapies belonging to BM.

Socio-Structural Features

This chapter will focus on the provenience of the writers, their gender, age and their spectrum of illnesses. Statements about education levels and professions cannot be made because this information was only revealed in a few cases.

To get information about regional differences, the next chart illustrates the total number of the writers' origins according to the sixteen Federal States of

---

28 Zilgrei is an exercise therapy developed by the German orthopedist and chiropractor Hans Greissing and his Italian patient Adriana Zillo in 1978. It is applied for self-treatment or prevention of muscle pain, joint pain and neuralgia. Cf. Zilgrei (2008).

Germany in proportion to their number of inhabitants.[29] For reasons of clarity and comprehensibility each proportion is presented with the help of the 'alpha-factor'. This factor is calculated by dividing the number of letters per Federal State by the number of its inhabitants and then multiplied by 1,000,000.

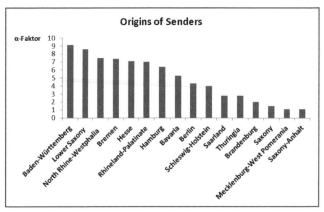

Number of letters used: 499

Although it can be clearly shown that the service of VNM with its office in Bonn – North Rhine-Westphalia – was used throughout Germany, the proportion of writers to the number of inhabitants per each federal state varies enormously. Letters from federal states[30] situated in the territory of the former German Democratic Republic are significantly underrepresented. This can be explained by the fact that the work of VNM had been restricted to West Germany until the reunification in 1990. Moreover, – as shown by recent research into homeopathy[31] – CAM in the Soviet Occupation Zone and in the GDR was constrained by the government and academic circles there. As a consequence the popularity and the use of CAM in the newly formed German States were – in comparison to the old West German States – less common.[32] This aspect was also expressed in the letters to VNM: "How can one get hold of the naturopathic method you propagate, especially here in the East?"[33]

29 Five letters from abroad and eight letters of unknown origin have been excluded. Due to the fact that the number of inhabitants of each Federal State varied between 1992 and 2000, the figures for 1996 – marking the middle of the investigation period – were used. They are provided by Statistisches Jahrbuch (1998), p. 46.

30 The following five German federal states are situated on the territory of the former German Democratic Republic: Thuringia, Brandenburg, Saxony, Mecklenburg-West Pomerania, Saxony Anhalt.

31 Cf. Nierade (2012).

32 Cf. Nierade (2012), pp. 168–172.

33 "Wie kann ein Mensch, besonders hier im Osten, der von Ihnen propagierten Naturheilmethode teilhaft werden". IGM, VNM 10, Mrs V. R., 12.09.1992.

A valid und comprehensive explanation for the varying proportion of writers in the remaining federal states has not been found yet, but will be elaborated in the further course of the research project. Thereby, the level of awareness of VNM among the inhabitants of the different federal states, as well as the density of the respective medical network according to the availability of both academically trained and non-academically trained caregivers should be taken into account. Further subdivision of the writers' origins into smaller regional units will therefore be necessary.

Providing exact information about the age-structure is difficult, because only a minor part of the writers indicated their age.[34] In some cases the age could be reconstructed with the help of medical reports included in the letters. According to both, the information given by writers and medical reports, the vast majority of writers was 60 years or older. This may be due to the fact that people of pensionable age simply have more time to write letters than members of the working population. Furthermore, they are less mobile than younger people and might prefer to seek medical advice by letter instead of visiting a BM or CAM practitioner. Moreover, the 'elderly' as opposed to the 'younger' people are more frequently affected by chronic or degenerative illnesses that BM cannot cure but only alleviate.

It this context an analysis of the illnesses mentioned in the letters to VNM is required. The following chart illustrates the distribution of illnesses mentioned.[35] Some letters contain more than one illness. Therefore the total number of illnesses (n) exceeds the number of relevant letters.

---

34 Only 94 letters (around 18% of the sample) provide detailed information about the writers' age.

35 The spectrum of illness is presented by reference to the ICD-10 main categories. Cf. http://www.dimdi.de/static/de/klassi/icd-10-who/kodesuche/onlinefassungen/htmlamtl 2013/index.htm (last accessed on May 22, 2013). Statements about prevention and aftercare have been excluded.

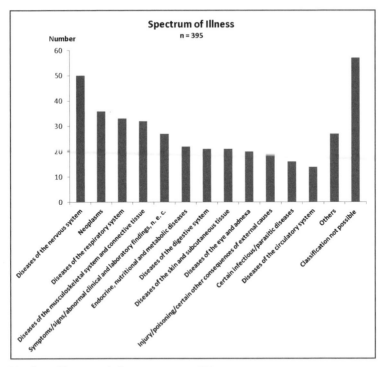

Number of letters including statements: 290

The spectrum of illnesses patients suffered from covers the whole range from mild to severe disorders. The majority of illnesses were chronic and had lasted for at least one year. Specific diseases most frequently mentioned were multiple sclerosis, cancer and allergies. Interestingly, many patients requested medical advice without providing an exact diagnosis but only symptoms, like for instance headaches, vertigo or various sorts of pain. This can be regarded as an indication that either an exact diagnosis could not been made by the therapist, or the patient had not consulted a health professional at all.

Concerning the gender ratio, the majority of writers – around 70% – are women.

This result is not surprising and it can still be assumed that women are generally more interested in health matters and turn more frequently to consulting organisations and institutions than men – a fact that has often been pointed out in research literature. This result also correlates with the fact that the majority (60%) of patients in doctor's surgeries are female as well.[36]

---

36 Cf. Dinges (2007), pp. 295–296. The fact that more letters were written by women than by men can also be influenced by the writers' age spectrum mentioned above. According to the gender specific age distribution in Germany the number of females exceeds significantly the number of males in the age group of 60 years and older. In 1994 for example females represent 61.2% of the German population above age 60. Cf. Statistisches Jahrbuch (1996), p. 62.

Having asked for the beneficiaries of each letter it turned out that the total number of women (99) who wrote for someone else instead of or besides themselves exceeds the number of men (38), whose letters contained this intention as well.[37] Considering the very high proportion of females among the writers to VNM in general, this result is not surprising. This fact can be seen as an indication that women writing to this organisation still adopt and accept the traditional role in the domestic environment at least with respect to higher responsibility in the context of health concerns.[38]

Another differentiation can help to change – at least to some extent – the traditional image of women as primarily feeling responsible for health concerns in their social environment. Regarding males and females separately, it turned out that the proportional distribution of writers who wrote for themselves and those who wrote for someone else does not confirm the claim made above. According to this differentiation, the percentage (62%) of those women writers addressing exclusively matters regarding themselves exceeds the percentage of men (55%). Consequently, when a male writer decided to turn to VNM, he wrote proportionally more often on behalf of someone else compared to his female counterpart. This result shows that a strict separation of gender-specific areas of responsibility in the context of health and illness does not exist.[39]

Considering the percentage distribution of both genders – as presented in the chart below – according to their relationship to the persons they wrote for, it becomes obvious that the social network of men was rather limited to the nuclear family, mostly encompassing their partner and children. Women instead had recourse to a broader social environment. Moreover, the tradition of the 18th and 19th century, where it was the husband or father who wrote letters for family members, seems to have continued at least rudimentarily until the end of the 20th and beginning 21st century.[40]

The following chart illustrates the distribution of beneficiaries according to the authors' gender. Two letters contain more than one sort of beneficiary. Therefore, the total number of beneficiaries (n) exceeds the number of relevant letters.

---

37 For this analysis only letters that contain clear information about the respective beneficiary of the request have been used – in total: 259 letters from women and 85 letters from men.

38 Cf. Grunow/Grunow-Lutter (2002).

39 In her study about the behavior of men in health matters between the 19th and the first half of the 20th century Nicole Schweig draws a conformable conclusion, cf. Schweig (2009), pp. 249–250. For the early 19th century cf. also Brockmeyer (2009), p. 139.

40 According to Michael Stolberg the practice that mainly men wrote letters in the name of their families started to decrease in the 18th century. Cf. Stolberg (2003), p. 94.

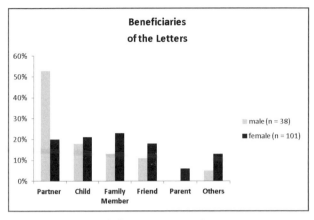

Number of letters including statements: 137

The Patient's View

Gathering Information

Another question concerned the way the writers gathered information about health-related aspects. Often the sources used were mentioned in the letters, because the writer hoped that VNM could certify or modify the preliminary information or provide suitable alternatives. An examination of the various sources of information the writers had used before they turned to VNM resulted in the following chart. Some letters contain more than one source of information. Therefore the total number of sources (n) exceeds the number of relevant letters.

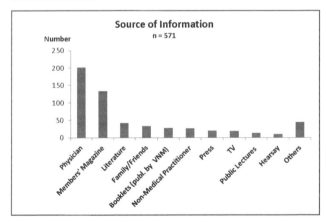

Number of letters including statements: 394

The most frequent source for questions dealing with health concerns was the academically trained care-giver. Even if the chart includes sources mentioned by patients who did not seek medical advice, a distortion of the physician-patient-relationship can be confirmed. In their letters patients often expressed their feelings of abandonment by and lack of confidence in the physicians who treated them. Some were even afraid of their doctor and the treatments. Moreover patients did not feel free to discuss CAM therapies with their doctors or were dissatisfied with the applied or suggested treatment. The following examples illustrate the distortions of the physician-patient-relationship:

> None of the physicians consulted could find the cause, if they were interested at all. Their diagnosis was always that I had to live with it.[41]

> I would really appreciate if you helped me in one way or another: With information or maybe with addresses of physicians [...] to whom I can turn confidentially. I lack the courage and unfortunately even the confidence to ask my gynaecologist.[42]

> I told my physician [...] about this therapy, but as an allopath he has got difficulties with getting involved with alternative treatments.[43]

> He's a well-known physician and maybe he's alright. Nevertheless I am afraid of those substances, whose effects I am not being able to judge as a layperson.[44]

The distorted physician-patient-relationship is surely one serious reason for patients to turn to VNM in particular and to turn to CAM in general. But an analysis of the way in which patients gather information reveals another issue worth mentioning. The patients did not exclusively rely on the medical advice of academically trained care givers. They also actively read health related literature – the members' magazine[45] of VNM was used most frequently –, involved their friends and families, contacted non-medical practitioners and made use of other media. Moreover, the category 'Others' in the chart above reveals a whole bunch of possibilities for patients to seek advice – e.g. self-help-groups, dieticians, health-related conferences and seminars. With regard to the claim of the 'informed patient' this fact indicates that those patients to some extent had developed strategies for coping with and making use of the versatile offers provided by a pluralistic medical market. This critical use of

---

41 "Alle konsultierten Ärzte haben nicht einmal die Ursache feststellen können, soweit sie sich überhaupt damit befasst haben. Diagnose stets, ich müsse damit leben". IGM, VNM 14, Mr W.R., 13.11.1992.

42 "Ich wäre Ihnen sehr dankbar, wenn Sie mir in irgendeiner Form helfen könnten: Mit Informationen oder möglicherweise auch Adressen von [...] Ärzten, an die ich mich vertrauensvoll wenden kann. Meine Gynäkologin danach zu fragen, dazu fehlt mir ein wenig der Mut und leider auch das Vertrauen." IGM, VNM 145, Mrs. H.R., 24.05.1996.

43 "Meinem Arzt [...] habe ich von dieser Therapie berichtet; als Schulmediziner hat er allerdings Schwierigkeiten, sich auf alternative Verfahren einzulassen". IGM, VNM 123, Mrs H.B., 31.03.1996.

44 "[Sic!] Er ist ein namhafter Arzt und vielleicht ist er O.K.: aber doch habe ich Angst für diese Präparaten deren Auswirkungen ich als Laie nicht kenne". IGM, VNM 145, Mrs C.R., 11.05.1996.

45 Cf. footnote 12.

information including the search for an independent second opinion can be regarded as an indication of maturity.

Why do patients use CAM?

Three types of CAM users could be classified: The patient who used CAM in addition to BM, the patient who used CAM instead of BM and finally the patient who used CAM when BM had nothing more to offer.

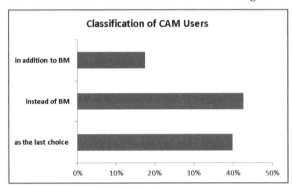

Number of letters including statements: 148

148 letters (29 % of the sample) contained information about the patients' use of CAM. In those letters the patients that used or wanted to use CAM instead of BM (about 43 %) were the majority but were directly followed by patients who regarded the use of CAM as the last chance to recover from their illness (about 40 %). Only a minority used or wanted to use CAM in addition to BM (about 18 %). Consequently, the larger part of patients did not turn to CAM, because BM had nothing more to offer. They turned to it, because they deliberately searched for an alternative or additional treatment. This result can surely not be applied to all CAM users in Germany, due to the fact that most writers only provided information for their specific situation. Therefore, no general statement can be made about their regular use within a longer period of time.

There are complex reasons involved in the decision-making process that eventually makes patients turn to CAM. The writers often emphasised the minor side-effects, gentle mode of action and holistic approach of CAM therapies that convinced them to try or to hold on to them. Another reason can be found in the family background of the patients. Writers to VNM often explained their dedication to CAM with the fact that they had been treated with it since childhood by their parents, family members or therapists. Mrs. B for instance explained her interest in naturopathy as follows:

> I have always been interested in naturopathy, because my parents who were allopaths educated themselves after graduation in the field of homeopathy and naturopathy. [...]

> For 17 years I have already been searching for a physician who works like my mother but have found no such physician here.[46]

The cost-factor played a minor role, however. Writers mostly referred to the lower costs of CAM in comparison to BM only when they complained about the alleged insufficient benefits of their private or compulsory health insurances.[47] The high costs of CAM were mentioned in those contexts, where the seriousness or efficiency of a certain therapy was doubted. All in all – with only a few exceptions – the writers to VNM were willing to pay for CAM offers as long as they believed in the competence of the practitioner and in the efficiency of the therapy.

Beliefs in the efficiency of CAM among the writers varied according to the individual illness. Considering the spectrum of illnesses as presented in the letters, where severe and chronic illnesses were predominant, the expectations of the writers usually were less optimistic. Most of them did not want to achieve complete recovery, but rather a stand-still, relief or partial improvement as the following examples show:

> Please, is there a possibility to alleviate this condition a bit with homeopathy?[48]

> I already know that even with naturopathy the chances to recover are very limited. But maybe it is still possible to stop the disease?[49]

> Please tell me in what way I can contribute to a standstill or improvement by myself.[50]

One serious reason that made patients turn to CAM could be found in the negative experiences they had with BM therapies and therapists. As mentioned above one factor was the distorted physician-patient-relationship. So, lots of writers contacted or wanted to contact a therapist offering CAM, because they expected or wished to find exactly those attributes that their physician did not possess. Other often mentioned negative experiences are the invasive methods, negative side-effects and ineffectiveness of BM. Many writers used or wanted to use CAM, because they tried to avoid an operation, get rid of the unbearable side-effects of pharmaceuticals or tried CAM, because BM had already given up. The following examples illustrate these three aspects:

---

46 "Ich interessiere mich schon immer für Naturmedizin, weil meine Eltern sich als Schulmediziner nach dem Studium auf dem Gebiet der Homöopathie und Naturheilkunde weitergebildet haben. [...] Seit 17 Jahren suche ich schon nach einem Arzt, der so wie meine Mutter behandelt, habe aber hier keinen solchen Arzt gefunden". IGM, VNM 124, Mrs H. B., no date (received on 01.02.1996).

47 In Germany the reimbursement policies of CAM vary according to the patients' individual insurance company and their insurance status. In most cases the statutory health insurances do not or only partially reimburse CAM.

48 "Bitte, gibt es eine Möglichkeit, mit Homöopathie diese Krankheit ein bißchen zu erleichtern?" IGM, VNM 144, Mrs E. R., 26.10.1996.

49 "Mir ist bekannt, daß die Heilungschancen auch mit Naturheilverfahren sehr gering sind. Aber vielleicht ist es noch möglich die Krankheit aufzuhalten". IGM, VNM 227, Mrs U. B., 20.08.1996.

50 "Bitte helfen Sie mir, wie ich zu einem Stillstand od. Besserung selbst beitragen kann". IGM, VNM 11, Mrs E. B., 10.10.1992.

My partner is consumed with the fear of a possible operation.[51]

Unfortunately, I am only treated with cortisone and chemo-therapy. Neither is doing me any good.[52]

According to my friend, allopathy has no cure. This is a shattering statement, of course.[53]

These three statements cannot deny the fact that many writers did not regard BM and CAM as incompatible opposites that can only be used separately. Some claim that they have a harmonious relationship with their BM physicians and with their non-academically trained care-givers and that they contact each of them depending on their respective health concerns. The reasons for using CAM can therefore not be explained solely with negative experiences patients had with BM therapies and therapists.

Self-medication and self-responsibility played a leading role in the decision-making process of patients. In their letters the patients explicitly articulated their desire to contribute to the preservation and restoration of their health and they wanted to take responsibility for their bodies instead of completely passing it over to a therapist – academically trained or not. This fact can also be regarded as an indication of maturity. Expressing the wish to contribute to his recovery Mr R. wrote the following lines: "I don't want to rely exclusively on the fact that my thyroid is being checked every four to five weeks. I want to contribute actively and with all means to my recovery."[54]

Having outlined some of the possible reasons that influenced the decisions of patients to turn to CAM shown by the letters to VNM, it is still difficult to provide a general judgement about what reasons played a minor and what reasons played a major role, because each writer presents his or her own individual attitudes and experiences. However, concerning the frequency and detailed descriptions of many writers about their negative experiences with BM practitioners and therapies and their strong desire to take responsibility for their own health and body, one can conclude that these two reasons – dissatisfaction with BM and the search for more autonomy – contribute to a large degree to the increasing use of CAM.

51   "Mein Lebensgefährte wird aus Angst vor einer möglichen Operation zerfressen". IGM, VNM 11, Mrs J. B., 17.11.1992.
52   "Leider werde ich nur mit Cortison und Chemotherapie behandelt. Beides bekommt mir gar nicht". IGM, VNM 11, Mr R. B., 07.12.1992.
53   "Die Schulmedizin hat nach Aussage meiner Freundin kein Heilmittel. Das ist natürlich eine niederschmetternde Aussage". IGM, VNM 11, Mrs R. B., 15.11.1992.
54   "Ich will mich nicht allein darauf verlassen, dass alle 4 – 5 Wochen der Status der Schilddrüsenwerte ermittelt wird. Ich möchte aktiv und mit allen Mitteln an einer Gesundung mitarbeiten". IGM, VNM 145, Mr H. R., 16.08.1996.

Summary

Although the sample used for this essay includes the total number of 512 letters, the results cannot be applied to the whole group of German CAM patients without reservations. Even if the letters represent a large number of patients who used or wanted to use CAM, those patients share distinct features other users do not possess.

It was the task of this essay to examine the patient's perspective in a pluralistic medical market. First of all, it provided an overview of selected research literature on this topic. Although these works can be distinguished by their different fields of research, methods and key aspects, their results show some common characteristics of patients who use CAM. Those patients share for example a higher education and financial status compared to the average German; their chosen CAM therapy corresponds to their personal life-style and they appreciate CAM because of its minor side-effects, gentle mode of action and holistic approach. Furthermore, this essay showed that an examination of the letters to VNM can provide new and different impulses to this research field due to the uniqueness of the letter as a source for contemporary history.

Secondly, analysis of the geographical distribution and the socio-structural features of the writers has shown that writers from the newly formed German states were underrepresented, that mainly older and female patients turned to VNM and that they suffered from various different, mostly chronic illnesses. According to the beneficiaries of the letters, it turned out that men proportionally more often wrote for their partners and children than women. Women, however, had recourse to broader social networks. Furthermore, with regard to the total number of female writers, the claim that women accept and take over the role of being responsible for health issues could be verified in general. When a male writer, however, decided to turn to VNM, he – unlike his female counterpart – wrote proportionally more often on behalf of someone else.

Thirdly, the patient's perspective was taken into account. In the first instance the sources of information used before writing to VNM were analysed. This revealed that the primary source according to health issues were academically trained physicians. This fact can be seen as indication for both a distortion of the physician-patient-relationship and a form of patient maturity. The patients who wrote to VNM did not rely exclusively on the judgement of the academically trained care-giver, but wanted to obtain a second opinion provided by the organisation. Moreover, the fact that patients referred to very different information sources is an indication that they actively and critically tried to cope with and make use of the various offers provided by a pluralistic medical market.

Regarding the question as to why patients use CAM, a classification of types of users has been made. This classification shows that the majority voted for CAM because they wanted a substitute for or an addition to BM treatments. Patients who voted for CAM because BM had nothing more to offer were a minority. As far as the letters to VNM are concerned, a large part of the patients used or wanted to use CAM because they had made negative experiences with BM therapies or practitioners on the one hand and because they actively wanted to contribute to the process of recovery on the other.

To summarize, the letters to VNM are perfectly suited to an approach towards a better understanding and comprehensive analysis of the patient's perspective. As a part of ongoing research towards a PhD thesis this essay is limited to the aspects discussed above and could therefore only provide a rather sketchy and provisional approach to the complex topic of 'Medical Pluralism in the Patient's Perspective'. Further investigations in the context of the dissertation will provide new results and may modify those presented above.

Bibliography

Archival Sources

Institute for the History of Medicine of the Robert Bosch Foundation, Stuttgart (IGM)

VNM 10,	Korrespondenz mit Mitgliedern (Ra-Re),	Laufzeit 1992–1992
VNM 11,	Korrespondenz mit Mitgliedern (A-D),	Laufzeit 1992–1992
VNM 14,	Korrespondenz mit Mitgliedern (M-R),	Laufzeit 1992–1992
VNM 15,	Korrespondenz mit Mitgliedern (S-Z),	Laufzeit 1992–1992
VNM 16,	Korrespondenz mit Mitgliedern (A-D),	Laufzeit 1992–1993
VNM 19,	Korrespondenz mit Mitgliedern (O-Sch),	Laufzeit 1992–1993
VNM 20,	Korrespondenz mit Mitgliedern (St-Z),	Laufzeit 1992–1993
VNM 123,	Korrespondenz mit Mitgliedern (B),	Laufzeit 1996–1996
VNM 124,	Korrespondenz mit Mitgliedern (B),	Laufzeit 1996–1996
VNM 125,	Korrespondenz mit Mitgliedern (B-D),	Laufzeit 1996–1996
VNM 142,	Korrespondenz mit Mitgliedern (N-P),	Laufzeit 1996–1996
VNM 144,	Korrespondenz mit Mitgliedern (R),	Laufzeit 1996–1996
VNM 145,	Korrespondenz mit Mitgliedern (R),	Laufzeit 1996–1996
VNM 146,	Korrespondenz mit Mitgliedern (R-S),	Laufzeit 1996–1996
VNM 152,	Korrespondenz mit Mitgliedern (St-T),	Laufzeit 1996–1996
VNM 153,	Korrespondenz mit Mitgliedern (T-V),	Laufzeit 1996–1996
VNM 227,	Korrespondenz mit Mitgliedern (B),	Laufzeit 1996–1996
VNM 326,	Korrespondenz mit Mitgliedern (B),	Laufzeit 2000–2000
VNM 327,	Korrespondenz mit Mitgliedern (B),	Laufzeit 2000–2000
VNM 342,	Korrespondenz mit Mitgliedern (O),	Laufzeit 2000–2000
VNM 344,	Korrespondenz mit Mitgliedern (R),	Laufzeit 2000–2000
VNM 349,	Korrespondenz mit Mitgliedern (T),	Laufzeit 2000–2000

Internet Links

http://www.ifd-allensbach.de/uploads/tx_reportsndocs/prd_0914.pdf (last accessed on May 22, 2013)

http://www.bundespraesident.de/DE/Die-Bundespraesidenten/Karl-Carstens/karl-carstens-node.html (last accessed on May 22, 2013)

http://www.bundespraesident.de/DE/Die-Bundespraesidenten/Karl-Carstens/Veronica-Carstens/veronica-carstens-node.html (last accessed on May 22, 2013)

http://www.dimdi.de/static/de/klassi/icd-10-who/kodesuche/onlinefassungen/htmlamtl2013/
   index.htm (last accessed on May 22, 2013)
http://www.naturundmedizin.de/wuu/presse/NaturundMedizin_Presskit.pdf (last accessed on
   May 22, 2013)

Literature

Becker, Raymond et al. (eds.): "Neue" Wege in der Medizin. Alternativmedizin – Fluch oder
   Segen? Heidelberg 2010.
Brockmeyer, Bettina: Selbstverständnisse. Dialoge über Körper und Gemüt im frühen 19.
   Jahrhundert. Göttingen 2009.
Cant, Sarah; Sharma, Ursula: A new medical pluralism? Alternative medicine, doctors, pa-
   tients and the state. London 1999.
Coulter, Angela; Magee, Helen: The European Patient of the Future. Maidenhead 2004.
Dinges, Martin: Medizinkritische Bewegungen zwischen "Lebenswelt" und "Wissenschaft".
   In: Dinges, Martin (ed.): Medizinkritische Bewegungen im Deutschen Reich (ca. 1870-ca.
   1933). (=Medizin, Gesellschaft und Geschichte, Beiheft 9) Stuttgart 1996, pp. 7–38.
Dinges, Martin: Immer schon 60 % Frauen in den Arztpraxen? Zur geschlechterspezifischen
   Inanspruchnahme des medizinischen Angebots (1600–2000). In: Dinges, Martin (ed.):
   Männlichkeit und Gesundheit im historischen Wandel ca. 1800-ca. 2000. (=Medizin, Ge-
   sellschaft und Geschichte, Beiheft 27) Stuttgart 2007, pp. 295–322.
Dinges, Martin; Barras, Vincent: Krankheit in Briefen: Einleitung. In: Dinges, Martin; Barras,
   Vincent (eds.): Krankheit in Briefen im deutschen und französischen Sprachraum. (=Medi-
   zin, Gesellschaft und Geschichte, Beiheft 29) Stuttgart 2007, pp. 7–22.
Dinges, Martin: The next decade for homeopathy: Any lessons from the last decades? In:
   Homoeopathy for Public Health: Proceedings of 66th LMHI Congress. Delhi 2012 [forth-
   coming].
Eckart, Wolfgang Uwe; Jütte, Robert: Medizingeschichte. Eine Einführung. Köln; Weimar;
   Wien 2007.
Faltermeier, Toni: Gesundheitsbewusstsein und Gesundheitshandeln. Weinheim 1994.
Grunow, Dieter; Grunow-Lutter, Vera: Geschlechterspezifische Formen von Selbstvorsorge
   und Selbsthilfe. In: Hurrelmann, Klaus; Kolip, Petra (eds.): Geschlecht, Gesundheit und
   Krankheit. Frauen und Männer im Vergleich. Bern 2002, pp. 548–564.
Günther, Martina: Der homöopathische Patient in der niedergelassenen Arztpraxis – Ergeb-
   nisse einer vergleichenden Patientenbefragung in konventionellen Arztpraxen und
   homöopathischen Privat- und Kassenpraxen. In: Medizin, Gesellschaft und Geschichte 18
   (1999), pp. 119–136.
Klusen, Norbert; Fließgarten, Anja; Nebling, Thomas (eds.): Informiert und selbstbestimmt.
   Der mündige Bürger als mündiger Patient. (=Beiträge zum Gesundheitsmanagement 24)
   Berlin 2009.
Köntopp, Sabine: Wer nutzt Komplementärmedizin? Theorie, Empirie, Prognose. Essen
   2004.
Kofahl, Christopher; Nickel, Stefan; Trojan, Alf: Gesellschaftliche Trends und gesundheit-
   spolitische Herausforderungen für die Selbsthilfe in Deutschland. In: Meggeneder, Oskar
   (ed.): Selbsthilfe im Wandel der Zeit. Neue Herausforderungen für die Selbsthilfe im Ge-
   sundheitswesen. Frankfurt/Main 2011, pp. 67–105.
Leonhard, Joachim: Motive zum Heilpraktikerbesuch. Eine empirische Untersuchung über
   die sozialen Aspekte und die Krankengeschichte als Hintergrund eines Entscheidungsprozesses. Konstanz 1984.
Maddalena, Stefano: Alternative Medicines: A Comparative Legal Analysis in Western Countries. Bern 2005.

Michl, Susanne; Potthast, Thomas; Wiesing, Urban (eds.): Pluralität in der Medizin. Werte – Methoden – Theorien. (=Lebenswissenschaft im Dialog 6) Freiburg/Brsg.; München 2008.

Nierade, Anna: Homöopathie in der DDR: die Geschichte der Homöopathie in der Sowjetischen Besatzungszone und der DDR 1945 bis 1989. (=Quellen und Studien zur Homöopathiegeschichte 16) Essen 2012.

Reinders, Marlis: Häufigkeit von Namensanfängen. In: Statistische Rundschau Nordrhein-Westfalen 11 (1996), pp. 651–660.

Schäfer, Daniel et al. (eds.): Gesundheitskonzepte im Wandel. Geschichte, Ethik und Gesellschaft. (=Geschichte und Philosophie der Medizin 6) Stuttgart 2008.

Schnalke, Thomas: Medizin im Brief. Der städtische Arzt des 18. Jahrhunderts im Spiegel seiner Korrespondenz. Stuttgart 1997.

Schweig, Nicole: Gesundheitsverhalten von Männern. Gesundheit und Krankheit in Briefen 1800–1950. Stuttgart 2009.

Schweiger, Matthias: Medizin – Glaube, Spekulation oder Naturwissenschaft? Gibt es zur Schulmedizin eine Alternative? Eine historisch-philosophisch begründete Auseinandersetzung zwischen Schulmedizin und alternativer Medizin. München; Wien; New York 2003.

Stange, Rainer; Amhof, Robert; Moebus, Susanne: Naturheilverfahren, Komplementär- und Alternativmedizin im Bewusstsein und Handeln von niedergelassenen Ärzten. In: Böcken, Jan et al. (eds.): Gesundheitsmonitor 2006. Gesundheitsversorgung und Gestaltungsoptionen aus der Perspektive von Bevölkerung und Ärzten. Gütersloh 2006, pp. 208–232.

Statistisches Bundesamt: Häufigkeit von Familiennamen und ihren Anfangsbuchstaben. In: Wirtschaft und Statistik 7 (1977), pp. 450–453.

Statistisches Jahrbuch 1996 für die Bundesrepublik Deutschland. Wiesbaden 1996.

Statistisches Jahrbuch 1998 für die Bundesrepublik Deutschland. Wiesbaden 1998.

Stolberg, Michael: Homo Patiens. Krankheits- und Körpererfahrung in der Frühen Neuzeit. Köln; Weimar 2003.

Wiesing, Urban: Pluralität in der Medizin. Ein Plädoyer für zielorientierte Paradigmenvielfalt aus ethischen Gründen. In: Michl, Susanne; Potthast, Thomas; Wiesing, Urban (eds.): Pluralität in der Medizin. Werte – Methoden – Theorien. (=Lebenswissenschaft im Dialog 6) Freiburg/Brsg.; München 2008, pp. 459–470.

Willich, Stefan N. et al.: Schulmedizin und Komplementärmedizin. Verständnis und Zusammenarbeit müssen verstärkt werden. In: Deutsches Ärzteblatt 101 (2004), no. 14, pp. 1314–1319.

Zilgrei. In: Lexikonredaktion des Verlags F. A. Brockhaus (ed.): Der Brockhaus Alternative Medizin. Heilsysteme, Diagnose- und Therapieformen, Arzneimittel. Leipzig; Mannheim 2008, p. 507.

Medical Pluralism in a Slum in Delhi: Global Medicine in a Local Garb?

Nupur Barua[1]

The burgeoning 80 million urban poor in India struggle for basic services like housing, water and sanitation. The links between these contextual forces and health outcomes is manifest not only in the striking differentials in health among urban poor and non-poor groups but in health indicators of the urban poor which have recently been found to be worse off than the poor living in rural areas of the country.[2]

With a population of more than 17 million, nearly half of Delhi, the capital city and one of the richest regions in the country, is estimated to be living in poor habitations. These habitations range from well-defined slum settlements, government-run shelters, and construction sites to precarious pavement dwellings. Despite the ambiguity that persists regarding the actual size of the urban poor population in the city, the abysmal critical health indicators among them indicate the multiple vulnerabilities that they face. Neo-natal, infant and child mortality rates among the urban poor in the city are among the highest in the country.[3] There are several outbreaks of preventable diseases. More than 35 percent of children living in slums in the city are malnourished. 25 percent of those who had completed one year were found fully immunized. Ante-natal coverage is low. Only one-third of the pregnant women receive three or more antenatal check-ups. Total fertility rate is high. Malaria prevalence is more than double that of urban high-income groups and tuberculosis prevalence is more than double that of the urban average.[4]

The latest UNICEF report on the "State of the World's Children" (2012) draws attention to the hardships endured by children in poor urban communities. Statistical averages tend to mask the inequities faced by different urban groups and the exclusion of children from essential services in particular remains 'concealed'. The report also reiterates that the urban situation is in itself a social determinant of health. Physical proximity to better health infrastructure in urban areas does not ensure actual utilisation of facilities. Social exclusion as we will see later in the paper is a powerful determinant.

India has been reported to have one of the largest private sectors in the world. It is not surprising, therefore, that in Delhi, despite the presence of a large number of hospitals and health facilities, there exists a burgeoning pri-

1   The author is Research Adviser with the South Asia Research Hub, UK Department for International Development, New Delhi. This paper is not related to her current position but is drawn from field work carried out partly during, and mostly after, a research project on the urban poor in New Delhi.
2   Statement made by the Parliamentary Standing Committee on Health and Family Welfare in 2012, reported widely in the media in India, e.g. in the *Times of India*.
3   UNICEF (2012).
4   Urban Health Resource Centre / Ministry of Health and Family Welfare (2007).

vate health sector. The private sector that the poor access may be thought of as consisting of three wings: (i) the fully-organized-and-fully-qualified, (ii) the fully qualified private providers that operate in less than well-to-do neighbourhoods where the slum population go too, and (iii) the 'less-than-fully-qualified' practitioners in the slum.[5] While many of these private facilities are beyond the reach of the poor, their first point of contact with the health system is invariably individual private practitioners, both qualified medical doctors as well as unlicensed health care providers who run clinics in and around slum settlements.[6]

A multi-disciplinary multi-country project was carried out during 2004 2008 in south and south-east Asia to study the private health sector in poor urban neighbourhoods.[7] In Delhi, the project studied the health-seeking behaviour and health expenditure patterns of households in a slum settlement and conducted an ethnographic study of private health practitioners who run clinics in and around the settlement. This paper is drawn from fieldwork carried out by the author in 2008 in a private clinic run by a homeopath in the slum. While contact with the homeopath was established during the project, this paper presents data from clinical interactions and exit interviews in the clinic after the project closed.[8]

Multiple vulnerabilities in Midanpuri

Midanpuri is a slum settlement in south Delhi.[9] Located near one of the city's most affluent neighbourhoods, it has an estimated population size of around 25–30,000, and is composed almost entirely of migrants from neighbouring villages and from rural areas of Uttar Pradesh, Rajasthan, Bihar, Haryana, Madhya Pradesh, Uttaranchal, Kerala, Karnataka and Andhra Pradesh.[10] A typical area of "concentrated disadvantage"[11], the settlement has densely packed shelters; many built with concrete and tin roofs but a majority with flammable roofs. Single room hutments of approximately 50 sq m each, they

---

5   The last group, to borrow Berman's (1998) label, comprises practitioners who are either untrained or minimally trained in any system of medicine or trained in one system and practise another. It is estimated that these untrained, unlicensed practitioners in the country outnumber qualified medical doctors by at least 10:1. Although a large majority of them operate in rural areas, urban areas too are witnessing increasing numbers of these untrained practitioners.

6   Barua/Seeberg/Pandav (2009); Kamat (2001); Bhat (1999).

7   This project was funded by Danida's Council for Development Research, Denmark.

8   The author wishes to acknowledge the following: Jens Seeberg for conceptualising the multi-country study; Chandrakant Pandav for his support in carrying out the study in Delhi; Harish Naraindas for his critical review of the paper; and above all Dr VS and other respondents who made this fieldwork possible.

9   The name of the settlement as that of all respondents have been changed to maintain anomity.

10 Barua/Seeberg/Pandav (2009).

11 Vlahov et al. (2007).

have high occupancy rates of an average of six persons per household. They serve as an all-purpose room generally demarcated into a sleeping area and a cooking area. All the houses are served by illegal electricity connections provided by a local 'contractor' for a monthly fee. There is no regular water supply in the settlement. The inhabitants are dependent on two communal water sources which provide water for two hours in a day and on water tankers that come once a day, and often in the summer once in two days, from the Delhi Water Supply department.[12] There are no toilet facilities inside the slum and the people use the open fields and surrounding scrub areas behind the slum to defecate. There is virtually no drainage in the settlement and during heavy rains the main entrance gets blocked. The urban environment is itself a social determinant of health.[13]

The inhabitants of Midanpuri are mainly wage labourers; they work as cleaners, auto-rickshaw drivers, guards in private offices, vegetable vendors and carpenters, with a striking majority of the women working as domestic help in the neighbouring areas. The lack of basic infrastructure impacts all aspects of the inhabitants' life in the settlement. As in other areas of urban poverty, the high population density, waste collection pits, open sewers, absence of toilets, and the lack of regular water supply contribute to the high reporting of illness. At least one member from the 25 households that were followed over the two-year period of the project was found to visit a health care provider once every five days.[14] During the summer months there was a surge in epidemic prone infections. Although there was general awareness about sexually transmitted diseases and HIV/AIDS, knowledge regarding its methods of transmission was very poor. A large number of mental conditions, many of them undiagnosed, were reported by the respondents. Very high alcohol consumption, drug use, sedatives, and extensive use of powdered tobacco were recorded. Although the women were reluctant to talk about domestic violence, almost half of them were found to be victims of physical violence.[15]

There was no government health centre inside the settlement with the two closest dispensaries being located approximately three kilometres away.[16] There were, however, more than 27 clinics run by private health care providers located inside the slum. These, and other individual clinics run by private practitioners in a market hub one and a half kilometres away, were found to be the first point of resort for more than 90 percent of the slum dwellers. There was an almost exclusive dependence on these practitioners in particular for "everyday illness conditions" like cold, cough, fevers, headache, joint

---

12   During the course of fieldwork, the research team was witness to stampedes in the area to collect water when these tankers arrive. A child of five was killed in such a stampede in May 2005.
13   UNICEF (2012).
14   Barua/Seeberg/Pandav (2009).
15   Barua/Seeberg/Pandav (2009).
16   The need to commute to the dispensary, the long waiting time and the lack of medicines in the dispensary were cited as deterrents to visits to the dispensary.

pains, and minor injuries. For conditions which required "further treatment", private practitioners in the neighbouring areas were consulted. Government hospitals were invariably cited as the main option in connection with conditions which were either considered to be "serious" or those that required inpatient care and surgical intervention. Unlike studies in slums elsewhere[17], there was little mention of traditional healers; the only exceptions being in connection with male sexual health and in cases of mental illness. As Subba et al. found in their study of slums in central Delhi[18], lack of awareness regarding mental disorders prevented them from seeking formal medical treatment.

Doctor Sahib

'Sharma Clinic' is one of the most popular clinics in the settlement. Vijay Sharma[19], a 48 year old homeopath, had been practising as a physician for the past 23 years when I interviewed him. He set up his clinic in Midanpuri five years ago after having worked in a private polyclinic in another part of Delhi. After he graduated from college, he attended a diploma course in homeopathy and trained under his father who was a homeopath in the town of Shahranpur in Uttar Pradesh (UP). For the first six years he worked as an assistant to his father in Shahranpur before leaving for Delhi in search of a more lucrative practice. He "became a doctor", he says, because this was "something [he] always wanted to be". He enjoys being addressed as "doctor sahib".[20] Motivated by the fact that at that time there were very few health practitioners in the area, VS felt that opening a clinic in the areas would mean lucrative business.

Doctor VS sees an average of 10–15 patients a day in his clinic. His clinic is small, approximately 6x8 feet, with just enough space for his desk and chair and a wooden bench for waiting patients. On one side of the wall is a wooden cabinet filled with glass bottles with biochemic medicines and small glass vials of homeopathic pills. The room is partitioned into two by a green curtain behind which there is a narrow wooden table which serves as a bed to examine patients. The 'bed' is covered with a stained white sheet. The signboard that marks the clinic says "Sharma Clinic" in both English and Hindi, the local language. Below that in Hindi, it says "Homeopathic and other treatment for all diseases. Specialise in fever, cold, cough, BP [blood pressure], headache, allergies, piles, diarrhoea, heavy bleeding, tension, children's illnesses".

His clinic timings are from 0900–1300 and 1600–2100 hrs. Almost all his patients are from Midanpuri with a sprinkling of cases from temporary dwellings nearby at a large construction site. He treats his patients with respect and listens to their narratives with patience. About one-third of his patients are

---

17   Awasthi/Srivastava/Pant (2008); D'Souza (2003); Papreen et al. (2000).
18   Subba/Joshi/Nagesh (2004).
19   Hereafter Vijay Sharma will appear in the narrative as VS or Doctor VS.
20   The word *Sahib* is an honorific suggestive of respect, rank or status.

children who are accompanied largely by their mothers. There is a clear difference in his prescription practices between children and adults. The maximum patient load is observed in the afternoon/evening shift. The doctor-patient interactions depend on the symptoms that are reported by the patient. An average interaction lasts for about five minutes and in approximately one-third of cases, the practitioner spends about 10 minutes with a patient. A typical interaction includes a narration of symptoms by the patient, a checking of the patient's pulse and examination of the afflicted area by the practitioner with a stethoscope. In some cases, especially when acute pain is reported, the patient is physically examined in the partitioned section.

A majority of cases include fevers (of indeterminate origin), headaches, body pain, persistent nausea, respiratory disorders, diarrhoea, fatigue and 'BP', and long term cases of tuberculosis (TB). It is not uncommon to see patients directly requesting specific medicines; the most common among them being painkillers such as Ibuprofen, tranquilisers such as alprazolam and 'medicines for BP'. A large majority of cases appear to be mental disorders most of which have not been medically diagnosed.

Drug dispensation

There was no system of prescribing drugs. The core of the clinical interaction was drug dispensation which was clearly the most profitable activity. Dispensation patterns, however, were predictable. Although in approximately one-third of the cases, loose medicines without counterfoils which were administered made it difficult to assess each category, virtually all prescriptions had multi-drug combinations, the most common combination of drugs being antibiotics, analgesics and multivitamins. Although making a prescription audit was impossible, observations revealed that there was excessive use of antibiotics and injections. While VS used anti-tuberculosis drugs to treat TB patients, he was not aware of the National TB Control guidelines. Many of the injections he administered were largely administered with corticosteroids. Pain killers were commonly prescribed. What was particularly interesting was that in three-fourths of cases, he gave a vial of homeopathic pills along with the tablets.

VS gave clear instructions on how to "take the tablets". Loose medicines were explained in detail according to colour, size and shape and doses were packaged in *pudiyas* (small individual paper packets). Generic descriptions were provided with medicines being specified as "for heart", "for bones", "for tension", "for sadness", "for BP".[21] Similar trends have been observed by Kamat in a slum in Mumbai.[22] Doses were given according to the amount of money in hand; if the -lack of cash was not cited by the patient, doses would be given for two days at a time. The sale of partial doses of medicine in par-

21   Barua/Seeberg/Pandav (2009).
22   Kamat (2001).

ticular was cited as a huge boon by a majority of patients who were dependent on daily wages. The only cases where homeopathic pills were administered were for children under five years – mostly for diarrhoea, worms, allergies and respiratory disorders.

> The function of medicine is to cure. My patient comes and tells me that he or she has a problem and wants a quick cure. While I would like to ideally give them just a homeopathic combination, it is not about me, it is about my patient. And if they want high powered medicines, I give them that. But very often I give homeopathic medicines also – together with tablets – it is a very effective combination and works far better than giving either allopathic or homeopathic medicines exclusively.
>
> For young children it is different – they don't have the urgency to get back to work! Mothers are also willing to wait longer for a cure and so I can give homeopathic pills. Homeopathic medicines in any case work better in children…

Many of VS' patients had already consulted other qualified medical practitioners and visited him for follow-up consultations. VS would often scrutinize the prescriptions given by qualified doctors and dispense the same set of medicines. Often, he retained the prescription and administered the same cocktail of drugs to other patients who reported similar symptoms!

There was no system of recording patient histories or of specific cases. Agents from pharmaceutical companies routinely visited with samples of medicines. These medicines are not meant to be sold but in fact were dispensed at the clinic. The payment system was flexible and ranged between INR 25–40 (~35–60 cents), depending on the amount of tablets or injections administered. For injections, there was a flat fee of INR 50 (~70 cents). VS insisted that there was no consultation fee and that he charged only for the medicines that he administered. The reality, however, was that the consolidated amount of money that was charged included consultation as well as the medicines. Notwithstanding the actual breakup, fee levels were kept low but he ensured that there was some profit after paying for capital costs.

Exploring mechanisms beyond patterns

Although the drugs administered were predominantly biomedical dugs, the underlying logic that drove the manner in which the medicines were administered borrowed quite heavily from some of the principles of homeopathy. Based on the doctrine *similia similibus curentur* (like may cure like), homeopathy is based on the principle that substances which produce specific symptoms in healthy individuals can also cure the same symptoms in someone who is sick although the symptoms may have arisen from another cause like bacteria, viruses, and so on.[23] What differs markedly from biomedicine (or allopathy as it is commonly referred to in India) is that the symptom complex in allopathy, in most cases, is seen as indicating the disease per se unlike with the principles of homeopathy where it is believed to be the reaction of the defence mecha-

23   Vithoulkas (1983).

nism mobilized by the body to counteract the influence caused by a specific stress such as bacteria or virus or non-specific stress like environmental factors.[24]

Most of the explanations offered by Dr VS to explain causality of illness conditions were based on the broad category of 'infection'. However, its rationalization was often translated by him into a coherent body of description which drew from references to human physiology or was based on a humoral explanation. Causation in most cases was attributed to either non-specific stresses such as climatic changes, environmental pollution, mental and emotional disturbances and so on, or specific stress as defined by a broad category – infection – which was explained in terms of bacteria. But it was an innovative mix. Rather than the homeopathic explanation where the symptoms are held to be the means through which the body tries to regain its homeostasis, attributions were based on a grid that drew from the vitiation of the humours, either because of external factors – the environment as defined by the weather, air pollution, lack of sanitation in the slum – or internal factors as defined by the impaired ability of the body to cope with these external factors. The explanation used for almost all cases of ill-health was poverty or the state of chronic crisis experienced by patients on an almost daily basis.

> The allopathic medicines attack the symptom and the homeopathic medicines restore the balance. You see, it is too much hardship that causes most of the ailments… that is [the poor patients'] fate. How can they be healthy and strong when they have to live lives based on such drudgery? Have you seen how they live? Their children defecate outside their houses, women have to walk for half a kilometre to go to the scrub jungle… instead they urinate outside their houses at night. You have to give medicines that fit well with the culture here [in the slum]. In slums, it is not about where you are from – that you are Bihari, or Tamil or Bengali – the conditions here bind you in a unique culture that is very different from anywhere else…

On being asked how he reconciled this kind of treatment mix with his original training as a homeopath, he was very clear that he was merely responding to what was needed for his patients. I asked about the basic principles of homeopathy which is based on the assumption that the body is a vital force which is essentially self-healing and whatever causes the disturbance of this vital force is believed to hold the cure. Thus, administering substances which will produce symptoms similar to those which the patient experiences is held to stimulate the body's capacity to cure itself.

> That is true. That is how I was trained to understand the body and what causes disease. But with homeopathic medicines, sometimes the symptoms of the patient get worse in the beginning. Of course, this is an indication that the medicine is working. But in these kinds of patients, if they see that the symptoms are getting worse, they will immediately jump to the conclusion that they are getting worse and they will go to another doctor looking for a cure. So if I don't give them tablets, the next doctor will… so what is the difference? I might as well give them the right combination based on my knowledge of homeopathy and allopathy…

---

24 Vithoulkas (1983).

Bhardwaj, while pointing out that various indigenous medical practitioners are not necessarily purists, stresses the importance of recognizing the varieties of pluralism in different parts of India and the relative importance of homoeopathic and indigenous physician's constituencies as well as the behavioural response of health seekers.[25] Extending the regional focus to that of (the urban) context, we see a pragmatic integration of concepts and what appears to be a shrewd assessment of what is needed for a successful practice in this context.

> There is decent work in the colony. But there is a big problem here – people just don't want to part with money. They will come for treatment but when it's time to pay, they say "I will pay you later" and often they don't come back. But I don't refuse to treat them. If I don't give them medicines, they will simply go to another doctor in the locality... At least they come back if I treat them successfully.

A question of competence?

This kind of treatment cocktail[26] seemed to sit well with the patients. The explanatory grid that the practitioner offered reflected the particular stresses that they confronted as a result of their experiences of acute poverty in their lives as migrants. Competence in public facilities was clearly considered to be higher by the patients but long distances to these facilities, circuitous and time-consuming registration procedures, waiting time, loss of wages, bribes that sometimes had to be paid to hospital staff, and disrespect shown by the staff and sometimes the doctor were deterrents. However, competence, as Jenkins has pointed out[27], is socially constructed and ascribed. It is a multi-layered concept. Variables like 'experience' were often used to calibrate these local practitioners, especially if the patients had an established and positive relationship with him. Hierarchies of competencies were arranged along notions of efficacy vis-à-vis what was perceived as working *under the circumstances* and what was not. The local models of competence that are built are clearly context-dependent and not based on a biomedical index.

A 42 year-old woman, diagnosed with TB, made a clear distinction between quality of care by Dr VS and a well-known biomedical doctor (Dr X) who runs a clinic in a market hub outside the settlement.

> Dr X... see what he does... people say he is a big doctor, but he gave me tablets... I didn't even get well, and when I went back after 10 days, he says loudly "you have TB, go get it checked"... in front of so many people and then calls out "next" to the other patients... [The husband, during a subsequent interview, justifies the reason why the wife prefers to continue with Dr VS instead.] When she visits him [VS], he gives her injec-

---

25 Bhardwaj (1980).
26 This kind of treatment cocktail is reminiscent of what Naraindas (2011) has called poly-therapeutics in the context of his study of the German Heilpraktiker, where too it seems to be partly propelled by patients' needs but in a very different socio-economic context.
27 Jenkins (1998).

tions, she is able to get back to work... his treatment is very good... and now whenever she feels sick she goes to him... he listens to her... understands. That is also important, isn't it?

There is no one particular grid for defining competence of a practitioner and the list of capabilities was usually drawn from previous experiences with the same practitioner or personal testimonies of neighbours, friends or kin. The level of certification of the practitioner was seldom found to be a deterrent to choice.

> He [Dr VS] may not have big degrees, may not speak good English, but is that important...? He knows what to do... has close to 20 years experience, he is better than many bada [big] doctors...

As far as the patients' demands were concerned, there was a clear preference, however, for allopathic medicines over homeopathic combinations. The 'tablets', as biomedical drugs were generically referred to, were considered to be 'strong' with the ability to induce 'immediate action'. The more dramatic the effect of the medicine, the more effective it was considered to be in curing an illness condition. Homeopathic medicines, in contrast, were believed to be helpful for 'general health' but were not considered to possess the same degree of 'power'.

Why private practitioners?

For the patients, the obvious benefits associated with having a responsive medical help at hand determining their choice of the practitioner, even if the people are aware that he might not possess the 'best' qualifications. As one of the key respondents, said:

> Of course they [the private practitioners in the slum] are not big doctors. But how is that important? Will a big doctor set up his clinic here? There are 25,000 people and no [government] dispensary. So what do we do? Wait for these big doctors to come and save us...? At least these doctors are here when we need them, and they know about medicines... they are good enough for us.

Different versions of the same sentiment were recorded time and again throughout the duration of the fieldwork. Thus, despite the much wider variety of options in an urban setting, access of the poor to qualified health care practitioners is severely compromised by their socio-economic status and private health care providers, especially the local practitioners, are invariably the practitioners of choice. The personal attention received in these clinics was a recurrent theme in their narratives.

A 48-year old construction labourer, and father of four children, said:

> It is all right for the hoardings to be screaming about AIDS... you only know what happens when it happens to you. I got myself tested and they told me that I had AIDS. Only my wife knows... how can we tell other people? I have seen what happened to Gunaram [his neighbour] the moment his neighbours found out that he had AIDS... that was it! They don't even want to drink tea with him in the evenings... so will I risk my wife and

my daughters in the locality…? In the public hospitals you go to the AIDS clinic, and everyone will know you have AIDS. Sooner or later somebody will see you there… then it is all over… and these people in these [government] clinics… how they treat you… like diseased dogs in the street… like you are a criminal… so I prefer to go to [Dr VS]… at least I am able to sit inside his clinic without being told to leave after my consultation is over, he talks to me properly and he gives me the right medicines that I need.

For people subsisting on daily wages, time is a crucial factor as time, among other things, translates into wages; and wages as opposed to pay are won and lost on a daily basis.[28]

> We get harassed when we go to these big places… We have to go stand in queue early in the morning to get a parchi [patient card] done. Sometimes it takes many days to get just that done. And the doctors are so rude. They spend 2 minutes with us – just write names of medicines, we buy the medicines from outside. If we have to get tests done, wait endlessly to show the results. They don't even listen to us… What's the point in all this?

> These sarkari [government] places are the last places where you must go. They are good if you need to have an operation. Not much cost. But these things… at least a week… And who can afford to lose wages for that much time… That's why I come here [to Dr VS' clinic] when I am ill.

This 'quick-fix, quick profit mentality' of private practitioners in the locality, as in the case of VS, is stoically accepted by the patients.[29] While many of the inhabitants of Midanpuri were aware of the fact that these *daktars* (doctors) did not possess the "right qualifications" (and one must not forget that Dr VS administers biomedical drugs without adequate training and without an appropriate license), and they often differentiated between a *bada daktar* (big doctor) and "these doctors", they were at the same time convinced that these practitioners had "knowledge about medicines" and were a pragmatic solution for "ordinary" or "not so serious" conditions like fevers, body ache, stomach disorders and cough and cold.[30] This concurs with Kamat's finding in his study of the role of private practitioners in the management of malaria in Mumbai, India, where patients were clear that they visited these practitioners primarily to "get medicines" and their expectations of these visits did not extend beyond finding an immediate solution to their problem.[31]

However, in conditions that required more attention, maintaining dignity and confidentiality of the patient emerged as a recurrent theme. Narratives of care-seeking for reproductive tract infections in particular were dominated by the need for sensitivity on the part of the health care provider. Reproductive tract infections are largely believed to occur among sexually-promiscuous adults. Thus, the need for discretion drove the patients to private practitioners such as VS who offered them a reprieve from the ridicule that they often faced in government hospitals. As a 33-year old woman summed up:

28   Barua/Seeberg/Pandav (2009).
29   Kamat/Nichter (1998).
30   Barua/Pandav (2011).
31   Kamat (2001).

Everyone will say the same thing... there is nothing new in what I am saying. You go to a government hospital, you are treated like an animal... they treat you badly because they think you are a loose woman just because you are a poor woman and live in a slum. I was told by a member of staff in the [government] hospital as she wrote the names of medicines on the parchi, "first clean up your habits and then come back here [to VS' clinic] for treatment". There were at least 30 people in the room with me. I felt like a dirty woman and couldn't look at the other women around me. Why should I ever go back there? Do they have a right to treat you like this just because you are poor...?

During a group discussion, the respondents emphatically said that they did not "get what [they] need in public facilities". They were almost always "made to run from department to department with long queues at each point". Indifference and a total lack of concern were encountered everywhere, especially from the clerical and other non-medical staff. Senior doctors were often not approachable and the younger, inexperienced doctors were brusque, generally did not listen to what the patient had to say and issued orders. Under the circumstances, there was an unambiguous preference for "better care" by the neighbourhood practitioners, who might be less-than-fully-qualified, in comparison to inadequate or "no care" in a government facility.[32]

Discussion

While patients' interests in, and the decision to seek, traditional or alternative systems of medicine – most notably ayurveda and homeopathy – may indeed be growing in most European countries or in the Americas, the slums of big metropolitan cities in India such as Delhi tell a story which is starkly different. Slum settlements are micro-universes of burgeoning population groups – mainly migrants – that have congregated in the city from different states in the country, primarily in search of jobs. A majority of these people are engaged in the informal sector and live a hand-to-mouth existence subsisting on daily wages in the most compromised living spaces. The high incidence of morbidity imposes a costly toll on most households. In the event of an illness, not only do medical costs deplete their already precarious financial condition, but the inability to earn during the period inflicts a double burden which often pushes them into debt traps with catastrophic consequences.

In the absence of a structured urban primary health care system, and with the critical lack of qualified health providers in burgeoning slum settlements, private health providers such as VS are invariably the first point of resort for a majority of inhabitants of slums such as Midanpuri. Notwithstanding antagonism from the formal medical establishment, private practitioners like him run flourishing clinical practices in and around slum settlements for a well-established clientele. Alternative epistemologies are modified to suit the particular context in which they operate. At a fundamental level, this approach may present an ontological challenge, and more importantly carry serious, and of-

32 Berman (1998).

ten dangerous, health consequences. It could also be seen as a form of 'forced pluralism'[33] that people in impoverished contexts are subjected to. Notwith-standing these arguments, for the patient in a pragmatic search for a 'cure', this is a strategy that 'works'. Despite the realization by patients that these practi-tioners are not 'as qualified' as formally trained doctors, proof of knowledge and effectiveness of their practice is defined by the 'powerful' medicines that they dispense. It is the perceived efficacy of these medicines, among other things, that brings the patients back to them. The neighbourhood practition-ers, in turn, demonstrate shrewd business acumen as they structure their prac-tice to suit the requirements of the population around them. The pluralism that one witnesses must be understood, therefore, in the context of one of the most densely populated and compromised population groups for whom the main imperative is to return to work as quickly as possible, driven as they are by the crippling insecurities of income and tenure.

VS's practice does not suggest any significant modification to basic ho-meopathic philosophy. What is interesting, however, is his integration of ho-meopathy with allopathy to fit the local context which both he and his patients inhabit. In a context that is marked by multiple and acute vulnerabilities, it is not surprising that to these patients, the neighbourhood private practitioners appear as a boon. In the absence of any other options within the immediate environment, they offer the most attractive and responsive option. Attendant social and locational advantages contribute to their acceptance by the com-munities they serve and over time they come to represent the healing ortho-doxy within that particular context. Whether it is time spent waiting in a queue to get the *parchi* done; or time spent on getting the tests done; or on a com-pletely different register, the amount of time the doctor spends with the pa-tient, which is a time of care, attention and the possibility for playing out a moral drama as, at times, the seeking of a cure may be an end in itself. On all these counts, the dice obviously rolls in favour of private *daktars* (physicians).

Bibliography

Awasthi, Shally; Srivastava, Neeraj Mohan; Pant, Shubha: Symptom-specific care-seeking be-havior for sick neonates among urban poor in Lucknow. In: Journal of Perinatology 28 (2008), pp. S69-S75.

Barua, Nupur; Pandav, Chandrakant: The allure of the private practitioner: Is this the only alternative for the urban poor in India? In: Indian Journal of Public Health 55 (2011), pp. 107–114.

Barua, Nupur; Seeberg, Jens; Pandav, Chandrakant: Health of the Poor and the Role of Pri-vate Practitioners: The Case of a Slum in Delhi. New Delhi 2009.

Berman, Peter: Rethinking health care systems: private health care provision in India. In: World Development 26 (1998), pp. 1463–1479.

33 Sen/Iyer/George (2007).

Bhardwaj, S.M.: Medical pluralism and homeopathy: A geographic perspective. In: Social Science & Medicine 14 B (1980), pp. 209–216.

Bhat, Ramesh: Characteristics of private medical practice in India: A provider perspective. In: Health Policy and Planning 14 (1999), no. 1, pp. 26–37.

Census of India 2011. Provisional Population Totals. Ministry of Home Affairs, URL: http://www.censusindia.gov.in (last accessed on May 22, 2013).

D'Souza, Rennie M.: Role of health-seeking behaviour in child mortality in the slums of Karachi, Pakistan. In: Journal of Biosocial Science 35 (2003), pp. 131–144.

Jenkins, Richard: Culture, classification and (in)competence. In: Jenkins, Richard (ed.): Questions of Competence: Culture, Classification and Intellectual Disability. Cambridge 1998, pp. 1–24.

Kamat, Vinay R.: Private practitioners and their role in the resurgence of malaria in Mumbai (Bombay) and Navi Mumbai (New Bombay), India: serving the affected or aiding an epidemic? In: Social Science & Medicine 52 (2001), pp. 885–909.

Kamat, Vinay R.; Nichter, Mark: Pharmacies, self-medication and pharmaceutical marketing in Bombay, India. In: Social Science & Medicine 47 (1998), no. 6, pp. 779–794.

Naraindas, Harish: Of relics, body parts and laser beams: The German Heilpraktiker and the Ayurvedic spa. In: Anthropology and Medicine 18 (2011), no. 1, pp. 67–96.

Nichter, Mark: Pharmaceuticals, the commodification of health care – Medicine use transition. In: Nichter, Mark (ed.): Anthropology and International Health. 2nd ed. Amsterdam 1996, pp. 265–326.

Papreen, Nahar et al.: Living with infertility: Experiences among urban slum populations in Bangladesh. In: Reproductive Health Matters 8 (2000), no. 15, pp. 33–44.

Sen, Gita; Iyer, Aditi; George, Asha: Systematic hierarchies and systemic failures: Gender and health inequities in Koppal district. In: Economic and Political Weekly 42 (2007), no. 8, pp. 682–690.

Subba, Sonu Hangma; Joshi, Hari; Nagesh, Shubha: Health seeking behaviour regarding psychiatric disorders in mothers of children in an urban slum. In: Indian Journal of Preventive and Social Medicine 35 (2004), pp. 121–126.

UNICEF: The State of the World's Children: Children in an Urban World. New York 2012.

Urban Health Resource Centre; Ministry of Health and Family Welfare: State of Urban Health in Delhi. New Delhi 2007.

Vithoulkas, George: Homeopathy. In: Bannerman, Robert H.; Burton, John; Wen-Chieh, Chen (eds.): Traditional Medicine and Health Care Coverage. Geneva 1983, pp. 110–115.

Vlahov, David et al.: Urban as a determinant of health. In: Journal of Urban Health 84 (2007), pp. 16–26.

Pluralism, Popularity and Propaganda: Narratives of Lay Practices of Homeopathy in India

Krishna Soman

'Pluralism' in health care

'Pluralism' in health care generally indicates the co-existence of a range of medical systems in human societies, regardless of their origin and organizations. In the current discourses in medicine however, it is more specifically known as 'medical pluralism' and characterized by a pattern where bio-medicine exerts dominance over alternative healing systems. This latter trend of coexistence has drawn attention from all quarters of medicine, driven largely by limitations of the allopathic system and growing awareness of the potential of homeopathic and Indian systems of medicine in ensuring healing and health in the human society.[1]

Such pluralism, however, revolves around a dialectic core of healer and patient in multiple spheres of the health care system. Like therapies, therapeutic institutions include an array of scale and organization, so do the healers associated with them. While there are folk practitioners such as midwives, bonesetters and others, there are also professionals associated with clinics, hospitals and associations. At times, health care is also provided by the patients themselves, their families, social networks and communities. Baer, presenting an Indian case study on 'Medical Pluralism' in an encyclopaedia of medical anthropology, has referred to the historical and ethnographic research conducted by the renowned anthropologist Charles Leslie in the 1970s. In his case study based on Leslie's work, Baer pointed out that the 'Indian dominative medical systems' in particular could be broadly delineated at five levels. These, in turn, involve a range of healers practising in the realms of biomedicine, indigenous medical systems, homeopathy, religious and folk healing in different institutional and social settings.[2] Baer added that anthropological research at a later stage, however, brought 'power relations' into the study of medical pluralism. Whereas, political economy of health, primarily takes note of the fact that societies are stratified and analyses how power and hierarchical relations influence 'medical pluralism' in societies.[3] Proponents assert that the hierarchical power relationships are based upon class, caste, racial, ethnic, regional, religious, and gender distinctions. While observing that the national medical system in India tends to be plural rather than pluralistic, Singer et al pointed out that bio-medicine enjoys the dominant status vis-à-vis other medi-

---

1   Elliott (1969); Illich (1975); Government of India (2008); Tibrewal (2013); Bhatia (2013); Malik (2013); Sachdeva (2011).
2   Baer (2004), p. 109. He referred to Leslie (1977).
3   Navarro (1986); Singer/Baer (1995), pp. 109–115.

cal systems. In such a scenario however, patients are capable of plural use of distinct medical systems.[4]

Homeopathy, although it originated in the West at the very end of the 18th century, has achieved its own distinct identity in close association with the Indian systems of medicine rather than allopathic medicine.[5] This is in spite of allopathic and homeopathic systems sharing a common origin in the west. In India, it was officially recognized along with the Indian systems of medicine through the establishment of a separate department in the Ministry of Health, in the year 1995. Later, in 2002, it became an integral part of the first National Policy on Indian Systems of Medicine and Homeopathy. Simultaneously, there has also been reorganization and expansion of the health infrastructures. Between the years 2000 and 2008, the strength of the Indian medical systems – Ayurveda, Yoga, Unani, Siddha and Homeopathy (AYUSH) grew more in the sphere of dispensaries than that of hospitals. In this, homeopathy per se made up around one-fourth and one-tenth of the AYUSH dispensaries and hospitals respectively.[6] Further, there was co-location of AYUSH in the Primary Health Centres (PHC). The Eleventh Five Year Plan had estimated that there was co-location in 3,528 of the total 23,291 PHCs. In an analysis of the data on homeopathic practices presented in a draft report published by the Indian government in 2008, Dinges indicated that a total of 6,030 PHCs made homeopathic services available to an average population of 170,480 per physician. In the nine years starting from 2000, while the total number of registered AYUSH practitioners increased by eleven per cent, homeopathy alone witnessed an increase of 23 per cent.[7] A recent report further shows that homeopathy constitutes 30 per cent of the registered AYUSH practitioners in India following the only larger presence of the Ayurveda practitioners that constitutes 60 per cent.[8] While this is a picture of the state of qualified homeopathy in formal public health care, it was earlier reported that the presence of homeopathy in government accounts extends to the private sphere of healing too. For instance, 675 of 1,220 dispensaries (i.e. 56 per cent) were run by local bodies in the state of West Bengal.[9] The state health-planning has hardly paid attention to how its people, particularly those at the periphery or fringe of the society, deal with their health or cope with ill-health. However, these government reports present no account of 'lay practices' of homeopathy which have been a reality in the Indian health culture.

Plurality of practices involving different systems of medicine has frequently surfaced in literature, although plurality within individual systems of medicine is rarely and only circumstantially discussed. However, like the for-

4   Singer/Baer (1995), pp. 109–115.
5   Government of India (2007), pp. 331–335; Singh/Yadav/Pandey (2005); Yadav/Pandey/
     Singh (2007); Priya/Shweta (2010).
6   Government of India (2011).
7   Dinges (2011).
8   Government of India (2011).
9   Government of India (2005).

mer, the latter is also a reality in the stratified Indian society. Within specific systems of medicine, this includes plural diagnostic and healing practices not only by qualified but also self-taught practitioners. Practices of the latter are referred to as lay practice, quackery or unqualified non-state provision.[10] Such practices have prevailed in homeopathy – an officially recognized medical system that has developed to the status of super-specialty care in India.[11] The forms or expressions, however, have changed over time. Bhardwaj circumstantially mentioned this phenomenon in his observations on the 'Naturalization process of homeopathy in India'.[12] This brought out yet another, then prevailing, similar kind of practice. During an early phase of the growth of homeopathy, qualified allopathic practitioners had turned to homeopathic practice. Such practice may now be referred to more precisely as 'cross practice'.[13]

Plurality within homeopathic practices has also been documented in the contexts of Europe and North America. A collection of essays edited by Jütte and others presented the historical perspectives of homeopathic medicine in these regions in the 19th and 20th centuries. Apart from the plurality in geographical contexts and their interweaving, the volume presents the evolution of homeopathy in its multiple dimensions including identities and socio-political relations.[14] Articles on the roles of laymen in the history of German homeopathy[15], the paradox of professionalization[16] and role of medical societies in the process of professionalization in Germany and the USA by Dinges[17] are worth mentioning here for their relevance.

This paper attempts to look into the social, cultural, economic and political dimensions of 'lay practices of homeopathy' in India, with a focus on pre- and post-colonial Bengal. This area of 'lay' or allied practices of homeopathy is yet to be adequately explored for policy making.[18] An attempt is being made here to put together a few narratives based on available literature, my own studies in social dynamics of health and healthcare in rural Bengal and some direct observations of social change across generations. The paper concludes with a discussion on 'lay practices of homeopathy' in the contexts of pluralism, popularity and propaganda.

10   Bhardwaj (1981); Palmer (2006); Sheehan (2009).
11   http://www.doctorcancer.org/index.php (last accessed on May 22, 2013).
12   Bhardwaj (1981).
13   Sheehan (2009).
14   Jütte/Risse/Woodward (1998).
15   Staudt (1998).
16   Jütte (1998).
17   Dinges (1998).
18   Soman (2003).

Lay Practices of Homeopathy in India: A View through Narratives

The history of homeopathy has been engaged largely in discourses on institutionalization and formalization of homeopathic education and practices. Lay practices of homeopathy however, have been rarely documented or analyzed, except by a few such as Morrell[19] and Staudt[20] in the British and German contexts respectively. Morrell revealed that Hahnemann's second wife, Melanie (1800–1878) and the Director of the Munster Botanic Garden, Carl von Bönninghausen (1785–1864), whom Hahnemann appreciated very much, were the first lay healers! While according to Morrell it was hard to find relevant information due to the thinly dispersed nature of the evidences that were either published or held by organizations, Staudt mentioned of the relevant information available in German publications of *Hahnemannia*, in particular.[21] Additionally, Petursdottir in an essay on patient's choice of homeopathic lay practices among the folk healers of Iceland emphasized upon patients' choice in health care.[22] Inquiry into the history of homeopathic lay practices in India, from the perspectives of the users or patients in particular, is a task yet to be initiated.

This section includes four narratives, which reflect on the multiple dimensions of homeopathic lay practices in 19th and 20th century India, with a focus on Bengal. Drawn largely from the historical essay of Bhardwaj, the first narrative attempts to trace the journey of lay practices as reflected in the account of 'naturalization' of homeopathy in colonial and post-colonial India.[23] The second narrative in this paper, aims at filling in the gap in literature through a sketch of the practices and related social relations that prevailed among the elite intellectual gentlemen of Bengal, during this time. It presents glimpses of the medical world of Rabindranath Tagore (1861–1941) – the Nobel Laureate for literature and founder of Santiniketan or Visva-Bharati – the world renowned university that became a meeting place of oriental and occidental scholars. This narrative reflects on how homeopathy was promoted and practised by persons from other disciplines or professions among the intellectual class and communities in Bengal in the wake of 'nationalism'. The concluding narrative included in this paper is located at the turn of the 20th century – that is after five decades of planning in health services development, including the official recognition of homeopathy at administrative and policy levels. Against the backdrop of transforming villages in Birbhum district of West Bengal – a state in eastern India, this narrative portrays the picture of health care prevailing in peri-urban villages. It maps out the social positioning of the lay practitioners, their practices and utilization of services by the villagers.

19   Morrell (1995).
20   Staudt (1998).
21   Dinges (2002). The introduction of the edited volume, however, indicates that there is more literature available on lay practices in Germany.
22   Pétursdóttir (2002).
23   Bhardwaj (1981).

As well as dealing with Tagore's interest in homeopathic practices and with some relatively contemporary aspects of homeopathy this paper also presents the narrative of a family. This narrative seeks to substantiate with additional insights into the knowledge of homeopathy and homeopathic lay practice as well as their cross-generational history within the Bengali patriarchal family of that time.

Narrative 1: Spread of Lay practices of homeopathy in India: A Sketch

Homeopathy was introduced to India in early 19th century by a few European physicians, missionaries and laypersons. While the physicians were practitioners of allopathic medicine, others were lay persons who travelled to India for other purposes and practised homeopathy either by themselves and / or encouraged others to do so. The essay by Bhardwaj gives an account of the arrival, naturalization and official recognition of homeopathy in India.[24] It circumstantially creates space for an argument on how 'lay practices' played an important role not only in the arrival of homeopathy in India but also during its growth and spread there. An article on homeopathy that was published in *The Calcutta Review* in 1852, made interesting observations about 'non-professionals' or 'amateurs' in homeopathic practices in India at that point in time. According to Bhardwaj, lay-homeopathy was practised in India as an 'amateur's hobby' by some Europeans even before that time. It was probably known to the Indians even before the establishment of a homeopathic hospital in 1847 by the then Raja of Tanjore in southern India. According to some influential homeopathic practitioners, Dr. Honigberger of Transylvania who had treated Maharaja Ranjit Singh in Lahore, Punjab during the 1830s, was responsible for introducing this medical system into India. He was an allopath, who included or turned to homeopathy in the course of his practice. He claimed that his system was the 'medium system'. Although he was primarily an allopath, he learnt the principles of homeopathy from Dr Samuel Hahnemann – the founder of the system – but did not wholeheartedly become a homeopath himself. However, as part of his 'medium system', he also dispensed homeopathic medicines in Calcutta in the 1850s and 1860s.

There were similar instances where trained European allopathic practitioners turned to homeopathic practices in India. For instance, a Madras Presidency surgeon, after his retirement in1846, had found employment in the homeopathic hospital, established in Tanjore in southern India. It is worth mentioning here that the British medical officials, who were appointed to the British Indian administration or the East India Company, had to have their training in modern allopathic medicine from reputed colleges in Britain. There is evidence that homeopathic treatment was used by such doctors in the General Military Hospital at Bombay, particularly in the treatment of cholera

---

24 Bhardwaj (1981). Unfortunately the recent history of homeopathy in India of B. Poldas is
    not translated into English.

in the 1840s. Another instance was that of a French doctor, C. Fabre Tonnerre, who served as the superintendent medical officer of the short-lived Calcutta Native Homeopathic Hospital in 1852.

In addition to this, there were European missionaries who, under certain circumstances, were engaged in homeopathic lay practices, mostly to serve humanity. Some missionaries had reported in publications and conferences that it was due to situations that often demanded medical relief that they had developed homeopathic practices as a hobby to adopt the 'novel and inexpensive system' and make it part of their 'do-good ethic'. Similarly, the Indian correspondent of the *Homeopathic World* reported from the Nilgiris in southern India in 1869 that he was 'often called upon to act the doctor' out there, 'where most people' were 'compelled to depend very much' on 'non-professional assistance' as they preferred 'homeopathic treatment'.[25] However, not all the missionaries were comfortable with these practices. A hint of their unease about their own lack of 'medical' credentials was expressed in the Allahabad Conference in 1872–73, in particular. This was revealed in the use, among themselves, of the term 'quacking' to describe their activities as 'self-employed doctors'. These self-doubts, were later however, overcome in favour of their lay practices. This was based on an argument that emerged in a wider denouncement by the Europeans pointing to the practitioners of the Indian systems of medicine as 'ignorant quacks'. At that point, missionaries argued that 'inexpert aid' in the form of lay practices was better than leaving the sick and the dying in the hands of local healers.[26]

In short, there were Europeans, who in various capacities had contributed to (if not enriched) the then prevailing culture of homeopathic practice in India through various kinds of lay practices. These contributors included trained practitioners of allopathic medicine, civil as well as military servants (as is shown by their ranks and titles), missionaries and traders. The Indians, however, were not far behind.

The Indians played important roles in naturalization or rather 'Indianization' of homeopathy. There were both, Hindu and Muslim gentlemen who, along with the Europeans, had donated to the Calcutta Native Homeopathic Hospital in the late 19th century. *The Calcutta Review* reported that the system of homeopathy was being practised intensely by amateurs. Calcutta – the capital of British India in Bengal – served as the hub for further growth or naturalization of homeopathy in the pluralist Bengali culture. A few influential Bengali elite, who were enthusiastic about homeopathy, made important contributions to this process of growth and naturalization. They identified courageous Bengali allopathic practitioners, and attempted to persuade them to engage in homeopathic practice. Lay homeopath Babu Rajendralal Dutta, a wealthy businessman, thus influenced an allopath and member of the medical faculty at the University of Calcutta – Dr Mahendralal Sircar – to take up homeopathy. In 1863 an allopath with an MD was thus introduced to the prac-

---

25 Bhardwaj (1981).
26 Fitzgerald (2001).

tice of homeopathy. With time, he changed his views and by 1867 had finally adopted the principles of homeopathy.[27] It was a process of conversion. He grew to be an example to the medical fraternity of Calcutta and a source of inspiration for other Indian allopathic practitioners to turn to homeopathy. Such was the influence of Indian 'lay' persons like Rajendralal Dutta who believed in the efficacy of homeopathy. This gradually paved the way for professionalization of homeopathy in India. However, this professionalization induced by conversion in turn led to the development of training curriculum and practices in homeopathy. The process of professionalization was uneven and marked by conflicts with the rival allopathic system which finally lead to a relationship of antagonism. It also placed homeopathy in a position subservient to allopathy. Amidst all these power struggles, the system continued to appeal to and influence the laypersons and the emerging educated elite of the society in favour of the homeopathic system.

The process of popularization and naturalization was facilitated through publications in vernacular languages, including Bengali. These involved Bengali translation of the *Indian Homeopathic Review* in 1890s followed by the *Hahnemann*, which was first published in 1917. Following the independence of India in 1947, the Homeopathic Inquiry Committee was constituted. The report of the committee had indicated low cost of homeopathic treatment compared to allopathic treatment, which implied that people would gain access to medical care. While an allopath excluded most common folk who were poor, an homeopath attracted and included them because of the low cost of treatment. By the end of the 19th century, homeopathy seemed to have been naturalized in India; the net result was confusing, though. According to the estimates of the Homeopathic Inquiry Committee, while there were 200,000–300,000 homeopathic practitioners in India in the year 1949, the number of the practitioners who had some sort of institutional training was not more than 5,000.[28] This tells a story of the social trend of lay practices of homeopathy in the 1950s. By then homeopathic lay practices had advanced to the villages of Bengal and penetrated the cultural norms of health care practices at family and community levels. Gradually, 'lay practices' in any medical system, have been viewed by the state as 'quackery', a term which includes even qualified physicians of various systems engaged in malpractices or negligence. An estimate by the Deputy Director of the Central Bureau of Health Intelligence claimed in the year 2007 that there were around 30,000 of 'quacks' in the capital city of Delhi alone.[29] The regulatory mechanisms presently involve the departments of health services in the states and the corresponding medical and AYUSH councils and legal establishments. To delineate an isolated picture of the 'lay practices' or 'quackery' in homeopathy itself requires a deeper inquiry, which is beyond the scope of this paper. It is worth noting here that the cultural connotation of 'lay practice' has been replaced by the medico-legal notion of

27   Bhardwaj (1981).
28   Bhardwaj (1981).
29   Kumar (2007).

'quackery' within the realm of health care. This can be interpreted as a repetition of history as the collection of essays mentioned earlier has revealed.[30] Dinges, in particular, brought insights regarding the role of the medical profession and societies in the similar yet distinct characters of the journeys of professionalization of homeopathy in the German and American contexts.[31]

In brief, a level of confidence had developed among the facilitators and lay practitioners of homeopathy. This probably gave rise to the hope that if even 'non-professional' people could achieve good results with homeopathic medicine, there was no doubt that when the professional men began practising, the result was likely to be even better'.[32] Further, it managed to survive the challenges of social, economic, cultural and above all, political transformation that India has gone through in the past hundred and seventy years. Planting and nurturing this confidence was probably a key to the development of the homeopathic system of medicine in Indian history.

Narrative 2: Rabindranath Tagore's medical world: Practices of Homeopathy

Nobel laureate Rabindranath Tagore was born in 1861 in a strictly monotheist family in Calcutta. Rabindranath declined formal education. Yet, besides having a great flair for poetry, he was also interested in science and its practical applications. He not only left behind a legacy of poems, stories, novels, plays and essays but also works on philosophy, philology, theosophy, physics and others. This versatile intellectual of the 19th and 20th centuries had an interesting hobby, which was medicine. This narrative was composed, borrowing largely from the essays contributed by Bagchi and Datta.[33]

The poet was a self-taught homeopathic practitioner until the 1930s. The main source of evidence for his interest in homeopathy was rooted in the small notebook of family expenses, which included records of expenditures on purchases of homeopathic medicines. The Tagore family used to seek homeopathic treatment from their personal allopath Dr Mahendralal Sircar, who started practising homeopathy in 1867, as well as from the man who convinced him of homeopathy, the wealthy businessman and a lay homeopath Babu Rajen Dutta. However, in his practising days, Tagore was found to occasionally consult his litterateur fourth sister Swarna Kumari Devi regarding diagnosis and treatment of ailing patients. It appears that the Tagore family did provide a homeopathy-friendly environment for its members and did not prevent them from taking amateur interest in applications of homeopathic knowledge or practice of Homeopathy.

Rabindranath, a voracious reader and owner of an analytical mind, was drawn to homeopathy by the work of Dr Mahendralal Sircar and his follow-

---

30 Jütte/Risse/Woodward (1998).
31 Dinges (1998).
32 Bhardwaj (1981).
33 Bagchi (2000); Datta (2002).

ers. His acquaintance with homeopathy was transformed into a kind of 'dependence' later in his life. During the late 19th and early 20th centuries he had to spend months in travelling alone on boats sailing on the river Padma in order to supervise the family estates in rural Bengal (now in Bangladesh). A chest of homeopathic medicines and books on how to diagnose and cure patients was his companion along with pen, ink and paper for his own writing. His interest in homeopathy grew further and he did not stop at treating just himself but made homeopathic treatment also available to his boatmen.

During his visits to the estates, he came face to face with the social oppressions and human sufferings of the socially and economically deprived. He observed the social structures and relations between the poor and the rich, the peasants and 'Zamindars' or the Landed Gentry in remote villages of Bengal. Similarly, he also formed his views regarding the difference between men and women prevailing in the Bengali elite that hindered the freedom of women. All this was eventually reflected in his writings.[34] It appears that all these experiences went to construct the 'interventionist' Rabindranath that manifested later in his experiments of 'rural reconstruction' in villages around Santiniketan. This attitude of 'intervention' or intention of bringing relief to human sufferings was also observed in his practice of homeopathy, particularly when he started living at Santiniketan.

Tagore was a homeopathic healer – even though a 'lay' healer! He successfully diagnosed and treated many of his associates and students as well as others at Santiniketan or other places of work, both friends and relatives, women and men alike. Once he treated Bonophul, a famous litterateur and author of "Memoirs of Tagore" (Rabi Smriti in Bengali) for piles, using *Sulphur* and *Nux-vomica*. In 1935 he also successfully treated Nirmal Kumari, the wife of the famous statistician Prasanta Mahalanabis, for pleurisy. Later, she wrote about this event in an article titled: "Chikitsak Rabindranath" (Rabindranath, the physician), which was published by the Government College of Arts and Crafts of Calcutta in the late 1970s. This is a summary of Tagore's ability for curing people using homeopathy. His capacity as a homeopathic healer touched many lives. He once treated a Japanese student at Santiniketan. He also cured the child of a Santhali (tribal) woman who was suffering from '*meningitis*'. While travelling, he used to carry a box of homeopathic medicines and dispensed them to the poor and sick in most of the places he visited in India. It is not that he was always successful. Whenever he failed to improve the condition of a patient, he would refer them to qualified doctors.[35]

Rabindranath Tagore's larger vision on homeopathy was to help more and more people, particularly the poor. He did not intend to keep himself engaged in diagnosis or treatment alone. He also wanted to bring in new practitioners who would serve the poor. Often he gave homeopathic books as presents to his patients, mostly with the intention of involving them further in the homeopathic world and empowering them to reduce human suffering. Ho-

34   Datta (2002).
35   Bagchi (2000).

meopathic treatment, according to him, was 'simple, rational and economic'. While treating litterateur Bonophul, he gave him the message that 'those drugs are very convenient; they are cheap. So, you can help many poor people'. This was very much a cultural initiative of Tagore towards the expansion and popularization of homeopathy in Bengal in the early 20th century. It is worth mentioning here that this was the period of 'nationalism' against colonial rule. This was also the time in the history of medicine when the Indian systems of healing such as Ayurveda and others were attempting a revival in the face of 'western modern' allopathic medicine. In this context, Tagore's initiative was an expression of 'patriotism', combined with notions of 'self-reliance'.

Rabindranath had declined formal education. Yet he had vast knowledge in many subjects. He had a great deal of respect for homeopathy. He had read books written by 'Lillienthal, Lupi, Allen, Boericke, Cowperthroat' and other famous authors. His great regard for this branch of medicine was reflected in many of his actions – to the extent that he sent his second son-in-law, the allopath Satyendranath, to study homeopathy in the United States. He was not only a healer but a trainer too. He taught homeopathy to a noted Sanskrit and Ayurvedic scholar – Pandit Kshitimohan Sen Shastri.[36] He also trained his associate, Sushil Kumar Bhanja Chowdhury, who was the Director of the music college of Visva Bharati. After receiving training, Sri Bhanja Chowdhury started a thriving practice of his own. Tagore always affectionately referred to him as 'amar daktar' (my doctor). This was the story of a lay homeopathic practitioner who never had any formal training in homeopathy.[37]

Narrative 3: Lay Practices of Homeopathy across generations:
the story of the Chatterjee family

In 1975, I (nee' Krishna Chatterjee) was pursuing undergraduate studies in human physiology in the city of Calcutta, when I had no idea of venturing into the history of medicine in future. At that time, my grandfather, Binoy Krishna Chatterjee, passed away at the age of 77 years, after suffering from brief bronchial illness. I miss him today. I miss his affection, his wisdom, his oneness with nature and, above all, his hair-raising stories of jungles – the wild elephants, spiders and *mohua*-intoxicated packs of bears surrounding the moonlit compounds of his forest bungalow... and so on. All these were after his retirement from the responsibilities of a Forest Conservator. After serving the British Indian government for decades, he retired around the 1950s – after national independence. Then he returned with my grandmother Maya Debi to the village of Malipota in Bengal where her father, i.e my great grandfather, was living at that time. They settled down in a small new house and nurtured beautiful orchards of mango, jack fruit, litchi, custard apple, and berries around our home. The villagers affectionately addressed my grandmother as

36   Maternal grandfather of Amartya Sen, the Nobel Laureate in Economics.
37   Bagchi (2000).

pishima or aunt.[38] I spent much of the formative years of my childhood in Malipota, under their wings.

My grandfather was a botanist and served as a conservator in the School of Forestry in Dehra Dun.[39] His postings were in the forests of Bihar and Orissa. Often he had to travel through jungles or sometimes he had to visit the Forest school at Dehra Dun, in connection with his job. Didu, my grandma, would often recall how dangerous and lonely it was for her to live in the official forest bungalows when her husband was away and the children were either small or sent to a residential school in Deoghar.[40] She also remembered the 'celebrations' that they used to have at home when my grandfather returned from tour – carrying books and periodicals she had chosen to keep her company when he would go on his next trip. Every evening after work, they spent time reciting poems together, singing songs and playing their favourite instruments – flute and Esraj. Both of them were creative and artistic, possibly because of their closeness to the tranquillity of nature. Whenever my grandfather was around he would always make a point of eating meals together with her. In the then dense forests of Keonjhar, Chaibasa, Koderma and others, they lived like friends, unlike many other patriarchal families in those days. However, while he was a government servant in British India, she was a 'Swadeshi' at heart. She insisted that her husband bring her booklets and periodicals about women, 'Swaraj' and the like. One name that I remember now, was '*Bharater Naari*' (Women of India). It was not mere coincidence that she, in those days, strongly resisted having any foreign products brought to their household. It was she who later sowed in me the ideas of 'self-reliance' and 'political economy' in the context of our village, Malipota.

They lived in remote areas where a 'doctor', with or without a degree or certificate, was a rare commodity. It is not very clear whether as a part of his own training at the Institute of Forestry or prompted by his own interest, grandfather – a 'lay man' – in the language of medical literature – became interested in homeopathic practice. I heard from my grandma that he was a support not only to her and the children but also to their cook or gardener in the forest bungalows. Once my grandparents discovered that one of their Bengali friends who used to manage a mica mine in Koderma where my grandfather was posted, was also a lay practitioner of Homeopathy.

I had seen him practising in our village Malipota, in post-retirement years. Having vast knowledge of Indian plants and herbs, he often used to read or refer to 'English' books on homeopathy that he kept on the shelf. My uncles who had grown up with the culture of homeopathic care in the family used to supply quality medicines from Calcutta. He used to treat his relatives and other residents in the village – the struggling migrant weavers from Tangail in then east Pakistan, toiling peasants, rickshaw pullers, fisher folks along with the formally educated school teachers or the village priest or the post master,

38   Father's sister.
39   Stebbing/Champion/Osmaston (2010).
40   Now in the state of Jharkhand.

at times. My grandmother played the role of his medical assistant. She would
take the patients' case histories, report them to grandfather and then dispense
the medicines prescribed by him. I saw him keeping his own notes for further
reference; there was no system of written prescription. He also sent patients to
Calcutta – to his eldest son – for modern medical treatment available in the
city. Once every month when he went to Ranaghat to collect his pension from
the post-office there, grandmother had the privilege of working independently
as the 'medical woman'. She often moved beyond the role of 'assistant' and
applied her own knowledge of homeopathic treatment to cure our domestic
animals – mother cow, Lali and her calf, Joba. As mentioned earlier, there was
no written prescription that the patient had to carefully store for the next visit.
Tiny bottles containing the 'magic' pills were alphabetically arranged in the
big 'double storied' wooden box. I had a lot of respect not only for my grandparents but also for the box for its age and experience. Like a poem, I had almost memorized and could understand the basic questions that grandma
would ask patients in order to report the signs and symptoms of their illnesses
to her husband for diagnosis and treatment. Later, I understood that this was
the method of his training; sitting in his chair, he always crosschecked whether
she was performing her job of history-taking and reporting with perfection
and precision. According to her, he considered his practice as an act of 'social
welfare', a way of helping others without asking anything in return. My pro-
active grandmother became directly involved in the lives of the villagers, particularly the poor. While trying to get them the benefits of the government
programmes, she became a direct witness of their sufferings and struggles.
This woman, who had earlier introduced me to the stars, flowers, butterflies,
colours and music of nature, also moulded me later to value human labour
and dignity. She taught me to appreciate hand woven cloths over the finished
products of the mills that were run by the 'rich' for larger profits. In the middle
of all this, I was naturally introduced to the world of homeopathy, too.

My mother Moitri Chatterjee, after marriage at the age of thirteen, came
to live with the family in Chaibasa as my father, after graduating in English
literature, was then completing a professional course in Veterinary Science in
the city of Kolkata. My mother was already familiar with biochemic medicines
as she saw her father dispensing the pallets to treat common ailments in the
joint family of around twenty five members. When she lived with her parents-
in-law for few years, mother became interested in the culture of homeopathic
remedies that prevailed in the family. When the grandparents were engrossed
in their homeopathic practice, she kept her eyes and ears alert. Later when she
came to Calcutta to live with her husband, my brother was born and I followed him after five years. I do not know how exactly it happened, but we,
along with our father and occasionally the domestic helps, became the subjects of her homeopathic apprenticeship whenever we were unwell. She me-
ticulously followed my grandmother's caution in advising patients to go to a
'doctor' if they did not improve. Like my grandmother, she was not sufficiently conversant with English to be able to pick every instruction from Eng-

lish books on homeopathic treatment but the difference was that my grand-mother was in direct contact with her trainer. However, my enthusiastic mother eventually found a Bengali book titled: "Homeopathic Paribarik Chikitsa" – a maroon-coloured hardback book on 'homeopathic treatment in the family' published by the M. Bhattacharyya and Company private Limited, Calcutta. She also managed to set up a stock of the commonly used medicines in a chest similar to that of my grandfather, but smaller in size. The tradition continued in the family.

My brother, even after he graduated in modern medicine and became a specialist in microbiology, often consulted my mother as the first resort for relief when he felt unwell. My mother never saw 'would be' homeopathic practitioners in us. She wanted to manage her nuclear family within her own means and with love and care. Like my grandmother, she often had to live with my brother and me as father went on his frequent official tours. She used her time to read homeopathic books and in reflections that she sometimes shared with me. I was fascinated by her sharp observations and understanding of our individual bodies, nature and habits. In the past thirty years, I have lived a bustling life, changing jobs, getting back to higher studies and research, shifting residences in three states in India. When I look back in time, I realize that I have turned to the trends of my foremothers – at least in taking care of myself and my husband or domestic help whenever they desire it. I have also been privileged to be able to associate with like-minded peer groups at places of work and elsewhere in order to learn more about the world of homeopathic remedies. When I travel, I feel confident if I carry a pouch with a few homeo-pathic medicines that, as I know from experience, work well on me. In this way, I not only carry on the tradition of 'lay practices', but also feel empow-ered to deal with my own body and mind if necessary. I go on searching for an alternative to either the total surrender to the aggressive profit-oriented world of allopathic medicine or the increasingly formalized set-up of homeopathic consultations, with simple complaints of common cold or indigestion. This is how 'lay practices of homeopathy' continued across generations in the Chat-terjee family. This has survived as a part of the health culture in time.

Narrative 4: Rural Health Care in Bolpur: The self-taught practitioners

Birbhum – a rural district in West Bengal in eastern India had a population of 30.1 Lakhs at the end of the 20th century.[41] It is constituted of four sub-divi-sions and fourteen administrative blocks. Bolpur, which existed as a small vil-lage of 163 mud houses at the beginning of the century[42] has grown into an administrative block with 168 census villages and a municipality, Bolpur town[43]. There have been three major harbingers of change in Bolpur adminis-

41 Government of India (2001).
42 O'Malley (1910), p. 35.
43 Government of West Bengal (1998), p. 5.

trative block. These include the naturally growing town and related urbanization, the national high way intersecting the block from south to north and connecting Bolpur with the district town Suri, neighboring districts and states; here, in 1927, the third harbinger of change, Visva-Bharati University was established by Rabindranath Tagore (1861–1941), the Nobel Laureate for literature. With time the villages of Bolpur have undergone a socio-economic transformation. Villages that are located in the closest proximity of these major harbingers of change show more indications of social change than others. Within the villages, the lives of women have changed following those of their men. In health care, while the district had a rich heritage of Ayurvedic treatment since the 11th century AD, the practice of the homeopathic system of treatment started much later, in 1905, probably through the missionaries. Both systems of medicine have contributed considerably to the development of related literature in the country.[44] However, the local health care system has been more influenced by the allopathic medicine that was introduced by the British during the epidemics earlier in the 19th century and was later institutionalized in independent India as the political powers were convinced of its value.

Adityapur is a village cluster located at a distance of seven kilometres to the north-east of Bolpur town, where the rural reconstruction unit of Visva-Bharati University had begun the experiment of health cooperatives in the late 1930s, under philosophical guidance of Rabindranath Tagore.[45] Seven decades after this, while the village still retains its rural and agricultural character, the production processes and social relations have changed. Within this larger transformation, the sources of health care have also changed. Health cooperatives have been replaced by a range of public and private health care institutions. At present, while the services provided by the state are delivered through the wide but inadequate governmental primary health care network, more powerful private medical care institutions have grown like mushrooms around the government health centres and hospital. A range of private practitioners tends to occupy the gap that exists between the villagers and the government health services. Private institutions however, are not all formal. While the formal institutions include qualified allopathic or homeopathic practitioners in private clinics located in and around the town, there is a range of healers who are self-trained. They practise either allopathy or homeopathy or both; there are others including folk and religious healers, serving particularly in areas and situations where the formal health care services are inadequate and inaccessible.

In 1992, two hundred and seventy-two families lived in Adityapur. Agricultural land, government service and businesses of varying scales and coverage were the principal sources of income. While there were waged labourers, share croppers and land owners in agricultural relations in the village, there were small and big business owning households too. Small business involved

---

44   Majumdar (1975), p. 18.
45   Tagore (1938).

small scale local productions primarily for sales and services in the village and its neighbourhood. This included the fish and milk sellers, jewellers, priests, grocers, a barber, a blacksmith, a goldsmith, a carpenter, a weaver, oil-pressers, potters and the like. Big business involved larger scales of production and sales, mostly catering to the needs of distant villages and/or the town. This included suppliers of fish, milk, rice and other products, owners of a shop in the town and one of the 'village doctors' practising in many villages. A census of the village cluster revealed that more than one-third (39 per cent) of the households were poor. They depended on waged labour alone or on waged labour plus a small piece of land.[46]

For health care, residents of Adityapur visited both government and private institutions, depending on the availability of and access to such services. However, the 'village doctors' were an important resource for care, particularly for the poor and women across all socio-economic categories. There were three such private practitioners in Adityapur, who combined their 'medical practices' with other occupations such as farming, private tuition or school teaching. These practitioners were either self-taught or trained by senior practitioners like them for the symptomatic treatment of common illnesses. Compared to the qualified practitioners who offered medical consultations largely in the town, these self-taught healers treated villagers at a lower cost – charging nearly one-tenth of the fee charged by the former. In addition, they also made medicines available to the patients at affordable prices and on loan, at times. While one of them who had been in profession for twenty years, practised allopathic medicine, there was a school teacher who practised homeopathy based on his knowledge gathered from various Bengali books that he had collected from book stalls set up in the local fair. Another practitioner, however, shifted his occupation from private tuition to lay practising as he found the latter paid more. He, however, practised both allopathic and homeopathic medicine – the latter preferably for children and chronic symptoms. All of them were men. As healers, these lay practitioners were accepted as a 'social support in need' by the villagers across socio-economic strata. There was yet another such medical man frequently visiting from a near-by village. He was quite popular among the poor socio-economic households for distributing medicines on loan. Briefly, the self-trained healing systems had their place in Adityapur, the traditional institutions of midwives or medical women had nearly withered away, though.[47] Similar pictures of health culture are found even today in the villages that are located in the closest proximities to the major harbingers of change. Surul, Binuria and Ballabhpur are three census villages of the latter type that reveal a more diversified economy and complex social relations and health culture.

Surul, Binuria and Ballabhpur together comprised 2,225 households in 1996. A survey of reported chronic illnesses and illness-care among the adult women and men living in 742 sample households, considering the preceding

46 Soman (1992).
47 Soman (1992).

year as the period of reference, revealed certain valuable insights regarding utilization of self-taught healers including homeopathic lay practitioners. Thirty three per cent of the 1,173 women and 1,147 men aged 15 years and above had suffered from chronic illnesses persisting for more than three months. Significant gender differentials were found in the disaggregated data. The gender gap increased as the position of households declined in the socio-economic hierarchy. The picture of the first source of health care contacted revealed certain patterns of utilization. In 24 per cent and 53 per cent of cases, primary care was sought from the public and private formal institutions respectively. Of the latter, only 15 per cent visited the qualified homeopaths in private clinics. The remaining 23 per cent of the total care was contributed by the informal institutions. This was the time when AYUSH or the Indian systems of medicine and homeopathy were yet to make their presence felt in the Primary Health Care network of Bolpur. However, various kinds of shifts from allopathic to homeopathic treatment were observed, in chronic illnesses in particular for economic and other reasons.

The informal sector was comprised of self-trained practitioners of allopathic, homeopathic and indigenous systems of medicine and others such as folk and religious healers. Of these the self-trained healers practising homeopathic and allopathic medicines constituted a larger portion amounting to 55 per cent (N=102). It was overwhelmingly the constituency of the poor and women as nearly two-third of the poor and a similar proportion of the women across all socio-economic categories sought their help. Among the women, those in the poorer households participated in such health care more than their better-off counterparts. They also found it useful for their children. It was not only a matter of low expenditure but also the convenient locations and timings suitable to their daily schedules of labour and leisure.

The data, while it reflects the degree of utilization of self-trained healing in allopathic and homeopathic systems of medicine, cannot pin-point the picture of homeopathic lay practices alone. Nevertheless, there are reports and there is evidence of such practices that prevail in the officially 'un-served or under-served' areas in districts of Bengal. The district health administration is yet to bring out an official estimate of these practices that are commonly seen in pockets of villages, at village bus stops or medicine stores and elsewhere. The bonds between such healers irrespective of the system of medicine they practice and the villagers are cultural. Villagers do recognize the 'situation and culture-specific' support extended by these healers; they often appreciate and take pride in them.[48]

Self-trained practice in these villages is dominated by allopathic medicine. Of the five such practitioners available in the census villages of Surul, Binuria and Ballabhpur, three were practising allopathic medicine. While one of them was a retired government 'health worker', another was educated up to the eighth standard in school and trained and certified by the block administration

48   Soman (1997); Soman (2002).

for treating domestic animals in the villages. There was yet another practitioner who was a graduate in chemistry and had experience of working in the 'lab to land' project run by Visva-Bharati. Apart from his degree, he also had a certificate dated 15 November 1984 from an organization (name sealed) of Calcutta, registered under the West Bengal Societies Registration Act, 1961. The seal on the certificate indicated that the organization was first registered in 1934 under the British Act XXVI of 1860, which was later revived under Act 26 of 1961. While these self-taught practitioners of allopathic medicine travel from village to village to find patients, offer treatment and sell medicines, the self-trained homeopathic practitioners are fewer in number and largely stationary and practise in make-shift clinics at convenient and commercial locations. They generally represent the middle socio-economic section of the village society and view their practice as a 'respectful' occupation, which also serves as a subsidiary source of income.

While the practitioners mentioned earlier in this narrative, mostly practised among the poorer and underprivileged households, I would like to end this narrative by presenting a swift sketch of a 'lay' homeopathic practitioner, Chandrachur Roy, who was able to attract even the well-off professors of Visva-Bharati. A gentleman of around seventy years of age, popularly known as 'Chandu Babu', has practised homeopathy in Surul village since 1960. At a distance of four kilometres from Bolpur town, the village is located in the vicinity of Visva-Bharati and well-connected with the district town by road. An ancestor of the waning 'Zamindars', Chandu Babu had some agricultural land and was employed as an office-assistant at Visva-Bharati but retired for more than a decade ago. He held his clinics twice a day for six days a week. While he kept the mornings for patients from outside the village, he treated the villagers preferably in the evenings. But emergencies were always an exception. This suited the village women in particular, who worked as wage labourers in the fields, on construction sites or in households at Santiniketan or in the town. His popularity as a healer reached beyond the village. Reflecting on his own evolution as a practitioner, Chandu Babu once said,

I took interest in healing as a gesture to my mother's death from cancer. There was a Bengali handbook of homeopathy at home – for home treatment of many ailments. I casually started off with that; and slowly it attracted patients from the neighbourhood. It is the people, who have made me 'god'!

But of those who had some experience of his treatment, not all accepted him as unique. However, he must be an assurance for some people at least for some of their health problems; they still manage to stand in the long queue waiting for consultation, even if they have to leave their home long before sunrise.

The 'low fees' (three Rupees per consultation) and 'doctor's ability for accurate diagnosis and cure' continue to attract patients even today; sometimes there are more than seventy per day. I recently had a conversation with a retired professor of Visva-Bharati, who has been his patient since the 1990s. Like many others, she has always praised his diagnosis and treatment of her digestive, reproductive and other chronic disorders. As she found it difficult to catch a place in the queue on her own, she managed to engage a local agent who, on payment of fifty rupees, would book her a convenient time and place in the long queue of patients waiting for consultation with Chandu Babu. This saves her time, energy and protects her 'social status' too. According to the Professor, his treatment is like 'Dhanwantari'. Dhanwantari is a supreme preacher mentioned in the ancient texts of Ayurveda. He was the founder of the distinct 'Dhanwantari system', which is believed to be older than that of Caraka.[49] The word 'Dhanwantari', however, is generally used in Bengali language to indicate the superiority and accuracy of any treatment leading to cure; it also describes a person who offers such quality treatment. The positive impact that Chandu Babu's treatment had on her have generated ripple effects among her friends and relatives. The most recent example is her post-graduate sister-in-law, Mitu, who visited Chandu Babu on 28 May 2011 with a history of 'chronic bronchosis'. According to Mitu, 'antibiotics not only failed earlier to cure her, they also spoilt her digestive power'. The impact of homeopathic lay practices on her was then yet to manifest, however.

Pluralism, popularity and propaganda: lay practices of Homeopathy

The history of homeopathic lay practices is as old as the history of homeopathy. In an exploration of 'the role of laymen in the history of German homeopathy', Staudt claimed that the spread of homeopathy in Germany, as seen in the late 20th century, was possible due to the powerful lobby of the lay organisations.[50] In the Indian context, homeopathy is modern yet traditional. In the array of medical systems, it is placed between the Indian and Allopathic systems of medicine; there has been more competition, however, from the latter than from the former. Rather, homeopathy continues to share with Ayurveda and Unani the common challenges of being 'dominated' by the allopathic system, even though the wave of 'pluralism' attempts to bring them together. Deviating from such a notion of pluralism between systems of medicine, this paper has attempted to explore 'lay practices of homeopathy' within the plurality of the homeopathic system itself. While it has been earlier documented in the European and North American contexts[51], this paper, in particular, has drawn insights from a few narratives in the Indian context. In the course of exploration, the narratives revealed continuities and changes in homeopathic lay practices enmeshed in the dynamics of social change and emerging consequences. This exploration, however, is limited by its geographical and cultural contexts in the plurality of India.

In the early 19th century, homeopathy arrived in India along with the European travellers, traders, officials and missionaries. Few of them were trained

---

49 Varier (2005), p. 28.
50 Staudt (1998).
51 Smith (2010); Jütte/Risse/Woodward (1998); Morrell (1995).

allopaths working in either the British medical mission in India in cities like Calcutta, Bombay and elsewhere or working independently in the royal institutions of Lahore in Punjab, Tanjore in southern India or in epidemic-stricken cities such as Calcutta. In the mid-19th century, however, the enthusiastic Indians followed the Europeans in this regard. In Bengal, the initiative came from the lay practitioner Babu Rajendralal Dutta, who represented the urban elite of Calcutta. He had influenced 'lay' individuals and planted the seed of homeopathy in the health culture of Bengali families and communities. Similarly, the allopaths were also influenced and inducted by him and other personalities such as Rabindranath Tagore into homeopathic practice through formal training and conviction. These new homeopaths, in turn, inspired others to practise homeopathic healing. In the first quarter of the 20th century, the influences of the 'pure' lay practice (not the cross or adapted practice promoted by the allopaths) were even found to touch the health cultures of the educated upper middle class Bengali families who lived in remote areas far from Calcutta, in connection with government jobs or family occupations. In brief, the key force of 'homeopathic lay practitioners' generated ripple effects in two directions through family and community networks; it manifested in both the social spheres – private and public. These two streams moved forward but produced different consequences. Social interactions between lay and other practitioners have been documented in North America. The coming together of lay and licensed homeopathic practitioners across generations, the reciprocity in their interactions and the involvement of members of their families with a common interest in serving communities have all been observed by Smith in his study of the dispensing regimes that prevailed in 19th and 20th century Canada.[52]

The bonding between homeopathy and allopathy that lasted almost for a century from the late 1790s, had contributed to the spread of homeopathy around the globe. India, by embracing it, had direct internal experiences. Since the arrival of homeopathy in India in the 1830s, homoeopathic lay practices continued to represent the system here almost until its professionalization in the late 19th century. This was in spite of the fact that homeopathy in general and the allopaths practising homeopathy in particular came under open attack in 1878. The *Indian Medical Gazette* had termed the system as 'positive quackery'. In the attempts at professionalizing homeopathy in India, however, the tie that had earlier developed between the two systems had turned sour for more than one reason. From a relationship of constructive coexistence, finally they ended up in a relationship of antagonism. Each attempted to belittle the other, citing examples from each other's practices. As a consequence, the homeopathic lay practices lost their facilitating role in the spread of homeopathy through the allopaths. However it continued its journey through the families and social networks.

---

52 Smith (2010).

At independence, the Homeopathic Inquiry Committee observed that the number of lay practitioners in India was around 40 to 60 times higher than that of the qualified homeopathic practitioners, while the total estimate ranged from two to three hundred thousand.[53] By then, lay practice had penetrated the core of the Bengali health seeking culture and found its place within the family. It started percolating down the generations in families of the educated middle class. While men took the initiative, women followed them and continued with their practices even when their men got distracted by allopathic medicine or engaged in other occupations. Women, who took an interest in the lay homeopathic practice in the domestic domain, appreciated it for empowering them with the skill of treatment in patriarchal families. According to one such woman, practice of homeopathy within the home often turns into an expression of love and care that the family demands from them. However, there are limits to the good effects of such love and care beyond which they do not hesitate to consult a qualified practitioner. Enquiring and purchasing a family kit over the counters of homeopathic medicine stores is a common scene in today's Kolkata. Internet sites also act as sources of information for the young techno-savvy women, responding to their queries regarding remedies and books. The trend that was set by the lay practitioners of homeopathy in some middle class families has been naturally adopted and nurtured in family health cultures in Bengal.

Lay practices of homeopathy have gone beyond the family to conquer the confidence of the communities at large. While this was initiated by the urban elite and intellectuals, for some it was routed through their respective families, as in the case of Rabindranath Tagore. Such practices in turn had generated ripple effects in the communities, by influencing the intellectual associates or even the enthusiastic patients irrespective of gender. Similarly, later it was also embraced by some other Bengalis of the middle class who lived in remote regions where quality medical care was rare. All this happened in the process of naturalization and professionalization of homeopathy in India, thus helping the spread of homeopathy in the communities in early decades of the 20th century and after.

Mostly influenced by the socialist models of development and allopathic medicine in the delivery of health care, Visva-Bharati – the university founded by Rabindranath Tagore engaged in rural reconstruction and introduced a health cooperative movement to the village communities in the 1930s. Thus the lay practice of homeopathy which was then the domain of the elite and the intellectuals, had to compromise on possibilities for taking it to a larger scale of organizations and operations in villages. Later, when the health cooperative movement started losing its ground, public health care institutions were established to cater for the health needs of rural Bengal in post-independent India. The emphasis however, was on allopathic medicine as the Indian planners – representing the elite – were convinced of its 'efficacy'. It is not very clear

---

53 Bhardwaj (1981).

though whether the compromise on the part of the lay practices was due to a demand of the western models and planners' conviction or a 'sense of playing safe yet being useful in a manageable manner' that had crept into the thoughts of the elite and intellectual lay practitioners of homeopathy. It is worth mentioning here that Rabindranath Tagore was later, in the 1930s, seen to be attracted by biochemical medicine. In the last years of his life, he had to submit himself to allopathic treatment since others insisted on it. Nevertheless, lay practices survived while shifting their class and community base in the villages.

In the fifties and sixties, it was almost a general trend that 'government servants' returned to their native village with pensions on retiring. Well informed and experienced lay practitioners like Binoy Chatterjee had followed this norm. Having access to standard books in English and Bengali advising on homeopathic practice, he started responding to the health needs of relatives and neighbours in his village of Malipota, which was far from the world of qualified medical services. This was possibly one way through which lay practices made an entry in some Bengal villages. There was yet another trend that had emerged later. As a consequence of the expansion of government institutions, men who had some formal education found employment in village schools or other institutions. They were exposed to information on homeopathic lay practices through booklets and other Bengali literature available at local fairs or with the hawkers selling books in local trains or railway stations. These are still found to be popular practices of lay homeopathic communication in these villages, while the character of communications and literature for the middle school educated lay practitioners representing the poorer or socio-economically marginalized section of the society are of a different design. However, the retired or primarily land-owning educated middle class in villages started the homeopathic lay practice to protect the health of their own families and neighbours who lived far from adequate public or private health care facilities. In time, this became the first point of medical care for many of the poor, particularly the women and children who were bound by domestic boundaries. Knowing that homeopathy sometimes required time to accurately diagnose and cure patients, the families were free to opt for any other system of healing that was available and accessible. Way back in the 1950s, a family-budget survey conducted in 1954 in the city of Calcutta, revealed that the urban population opted primarily for allopathic treatment as the first preference but chose homeopathy as the second source of care in ill-health.[54]

Glimpses of presently prevailing perceptions of lay and qualified practitioners engaged in teaching, research, manufacture, sales or publishing in Kolkata provide more dimensions to the picture of homeopathic lay practice. Dr. Rath, a faculty member of the National Institute of Homeopathy in the city, stated that Bengal has a history of family lay practices. It also maintained its presence at community level at a time when the primary health care network

---

54   Government of West Bengal (1954), p. 244.

was less developed.[55] He added that like mainstream homeopathy, such treatment also involved individual attention; it is cheap yet efficient. He also pointed out that unlike 'expensive' allopathic medicine 'our' (homeopathic) medicine does not have 'side effects'. Commenting on the relationship between contemporary practitioners of homeopathy and allopathy, he said: 'There are allopaths who recommend homeopathic treatment especially for babies and the elderly. Popular websites, now available for consultation with qualified homeopaths, reveal the presence of a modest note among the homeopaths too. While responding to the question whether a patient can combine allopathy with homeopathy in specific cases, these qualified homeopaths available on a number of websites are found to strike a balance between the two; they reflect on the benefits of tolerance and wisdom of plural existence. Can one then make a comment that in the social ambience of 'plurality', the relationship between the two systems of medicine is one of tolerance as opposed to the antagonism that persisted for a long time?!

Dr. Sanjay Bhattacharya, the manager of a popular medical shop and polyclinic recollected the propaganda that homeopathy had to face in Bengal even in the 1990s.[56] This was spread through little magazines and vernacular news dailies. According to him, such propaganda might confuse and demoralize those who were amateurs in homeopathy. Dr. Bhar, the Managing Director of the Hahnemann Publishing Company Private Limited in Kolkata, pointed out in one of his PowerPoint presentations that the basic question of 'whether homeopathy is a science' has been answered by the research-scientists in the areas of nano medicine, human toxicology and others.[57] Referring to the old issues of the Bengali periodical *Hahnemann* that his company published from 1917 to the end of the century, he expressed that the contemporary journalists have now taken up similar responsibilities by writing Bengali articles in local newspapers, which have a much wider readership, particularly in the rural areas.

The days of the 'family physician' making home visits are gone. Qualified medical services are yet to reach the marginalized village communities through the public health care system. The easiest and nearest resource in villages is a lay practitioner. In the users' perception, lay homeopathic practice is as safe as qualified homeopathy. When it comes to practice within the family, it is described as 'economic', 'handy and safe', 'simple, can be accommodated in family routines, women's chores', and 'confidence-boosting for both the practitioners and the users'. The rural better-off have for the most part the freedom of opting for qualified practitioners, if the situation demands it. Homeopathic lay practices being a forte of woman practitioners, families provide a potential site for sharing demystified medical knowledge that is essential for the first-hand home care of common ailments and preservation of health. This may also be a point of initiating the practice of pluralism within the purview of lay

---

55   Personal interview on April 5, 2011.
56   Personal communication on December 15, 2010.
57   Bhar (2011).

practices, through the convergence of different traditional or modern systems of medicine. In the German context, it has been noted that, although professional self-interests appeared to lie behind the negative response of regular medicine to medical sects (e.g. there were charges of 'promoting quackery' from the allopathic medical fraternity against the system of 'homeopathy' among others), there was also the move towards greater harmony among homeopaths and another indigenous healing system, that of hydropathy.[58] Both saw some merits in maintaining therapeutic unity and achieving institutionalization.

In spite of national planning, economic and political developments over the past seven decades, the picture of poverty in the Indian villages remains appalling. According to official estimates 22 per cent of the rural population in India and 24 per cent of the rural population in the state of West Bengal live in poverty.[59] More live at the fringes and are not included in the official statistics. Extent of poverty is reported to be higher in villages compared to urban areas. The socio-economically marginalized are not only poor but also deprived of the fruits of planned development. Lopsided growth of the national health services and inadequately regulated private health care sector coexist with higher prevalence and burdens of illness reported by the poorer as compared to that by the better-off. Although gender differential in reported illness against women cuts across socioeconomic strata, the gap is wider among the poorer households as compared to the better-off.[60] Self-taught 'lay' practitioners continue to be an important source of health care for the socio-economically marginalized in underserved areas, in particular. This is observed in villages that are located closest to the towns.

Villagers, particularly the marginalized, identify the self-taught 'lay' practitioners as a composite category of 'village doctors', selling medicines of different systems according to their own convenience. Health-related qualitative studies conducted in West Bengal between 1990 and 2002 pointed out that such practitioners serve as an immediate source of medical support for the ailing villagers in situations where the basic health services are inadequate and of poor quality.[61] As found in the narratives and other direct observations, the major source of information for these practitioners includes the medical stores in town or literature and books sold by shady registered societies operating in the city, some of which also offer organizational support. Under paid membership, such organizations issue certificates and relevant information and books to their members. The format of such a certificate reveals that one such institution has been operating since 1934 and it promotes not only 'lay' allopathic practices but also practices of other systems. While the self-taught practition-

---

58 Jütte (1998).
59 Government of India (2007), http://planningcommission.nic.in/news/prmar07.pdf (last accessed on May 22, 2013); Government of India (2004), http://www.planningcommission. gov.in/news/p.. (last accessed June 11, 2011).
60 Soman (2007).
61 Soman (2003).

ers in villages consider their practice as a source of income, their practices are vulnerable to the pressures of the hidden commercial networks that maximize profits and thrive on their vulnerabilities. Under the circumstances, regulation emerges as an important issue in the provision of quality health care to the rural population, particularly the socio-economically marginalized.

As mentioned earlier in the paper, the Indian regulatory mechanism involves primarily the department of health services in the states and the corresponding medical and AYUSH councils and legal establishments for monitoring, scrutiny and necessary action. Citing a composite picture of illegalities in medical practices (that include both qualified and lay practitioners), a government official in the Indian health ministry, Dr. Kumar, admitted that while regulation through legislation may be a direct measure in 'tackling quackery' in order to avoid consequential medical implications and health hazards among the Indian people, the public health care system has to be far stronger and far more efficient in dealing with today's health care practices or 'malpractices' as a whole.[62] Strengthening the public health care delivery system to ensure quality care to its people, will probably address the state's burden of dealing with 'quackery and mal practices', in turn. While the official reports confirm shortfalls in infrastructures and manpower in the health service system[63], the Eleventh Five Year Plan acknowledges: 'Despite constraints of human resources, practitioners of Indian Systems of Medicine (ISM), Registered Medical Practitioners (RMPs), and other locally available human resources have not been adequately mobilized and integrated in the system'.[64] A report on 'mainstreaming of AYUSH and revitalizing local health traditions under the NRHM' regarding an important aspect of the National Rural Health Mission[65], however, placed greater emphasis on the qualified Indian systems of medicine and homeopathy and the respective practitioners in the public health care system than the local health traditions of lay practices which is a social reality. As a consequence of inadequate provision of quality health care services by the state, they are subjected to a kind of 'forced pluralism' and users are often being left to choose from lay self-taught practitioners in homeopathy, allopathy or any other informal healing system that is available. Ensuring quality services and care by the state is also important if viewed from the perspective of those who are un-served or under-served, representing those who are socio-economically marginalized.

The history of health care planning and development in India has witnessed patchy attempts of empowering people to take care of their own health. India's signing of the Alma Ata Declaration in 1978 and its subsequent identification with the Asian Charter helped India to reinforce its earlier commit-

---

62 Kumar (2007).
63 Government of India (2011); http://mohfw.nic.in/NRHM/State%20Files?wb.htm (last accessed on August 23, 2011).
64 Government of India (2008).
65 National Health Systems Resource Centre (2009), p. 6.

ment to improve coverage and quality health care in the rural periphery.[66] This was through entrusting 'people's health in people's hands' where the medical and health establishment was specially required to promote self-reliance by providing training to representatives chosen by the community and offering them support in the form of referral facilities or conditions which needed advanced services. There was a basic shift in the approach towards development of health services that was introduced through a landmark scheme of Community Health Volunteers (Guides) in 1977, which became the link between the primary health centre and the community. But subsequent evaluation and analysis suggested that the highly medicalized, professionalized, bureaucratized and mystified superstructure had an adverse effect on the thrust of the programme. Promotion of democratization of health services that was the very essence of this programme was lost in the course of its implementation.[67] The blurred and neglected shades in the lay or self-taught health care practices in general reflect a grey area in social research and planning in India. It prevents the researchers and planners from using the potential that lives in the people at the periphery and their cultures.

It has been more than sixty years since India became an independent federal state. Economic and political planning is yet to meet the health needs of the people, particularly the socio-economically marginalized. The period of post-independence is marked by lopsided development. While the state is committed to uphold people's right to dignity, provision of quality health care is the responsibility of the government. Lay practice among the marginalized, which is a reality of today, is probably a social consequence of the fact that the state has failed to respect the rights of the people. It is unable to provide quality health care to the marginalized at the least. People, who are deprived, assert their rights to freedom of choice to ensure their own access to lay practices at the very least when they can still only dream of quality public health care. Drawing from the insights laid down by the physician and anthropologist Arthur Kleinman, it can also be said that those in the society, who live amidst uncertainty and dangers of various kinds, learn to help themselves from their day to day struggles for survival and associated experiences of life.[68] Seen against this background, lay practices are a socio-cultural response of the communities to their health needs given the socio-economic deprivations they live with.

---

66 World Health Organization (1980).
67 Banerji (1985), pp. 28, 279.
68 Kleinman (2006).

Bibliography

Internet Links

http://www.doctorcancer.org/index.php (last accessed on May 22, 2013)
http://planningcommission.nic.in/news/prmar07.pdf (last accessed on May 22, 2013)

Literature

Baer, Hans A.: Medical Pluralism. In: Ember, Carol R.; Ember, Melvin (eds.): Encyclopedia of Medical Anthropology: Health and Illness in the World's Cultures. Vol. I. New York 2004, pp. 109–116.

Bagchi, Asoke K.: Rabindranath Tagore and his medical world. New Delhi 2000.

Banerji, Debabar: Health and Family Planning Services in India: An Epidemiological, Socio-cultural and Political Analysis and a Perspective. New Delhi 1985.

Bhar, D.: Is Homeopathy scientific? Personal Communication. Power Point presentation, Kolkata 2011.

Bhardwaj, Surinder M.: Homeopathy in India. In: Gupta, Giri Raj (ed.): The Social and Cultural Context of Medicine in India. New Delhi 1981, pp. 31–54.

Bhatia, Manish: Can we take Allopathy medicine together with Homeopathy to cure PCOS. Currently I am taking Metformin 500mg with Homeopathy medicine, Is it OK?, URL: http://hpathy.com/ask-homeopathy-doctors/can-allopathy-medicines-be-taken-with-homeopathy-in-case-of-pcos/ (last accessed on May 22, 2013).

Datta, Pradip Kumar: Introduction. In: Datta, Pradip Kumar (ed.): Rabindranath Tagore's The Home and The World: A Critical Companion. New Delhi 2002, pp. 1–26.

Dinges, Martin: The Role of Medical Societies in the Professionalisation of Homeopathic Physicians in Germany and the USA. In: Jütte, Robert; Risse, Guenter B.; Woodward, John (eds.): Culture, Knowledge, and Healing: Historical Perspectives of Homeopathic Medicine in Europe and North America. Sheffield 1998, pp. 173–198.

Dinges, Martin: Patients in the History of Homeopathy. In: Dinges, Martin (ed.): Patients in the History of Homeopathy. Sheffield 2002, pp. 1–32.

Dinges, Martin: Der Versorgungsbeitrag der Homöopathie in Indien (Teil 1). In: Zeitschrift für Klassische Homöopathie 55 (2011), no. 1, pp. 4–18.

Dirghangi, G.: Homeopathic Philosophy. In: Hahnemann Jaistha 1325 (1917), pp. 36–40.

Elliott, J.: More Ways Than One: A Look at Pluralism in Health-care. In: Lancet 293 (1969), no. 7597, pp. 715–718.

Fitzgerald, Rosemary: Clinical Christianity: The Emergence of Medical Work as a Missionary Strategy in Colonial India, 1800–1914. In: Pati, Biswamoy; Harrison, Mark (eds.): Health, Medicine and Empire: Perspectives on Colonial India. New Delhi 2001, pp. 165–187.

Government of India: Populations Tables. Census of India. New Delhi 2001.

Government of India: Estimates of Poverty in India (2004), URL: http://www.planningcommission.gov.in/news/p.. (last accessed on June 11, 2011).

Government of India: AYUSH in India 2005. Programme & Implementation Cell, Department of Ayurveda, Yoga, & Naturopathy, Unani, Siddha and Homeopathy (AYUSH). Ministry of Health and Family Welfare. New Delhi 2005.

Government of India: National Policy. Annual Report of the Ministry of Health and Family Welfare 2006–07. New Delhi 2007.

Government of India: Five Year plan, Health and Family Welfare and AYUSH. In: Eleventh Five Year Plan (2007–2008). Social sector II. New Delhi 2008, pp. 57–123.

Government of India: Health and Family Welfare. In: Government of India: Statistical Year Book India. Ministry of Statistics and Programme Implementation. New Delhi 2011, URL:

http://mospi.nic.in/Mospi_New/upload/statistical_year_book_2011.htm (last accessed on May 22, 2013).

Government of West Bengal: Family Budget Enquiry in 23 Towns of West Bengal including Calcutta 1950–51. State Statistical Bureau. Calcutta 1954.

Government of West Bengal: District Statistical Handbook: Birbhum. Calcutta 1998.

Illich, Ivan: Limits to Medicine: Medical Nemesis, the Expropriation of Health. Bombay 1975.

Jütte, Robert: The Paradox of Professionalisation: Homeopathy and Hydropathy as Unorthodoxy in Germany in the 19th and early 20th Century. In: Jütte, Robert; Risse, Guenter B.; Woodward, John (eds.): Culture, Knowledge, and Healing: Historical Perspectives of Homeopathic Medicine in Europe and North America. Sheffield 1998, pp. 65–88.

Jütte, Robert; Risse, Guenter B.; Woodward, John (eds.): Culture, Knowledge, and Healing: Historical Perspectives of Homeopathic Medicine in Europe and North America. Sheffield 1998.

Kleinman, Arthur: What Really Matters: Living a Moral Life Amidst Uncertainty and Danger. New York 2006.

Kumar, Ashok: Regulation of Medical Practitioners in India, PowerPoint Presentation at the International Workshop "Strategies for Health Sector Reform in South and South-east Asia", Naresuan University, Thailand, 20–22 June 2007, URL: http://www.hum.au.dk/hsre/Docs/Presentations/4_Regulation-scope%20and%20limitations/1_Ashok_Kumar_Regulation.pdf (last accessed on May 22, 2013).

Leslie, Charles: Medical Pluralism and legitimation in the Indian and Chinese medical systems. In: Landy, David (ed.): Culture, disease and healing: Studies in medical anthropology. New York 1977, pp. 511–517.

Majumdar, Durgadas: West Bengal District Gazetteers. Calcutta 1975.

Malik, Nancy: Does Homeopathy go with any kind of other medicine like Allopathy or ayurveda?, URL: http://wiki.answers.com/Q/Does_homeopathy_go_with_any_kind_of_other_medicine_like_allopathy_or_ayurveda (last accessed on May 22, 2013).

Morrell, Peter: A Brief History of British lay Homeopathy. Paper presented at the 1st International Conference of the History of Homeopathy at the Robert Bosch Institute for the History of Medicine, Stuttgart, 4–6 April, 1995, URL: http://www.homeoint.org/morrell/articles/pm_lay.htm (last accessed on May 22, 2013).

National Health Systems Resource Centre: Mainstreaming AYUSH & Revitalizing Local Health Traditions under NRHM: A Health Systems Perspective: An Appraisal of the Annual State Programme Implementation Plans 2007–10 and Mapping of Technical Needs. New Delhi 2009.

Navarro, Vicente: Crisis, health and medicine: A social critique. New York 1986.

O'Malley, Lewis Sydney Steward: Bengal District Gazetteers: Birbhum. Calcutta 1910.

Palmer, Natasha: An Awkward Threesome – Donors, Governments and Non-State Providers of Health in Low Income Countries. In: Public Administration and Development 26 (2006), pp. 231–240, published online in Wiley InterScience (http://www.interscience.wiley.com, last accessed on May 22, 2013) DOI: 10.1002/pad.421.

Pétursdóttir, Sigrídur Svana: 'Patients don't care from where the cure comes': Patients' Choice of a Homoeopathic Lay Healer in Iceland. In: Dinges, Martin (ed.): Patients in the History of Homeopathy. Sheffield 2002, pp. 173–184.

Poldas, Samuel Vijaya Bhaskar: Geschichte der Homöopathie in Indien: von ihrer Einführung bis zur ersten offiziellen Anerkennung 1937. Stuttgart 2010.

Priya, Ritu; Shweta, A. S.: Status and Role of AYUSH & Local Health Traditions under the National Rural Health Mission. Draft Report of a survey for discussion at the National Health Systems Resource Centre. New Delhi 2010.

Sachdeva, Suchindra: Taking Homeopathy Along With Allopathy (2011), URL: http://health.indiatimes.com/articleshow/msid-979986.prtpage-1.cms (last accessed on June 11, 2011).

Sheehan, Helen E.: Medical Pluralism in India: patient choice or no other options? In: Indian Journal of Medical Ethics 6 (Jul.-Sep. 2009), no. 3, pp. 138–141, URL: http://web.archive.

org/web/20110622060521/http://issuesinmedicalethics.org/173AR138.html (last accessed on May 22, 2013).

Singer, Merrill; Baer, Hans A.: Critical medical anthropology. Amityville, NY 1995.

Singh, Padam; Yadav, R. J.; Pandey, Arvind: Utilization of indigenous systems of medicine and Homeopathy in India. In: Indian Journal of Medical Research 122 (2005), pp. 137–142.

Smith, Douglas W.: Potency and Provenance: An Inter-Generational Study of Homeopathic Practice in Ontario. In: Medizin, Gesellschaft und Geschichte 29 (2010), pp. 275–315.

Soman, Krishna: An Exploratory study of Social Dynamics of Women's Health in Adityapur village of Birbhum District. M.Phil Dissertation, Jawaharlal Nehru University, New Delhi 1992.

Soman, Krishna: Social Dynamics of Women's Health: A Study of Bolpur Block in the District of Birbhum. PhD. thesis, Jawaharlal Nehru University, New Delhi 1997.

Soman, Krishna: Rural health Care in West Bengal. In: Economic and Political Weekly 37 (2002), no. 26, pp. 2562–2564.

Soman, Krishna: Health Related Qualitative Data on West Bengal: An Analysis. Report submitted to DFID-UK, 18 July, 2003.

Soman, Krishna: Social Dynamics of Women's Heath: Reflections from India. In: Global Social Policy 7 (2007), no. 2, pp. 138–140.

Staudt, Dörte: The Role of Laymen in the History of German Homeopathy. In: Jütte, Robert; Risse, Guenter B.; Woodward, John (eds.): Culture, Knowledge, and Healing: Historical Perspectives of Homeopathic Medicine in Europe and North America. Sheffield 1998, pp. 199–216.

Stebbing, E. P.; Champion, H. G.; Osmaston, E. C.: The organisation and education of the staff of the Department, 1871–1900. In: The Forests of India: And the Neighboring countries. Delhi 2010, pp. 485–509.

Tagore, Rathindranath: Health Cooperatives. In: Institute of Rural Reconstruction Sriniketan/ Visva-Bharati, Bull. No. 25 (1938).

Tibrewal, Deepak K.: Homeopathy and Allopathy?, URL: http://web.archive.org/web/20120617214049/http://www.homeoclinic.in/homeopathy_bangalore.html (last accessed on May 22, 2013).

Varier, N. V. Krishnankutty: Classical Texts in Ayurveda. In: History of Ayurveda. (=Kottakkal Ayurveda Series 56) Kerala 2005.

World Health Organization: Charter for Health Development: A Milestone for WHO's South-East Asian Region. In: WHO Chronicle 34 (1980), pp. 171–174.

Yadav, R. J.; Pandey, Arvind; Singh, Padam: A study on acceptability of Indian system of medicine and homeopathy in India: results from the State of West Bengal. In: Indian Journal of Public Health 51 (2007), no. 1, pp. 47–49.

Looking Behind and Ahead

William Sax

Medical Pluralisms

It might seem unusual for a book to focus on the comparison of homeopathy and CAMs (Complementary and Alternative Medicines) in India and Germany, but it's actually a rather sensible thing to do. For complex but different reasons, both India and Germany are havens for complementary and alternative medicines of all kinds. Yoga and Ayurveda are rapidly gaining in popularity in Germany along with Traditional Chinese Medicine and other non-European medical traditions, while homeopathy has been very well received in India since shortly after its invention. By looking closely at the diversity of medical systems in both countries, the essays in this book point toward two important conclusions, both of which challenge certain widely held assumptions. The first of these conclusions is that medical pluralism is the standard human condition, and the second is that the forms it takes are much more diverse than previously realized. Let us examine them one at a time.

Many people assume that medical pluralism, where a number of different medical systems exist in the same social space, is a special feature of non-Western societies. Perhaps it is thought of as a temporary phase, which will come to an end after the older medical traditions have withered under the impact of modern biomedicine. Or perhaps it is an expression of cultural pluralism, where different ethnic groups, each with its own healing traditions have brought together artificial colonial borders. This perhaps explains why so many articles on the topic focus on medical pluralism in the "exotic" societies of Asia, Africa, and South America.

But in fact, medical pluralism is not at all exotic. It seems to be characteristic of most cultures, at most times and in most places. Certainly it is characteristic of contemporary Germany and the USA, as well as India. As Martin Dinges points out in his Introduction to the volume, the use of what are now called "Complementary and Alternative Medicines" was probably always quite high: it's just that it wasn't much noticed or commented on. Sylvia Waisse's delightful biography of Johann Honigberger also shows how medically plural Honigberger's Transylvanian homeland was in the first half of the 19th century, and this must have had an important influence on his own investigations, which were always open to new and useful ideas from non-European medical traditions. Marion Baschin's essay illustrates something similar: that is, how common it was for residents of 19th century Münster to "shop around" for various kinds of medical treatment. She concludes that in this "medical market", homeopathy was not really an "alternative" but was rather "complementary," by which she means that it was one of a range of treatments available under the medically plural system of the time. A similar situation may have obtained in the early days of homeopathy in Bengal where, according to Shinjini Das, "medical pluralism" was as much about mutual interactions between differing forms of medicine as it was about delineating a unique space for each medical tradition. Back in Europe, Sharma shows how legal attempts by the biomedical profession in the late 19th century to restrict the advertising of non-conventional healers failed, in part because the dominance of biomedicine was not yet well-established.

It is interesting to compare these results with those of Barua, who studied medical pluralism in an Indian slum. Her conclusion is that the demand for CAMs in the slum has utterly different causes than in Europe and North America. The poverty-stricken slum residents want powerful medicines because they cannot afford to miss a day of work: if they do so, they may not eat. As Barua puts it, "the main imperative is to return to work as quickly as possible driven by the crippling insecurities of income and tenure." Therefore, they choose to visit the "Quacks" (unlicensed healthcare providers) who work in the slums, and from whom they can easily obtain such medications. Moreover, the slum-dwellers feel that they are treated very badly by staff in public hospitals, and prefer the personal care they receive from Quacks who know them.

"Easy" and "Hard" Models of Medical Pluralism

Barua's argument leads us in the direction of a second conclusion, which also challenges a widely held assumption. The assumption has to do with what one might call the "easy coexistence" model of medical pluralism; in other words, the idea that the various medical systems co-exist with each other in a frictionless and non-competitive way. Such a situation may well obtain at certain times and places, and indeed the essays by Waisse and Baschin suggest that it was characteristic of parts of 19th century Europe. But this is not always the case. In fact, medical pluralism is rarely symmetrical: One or another of the various systems dominates the other politically, economically, scientifically, culturally, or through a combination of these. In the contemporary world, the overwhelming dominance of biomedicine is an undeniable fact, even though biomedicine itself may not be so monolithic as is sometimes supposed. This explains the conclusions reached by Eisele, who finds that most people writing letters in the 1990s to the independent patient organisation *Natur und Medizin* were seeking advice, or therapies, that were additional to, or an enhancement of, biomedicine, but not a replacement for it. The dominance of biomedicine affects the most basic terms that we use to discuss the matter: what, after all, do the CAMs "complement," and to what are they an "alternative," if not biomedicine? It is not particularly respectful to lump the multiple alternative medical systems together in the single "leftover" category of "Complementary and Alternative Medicines", but no doubt this is an accurate reflection of the current situation, in which Biomedicine is overwhelmingly dominant.

Because of its department of AYUSH[1], India is often held up as support-
ing medical pluralism in a unique way. Amita Machanda has pointed to the
popularity of CAMs in India, and Raj Manchanda has provided detailed statistics on history and uptake of homeopathy in Delhi. But as Dinges points out,
absolute levels of funding for these CAMs are remarkably low: they receive
something like nine times less funding than the dominant biomedicine. This is
another result of the asymmetries that exist despite "official" medical pluralism, and the volume provides other examples as well. Dusausoit's essay offers
an especially poignant example of the effects of the asymmetry on one particular practitioner. Naraindas examines in detail the consequences of biomedical dominance in the field of nosology, and even in the training of practitioners of CAMs in various countries. But he focuses on Indian case studies, and
examines practices of translation among the various systems, such practices
being also quite strongly affected by the epistemic dominance of modern biomedicine.

Another widespread assumption called into question by these essays is
that regulations upholding the dominance of biomedicine come after its scientific authority and/or therapeutic efficacy have been established. However,
some of the papers presented here point in the other direction, suggesting that
regulatory frameworks themselves were instrumental in confirming the scientific authority and/or therapeutic efficacy of biomedicine, and sometimes challenging it. I have already called attention to Sharma's nuanced discussion of
the failure of late-19th century attempts to regulate non-biomedical healers. In
the same essay, he points to the far-reaching and largely unexpected effects of
changing regulations: An attempt to roll back legislation affecting doctors led
to the opening up of the medical marketplace, exposing biomedical practitioners to new competition from non-biomedical healers.

Medical "Systems", Culture, and Class

One of the most interesting things about medical traditions of all kinds is how
they are infused with moral issues. Doctors and healers are typically confronted with suffering patients, and thus face a moral imperative to use their
knowledge for mitigating that suffering in the most optimal way. In this sense,
the "systematicity" of the medical traditions discussed in this volume is at least
partly mythical: what counts is what works, and committed healers are normally quite willing to use ideas and techniques from outside of their own tradition if they think that these are useful, or even to incorporate them within it.
Such processes are evident in three of the essays about India. Shinjini Das
shows that Indians insisted on the indigeneity of Homeopathy, claiming either
that it was compatible with Ayurveda, or that it actually originated in India,

---

1   AYUSH is the name of a Government of India Department responsible for administering
     complementary and alternative medicine. It is also an acronym standing for the various
     traditions that are recognized, viz., Ayurveda, Yoga, Unani, Siddha and Homeopathy.

ideas that came to be commonplace amongst Indian homeopaths. She also describes a number of attempts to synthesize the two systems into one. Naraindas begins his essay by noting that the naturopathy students he met in the 1990s "were not only not aware of Naturopathy's German roots (unlike homeopathy), but insisted that this system was a wholly Indian invention and all the remedies could be found in some canonical Indian text or other." Finally, Soman provides a truly charming account of homeopathy in several different settings, concluding with the development of lay homeopaths in India.

Social and historical contexts are decisive for health-seeking behavior, and one of the most important contextual factors is class, as Barua's essay on the Delhi slum dwellers so poignantly shows. Taken as a whole however, the essays in this volume caution us against the easy association of CAMs with the lower classes. They show, for example, that homeopathy in India is quite widespread, with perhaps slightly more adherents among the middle and upper classes. Sharma demonstrates that opposition to / support of "quackery" in late 19th-century Berlin did not break down along class lines. Indeed, many elite citizens defended the rights of "quacks". As Sharma puts it, "Medical Pluralism was a shared commitment that cut across class, party, and even confessional lines," but we sometimes lose sight of this because the "post-war hegemony" of biomedicine is so complete, making it "remarkably difficult to recognize other forms of medical knowledge as legitimate."

It is in this sense that the regulatory frameworks discussed above are (negatively) productive, since they tend to sharpen the distinction between the various traditions, enhancing their "systematicity" at the cost of their flexibility, thus producing the very distinctions that they enforce. So much is evident in the historical progression charted by the papers in this volume, from the "easy" medical pluralism of late-19th century Europe to the more rigidly-policed boundaries of the present.

Conclusion

The lessons of this volume are therefore both negative and positive. On the negative side, these essays make it clear that we should not assume (or, we should no longer automatically assume) that medical pluralism is a special feature of non-Western societies, nor that it disappears with the emergence of biomedicine, nor that it necessarily equates to a "live and let live" attitude amongst competing medical traditions, nor that the dominance of biomedicine is a direct result of its scientific authority and/or therapeutic efficacy, nor that medical "systems" are rigidly "systematic." On the positive side, we can assume that medical pluralism is the standard human condition, that medical systems may sometimes be in relations of competition and even hostility; and that they are often quite fluid and adaptable. Hopefully these points, both positive and negative, will guide future research on this topic.

Authors

Barua, Nupur, Ph.D., Research Adviser with the South Asia Research Hub, UK Department for International Development, New Delhi, India, e-mail: nupur_barua@yahoo.com

Baschin, Marion, Ph.D., Researcher, Institute for the History of Medicine of the Robert Bosch Foundation Stuttgart, Germany, e-mail: marion.baschin@igm-bosch.de

Chhatre, Leena V., Chief Medical Officer (Homeopathy), Directorate of ISM & Homeopathy, Govt. of Delhi, India

Das, Shinjini, Ph.D., Postdoctoral Fellow, Centre for Research in Arts, Social Science and Humanities, University of Cambridge, UK, e-mail: das.shinjini@gmail.com, sd591@cam.ac.uk

Dinges, Martin, Ph.D., Professor, deputy director, Institute for the History of Medicine of the Robert Bosch Foundation Stuttgart, Germany, e-mail: martin.dinges@igm-bosch.de

Dusausoit, Hugues, Ph.D., University of Namur, Belgium, e-mail: hugues.dusausoit@unamur.be

Eisele, Philipp, Ph.D. student, Institute for the History of Medicine of the Robert Bosch Foundation Stuttgart, Germany, e-mail: philipp.eisele@igm-bosch.de

Kaur, Harleen, Senior Research Fellow, Central Research Institute for Homoeopathy, Noida, India

Manchanda, Ameeta R., M.D.(H), Former Homeopathic Consultant, Holy Family Hospital, New Delhi; Associate Professor, Baksons Homeopathic Medical College and Hospital, Greater Noida, India, e-mail: ameetarm@gmail.com, ameetarm@yahoo.com

Manchanda, Raj Kumar, M.D., Director General, Central Council for Research in Homeopathy, New Delhi, India, e-mail: rkmanchanda18@yahoo.com, rkmanchanda@gmail.com

Naraindas, Harish, Associate Professor, Centre for the Study of Social Systems, School of Social Sciences, Jawaharlal Nehru University, New Delhi, India, e-mail: harish_naraindas@yahoo.com, harish-naraindas@uiowa.edu

Sax, William, Ph.D., Head, Department of Ethnology, South Asia Institute, University of Heidelberg, Germany, e-mail: william.sax@urz.uni-heidelberg.de

Sharma, Avi, Johnson Instructor in MAPSS and History, The University of Chicago, USA, e-mail: asharma@uchicago.edu

Soman, Krishna, Associate Professor, Public Health, Institute of Development Studies Kolkata, Salt Lake Campus, India, e-mail: healthykrishna@gmail.com, krishna.idsk@gmail.com

Tewari, Rahul, Medical Director, Dr. Vivekananda's Vision, A Chain of Homeopathy Clinics, Noida, Uttar Pradesh, India, e-mail: drrahultewari@gmail.com

Valavan, Ramachandran, M.D., Manager – Scientific Affairs, Dr. Willmar Schwabe India Pvt. Ltd., Noida, Uttar Pradesh, India, e-mail: drvalavan@yahoo.com

Verma, Surender Kumar, Deputy Director (Homeopathy), Directorate of ISM & Homeopathy, Govt. of Delhi, India

Waisse, Silvia, M.D., Ph.D., Prof., Post Graduate Program of Studies in History of Science/Researcher, Centre Simão Mathias of Studies in History of Science; Pontifical Catholic University of São Paulo (PUC-SP), Brazil, e-mail: swaisse@pucsp.br, dr.silvia.waisse@gmail.com

MEDIZIN, GESELLSCHAFT UND GESCHICHTE — BEIHEFTE

Herausgegeben von Robert Jütte.

Franz Steiner Verlag   ISSN 0941–5033

19. Claudia Stein
    Die Behandlung der Franzosen-
    krankheit in der Frühen Neuzeit
    am Beispiel Augsburgs
    2003. 293 S., kt.
    ISBN 978-3-515-08032-3
20. Jörg Melzer
    Vollwerternährung
    Diätetik, Naturheilkunde,
    Nationalsozialismus, sozialer Anspruch
    2003. 480 S., kt.
    ISBN 978-3-515-08278-5
21. Thomas Gerst
    Ärztliche Standesorganisation
    und Standespolitik in Deutschland
    1945–1955
    2004. 270 S., kt.
    ISBN 978-3-515-08056-9
22. Florian Steger
    Asklepiosmedizin
    Medizinischer Alltag in der römischen
    Kaiserzeit
    2004. 244 S. und 12 Taf. mit 17 Abb., kt.
    ISBN 978-3-515-08415-4
23. Ulrike Thoms
    Anstaltskost im
    Rationalisierungsprozeß
    Die Ernährung in Krankenhäusern und
    Gefängnissen im 18. und 19. Jahrhundert
    2005. 957 S. mit 84 Abb., kt.
    ISBN 978-3-515-07935-8
24. Simone Moses
    Alt und krank
    Ältere Patienten in der Medizinischen
    Klinik der Universität Tübingen zur Zeit
    der Entstehung der Geriatrie 1880 bis 1914
    2005. 277 S. mit 61 Tab. und 27 Diagr.
    ISBN 978-3-515-08654-7
25. Sylvelyn Hähner-Rombach (Hg.)
    „Ohne Wasser ist kein Heil"
    Medizinische und kulturelle Aspekte
    der Nutzung von Wasser
    2005. 167 S., kt.
    ISBN 978-3-515-08785-8
26. Heiner Fangerau / Karen Nolte (Hg.)
    „Moderne" Anstaltspsychiatrie

im 19. und 20. Jahrhundert
    Legitimation und Kritik
    2006. 416 S., kt.
    ISBN 978-3-515-08805-3
27. Martin Dinges (Hg.)
    Männlichkeit und Gesundheit
    im historischen Wandel ca. 1800 –
    ca. 2000
    2007. 398 S. mit 7 Abb., 22 Tab.
    und 4 Diagr., kt.
    ISBN 978-3-515-08920-3
28. Marion Maria Ruisinger
    Patientenwege
    Die Konsiliarkorrespondenz Lorenz
    Heisters (1683–1758) in der Trew-
    Sammlung Erlangen
    2008. 308 S. mit 7 Abb. und 16 Diagr., kt.
    ISBN 978-3-515-08806-0
29. Martin Dinges (Hg.)
    Krankheit in Briefen im deutschen
    und französischen Sprachraum
    17.–21. Jahrhundert
    2007. 267 S., kt.
    ISBN 978-3-515-08949-4
30. Helen Bömelburg
    Der Arzt und sein Modell
    Porträtfotografien aus der deutschen Psy-
    chiatrie 1880 bis 1933
    2007. 239 S. mit 68 Abb. und 2 Diagr., kt.
    ISBN 978-3-515-09096-8
31. Martin Krieger
    Arme und Ärzte, Kranke und Kassen
    Ländliche Gesundheitsversorgung und
    kranke Arme in der südlichen Rheinprovinz
    (1869 bis 1930)
    2009. 452 S. mit 7 Abb., 16 Tab. und 5 Ktn.,
    kt.
    ISBN 978-3-515-09171-8
32. Sylvelyn Hähner-Rombach
    Alltag in der Krankenpflege /
    Everyday Nursing Life
    Geschichte und Gegenwart /
    Past and Present
    2009. 309 S. mit 22 Tab., kt.
    ISBN 978-3-515-09332-3

33. Nicole Schweig
Gesundheitsverhalten von Männern
Gesundheit und Krankheit in Briefen,
1800–1950
2009. 288 S. mit 4 Abb. und 8 Tab., kt.
ISBN 978-3-515-09362-0

34. Andreas Renner
**Russische Autokratie
und europäische Medizin**
Organisierter Wissenstransfer
im 18. Jahrhundert
2010. 373 S., kt.
ISBN 978-3-515-09640-9

35. Philipp Osten (Hg.)
Patientendokumente
Krankheit in Selbstzeugnissen
2010. 253 S. mit 3 Abb., kt.
ISBN 978-3-515-09717-8

36. Susanne Hoffmann
**Gesunder Alltag im
20. Jahrhundert?**
Geschlechterspezifische Diskurse und
gesundheitsrelevante Verhaltensstile
in deutschsprachigen Ländern
2010. 538 S. mit 7 Abb., kt.
ISBN 978-3-515-09681-2

37. Marion Baschin
**Wer lässt sich von einem
Homöopathen behandeln?**
Die Patienten des Clemens Maria Franz von
Bönninghausen (1785–1864)
2010. 495 S. mit 45 Abb., kt.
ISBN 978-3-515-09772-7

38. Ulrike Gaida
**Bildungskonzepte der
Krankenpflege in der
Weimarer Republik**
Die Schwesternschaft des Evangelischen
Diakonievereins e.V. Berlin-Zehlendorf
2011. 346 S. mit 12 Abb., kt.
ISBN 978-3-515-09783-3

39. Martin Dinges / Robert Jütte (ed.)
**The transmission of health
practices (c. 1500 to 2000)**
2011. 190 S. mit 4 Abb. und 1 Tab., kt.
ISBN 978-3-515-09897-7

40. Sylvelyn Hähner-Rombach
**Gesundheit und Krankheit im
Spiegel von Petitionen an den
Landtag von Baden-Württemberg
1946 bis 1980**
2011. 193 S. mit 27 Tab., kt.
ISBN 978-3-515-09914-1

41. Florian Mildenberger
**Medikale Subkulturen in der
Bundesrepublik Deutschland
und ihre Gegner (1950–1990)**
Die Zentrale zur Bekämpfung der
Unlauterkeit im Heilgewerbe
2011. 188 S. mit 15 Abb., kt.
ISBN 978-3-515-10041-0

42. Angela Schattner
**Zwischen Familie, Heilern und
Fürsorge**
Das Bewältigungsverhalten von
Epileptikern in deutschsprachigen
Gebieten des 16.–18. Jahrhunderts
2012. 299 S. mit 5 Abb. und 2 Tab., kt.
ISBN 978-3-515-09947-9

43. Susanne Rueß / Astrid Stölzle (Hg.)
**Das Tagebuch der jüdischen Kriegs-
krankenschwester Rosa Bendit,
1914 bis 1917**
2012. 175 S. mit 6 Abb., kt.
ISBN 978-3-515-10124-0

44. Sabine Herrmann
**Giacomo Casanova und die Medizin
des 18. Jahrhunderts**
2012. 214 S. mit 8 Abb., kt.
ISBN 978-3-515-10175-2

45. Florian Mildenberger
**Medizinische Belehrung
für das Bürgertum**
Medikale Kulturen in der Zeitschrift
„Die Gartenlaube" (1853–1944)
2012. 230 S. mit 11 Abb., kt.
ISBN 978-3-515-10232-2

46. Robert Jütte (Hg.)
Medical Pluralism
Past – Present – Future
2013. 205 S. mit 3 Abb., kt.
ISBN 978-3-515-10441-8

47. Annett Büttner
**Die konfessionelle Kriegskranken-
pflege im 19. Jahrhundert**
2013. 481 S. mit 22 Abb., kt.
ISBN 978-3-515-10462-3

48. *in Vorbereitung*

49. Astrid Stölzle
**Kriegskrankenpflege im
Ersten Weltkrieg**
Das Pflegepersonal der freiwilligen
Krankenpflege in den Etappen
des Deutschen Kaiserreichs
2013. 227 S. mit 18 Abb., kt.
ISBN 978-3-515-10481-4